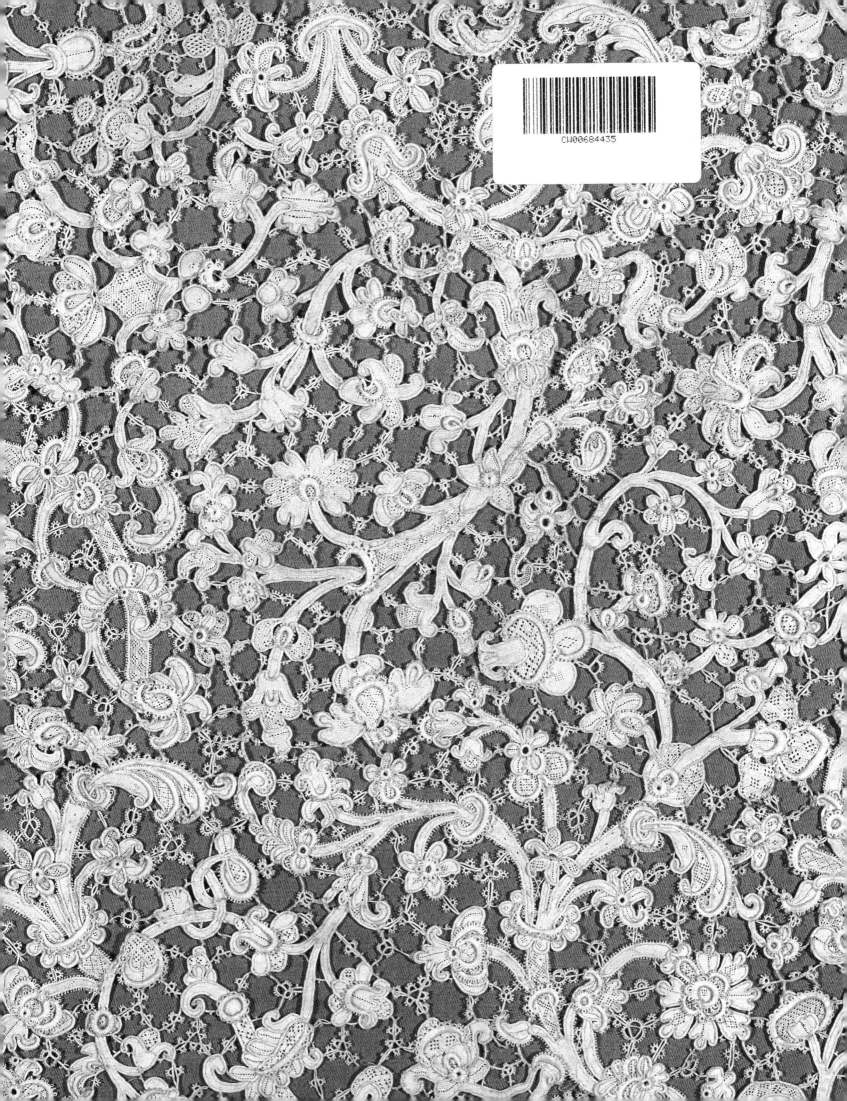

HOUSE
STYLE

HOUSE STYLE

FIVE CENTURIES OF FASHION AT CHATSWORTH

LAURA BURLINGTON & HAMISH BOWLES

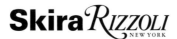

Skira RIZZOLI NEW YORK

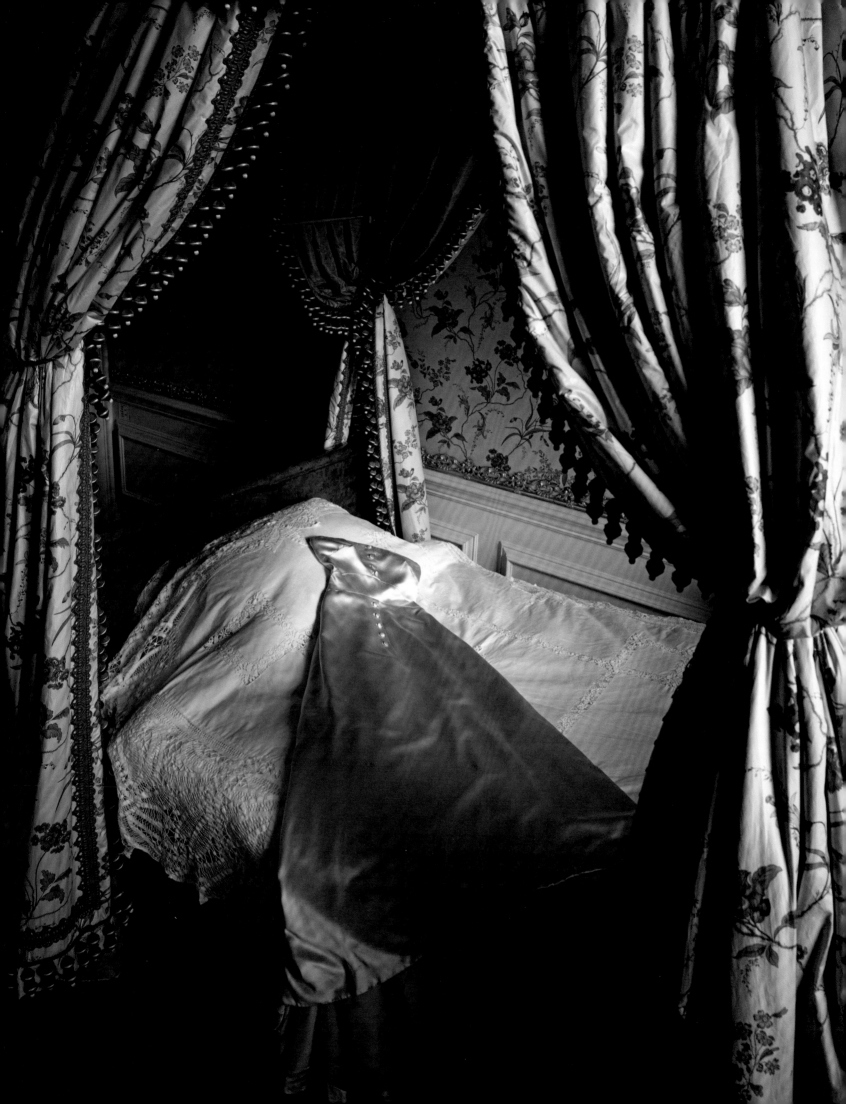

TABLE OF CONTENTS

CAVENDISH FAMILY TREE

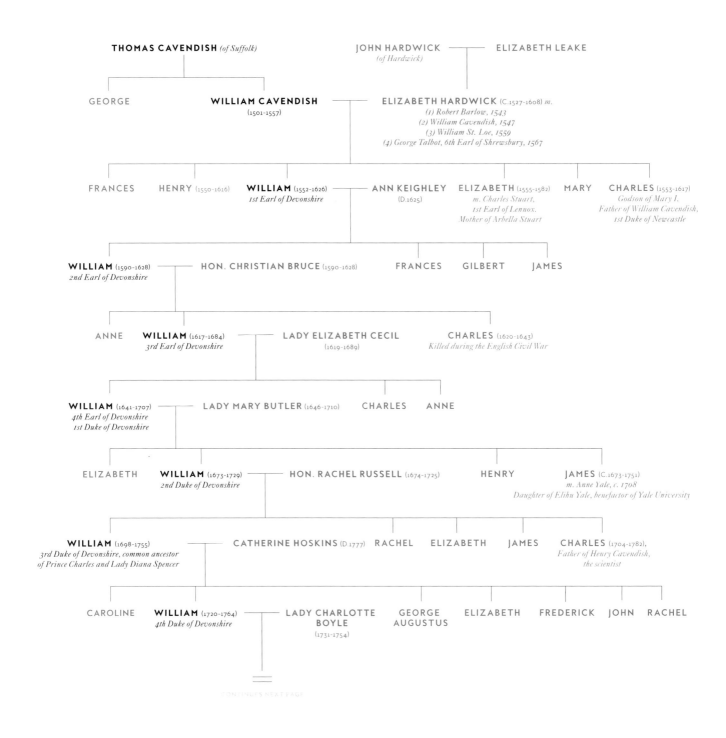

THOMAS CAVENDISH (*of Suffolk*)

JOHN HARDWICK (*of Hardwick*) — ELIZABETH LEAKE

GEORGE **WILLIAM CAVENDISH** (1501-1557) — **ELIZABETH HARDWICK** (C.1527-1608) *m.*
(1) Robert Barlow, 1543
(2) William Cavendish, 1547
(3) William St. Loe, 1559
(4) George Talbot, 6th Earl of Shrewsbury, 1567

FRANCES HENRY (1550-1616) **WILLIAM** (1552-1626) *1st Earl of Devonshire* — ANN KEIGHLEY (D.1625) ELIZABETH (1555-1582) *m. Charles Stuart, 1st Earl of Lennox, Mother of Arbella Stuart* MARY CHARLES (1553-1617) *Godson of Mary I. Father of William Cavendish, 1st Duke of Newcastle*

WILLIAM (1590-1628) *2nd Earl of Devonshire* — HON. CHRISTIAN BRUCE (1590-1628) FRANCES GILBERT JAMES

ANNE **WILLIAM** (1617-1684) *3rd Earl of Devonshire* — LADY ELIZABETH CECIL (1619-1689) CHARLES (1620-1643) *Killed during the English Civil War*

WILLIAM (1641-1707) *4th Earl of Devonshire 1st Duke of Devonshire* — LADY MARY BUTLER (1646-1710) CHARLES ANNE

ELIZABETH **WILLIAM** (1673-1729) *2nd Duke of Devonshire* — HON. RACHEL RUSSELL (1674-1725) HENRY JAMES (C.1673-1751) *m. Anne Yale, c. 1708 Daughter of Elihu Yale, benefactor of Yale University*

WILLIAM (1698-1755) *3rd Duke of Devonshire, common ancestor of Prince Charles and Lady Diana Spencer* — CATHERINE HOSKINS (D.1777) RACHEL ELIZABETH JAMES CHARLES (1704-1782), *Father of Henry Cavendish, the scientist*

CAROLINE **WILLIAM** (1720-1764) *4th Duke of Devonshire* — LADY CHARLOTTE BOYLE (1731-1754) GEORGE AUGUSTUS ELIZABETH FREDERICK JOHN RACHEL

CONTINUES NEXT PAGE

LADY GEORGIANA SPENCER — **WILLIAM** (1748–1811) — **LADY ELIZABETH FOSTER** (1759–1824) — DOROTHY — RICHARD — **GEORGE AUGUSTUS HENRY** (1754–1834) — **LADY ELIZABETH COMPTON**

(1758–1806) Daughter of 1st Earl Spencer — *5th Duke of Devonshire* — *Daughter of 4th Earl of Bristol* — *1st Earl of Burlington, 2nd Creation* — *(1760–1835) Daughter of 7th Earl of Northampton*

WILLIAM SPENCER (1790–1858) — GEORGIANA (1783–1858) — **GEORGE HOWARD** (1773–1848) — HARRIET — **WILLIAM CAVENDISH** (1783–1812) — **HON. LOUISE CALLAGHAN** (D.1863)

6th Duke of Devonshire — *6th Earl of Carlisle* — *Killed in a carriage accident* — *Daughter of Lord Lismore*

LADY CAROLINE HOWARD (1803–1881) — **RT. HON. WILLIAM LASCELLES** (1798–1851) — **LADY BLANCHE HOWARD** (1812–1840) — **WILLIAM** (1808–1891) — FANNY — GEORGE — RICHARD

Son of 2nd Earl of Harewood — *7th Duke of Devonshire*

EMMA LASCELLES (1838–1820) — **EDWARD CAVENDISH** (1838–1891) — FREDERICK — LOUISA — **SPENCER COMPTON** (1833–1908) — **COUNTESS VON ALTEN** (1832–1911)

8th Duke of Devonshire — *Formerly Duchess of Manchester*

VICTOR (1868–1938) — **LADY EVELYN FITZMAURICE** (1870–1960) — RICHARD — JOHN

9th Duke of Devonshire — *Daughter of 5th Marquess of Landsdowne*

EDWARD (1895–1950) — **LADY MARY CECIL** (1895–1988) — MAUD — BLANCHE — DOROTHY (1900–1966) — RACHEL — CHARLES (1905–1944) — ANNE

10th Duke of Devonshire — *Daughter of 5th Marquess of Salisbury* — *m. Harold Macmillan, 1929* — *m. Adele Astaire, 1932*

WILLIAM (1917–1944) — **ANDREW** (1920–2004) — **HON. DEBORAH MITFORD** (1920–2014) — MARY — ELIZABETH — ANNE

Marquess of Hartington. m. Kathleen Kennedy, May 1944. Killed in action — *11th Duke of Devonshire* — *Daughter of 2nd Lord Redesdale*

MARK (BORN AND DIED 1941) — LADY EMMA (B.1943) — **PEREGRINE [STOKER]** (B.1944) — **AMANDA HEYWOOD-LONSDALE** (B.1944) — VICTOR (BORN AND DIED 1947) — MARY (BORN AND DIED 1953) — LADY SOPHIA LOUISE SYDNEY

m. Hon. Tobias Tennant — *12th Duke of Devonshire* — *Daughter of Commander Edward Gavin Heywood-Lonsdale* — *B.1957 m. (1) Anthony Murphy (2) Alastair Morrison (3) Will Topley*

WILLIAM (B.1969) — LAURA MONTAGU (B.1972) — LADY CELINA (B.1971) — LADY JASMINE (B.1973)

Earl of Burlington — *m. Alexander Carter* — *m. Nicky Dunne*

LADY MAUD ELIZABETH CAVENDISH (B.2009) — LORD JAMES WILLIAM PATRICK CAVENDISH (B.2010) — LADY ELINOR MYRTLE CAVENDISH (B.2013) — JAKE EDWARD CARTER (B.1997) — ALFIE WILLIAM CAVENDISH CARTER (B.2000) — NED ARTHUR CAVENDISH CARTER (B.2002) — WILLA GRACE CAVENDISH CARTER (B.2005) — COSMO EDWARD WALKER DUNNE (B.2006) — BARNABY STOKER DUNNE (B.2008) — REGINALD THOMAS DREW DUNNE (B.2010)

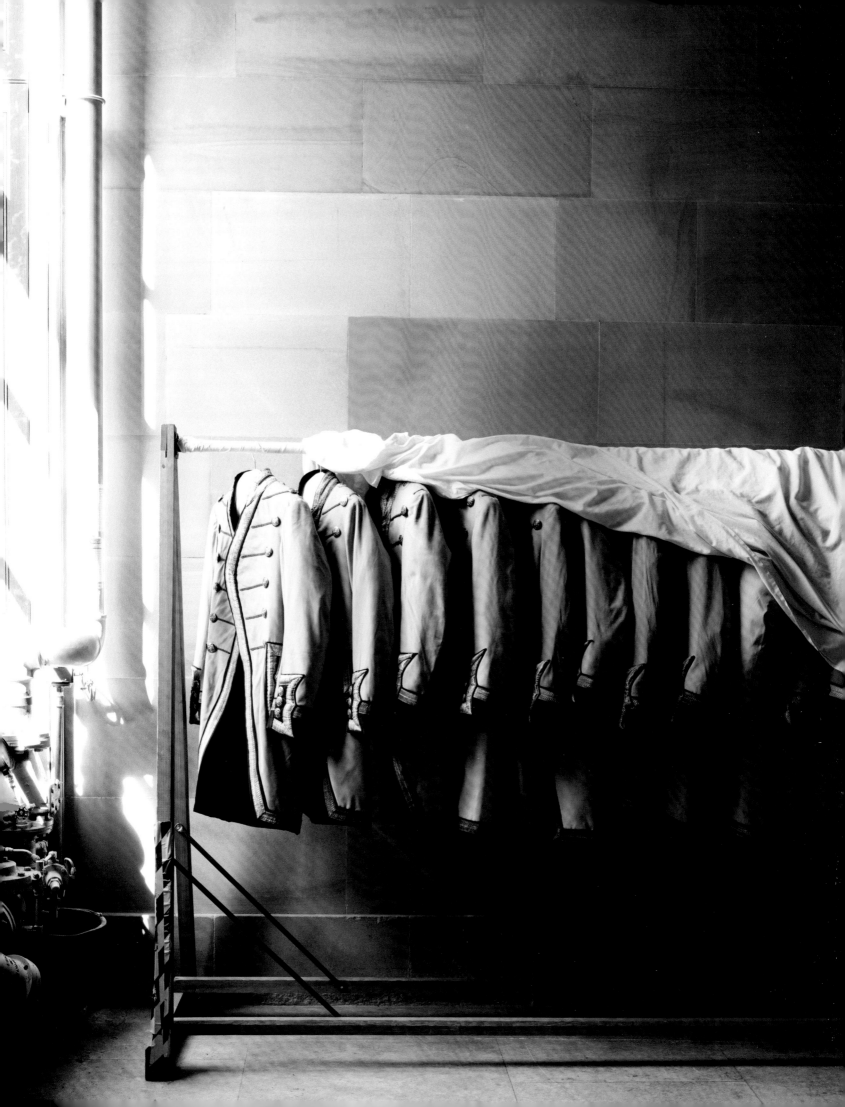

FOREWORD

THE DUKE OF DEVONSHIRE

Until our daughter-in-law Laura Burlington suggested an exhibition of costume, I hadn't properly realised how much 'fashion' there is at Chatsworth. Susie Stokoe, Textile Department Supervisor, and her team have discovered an incredible treasure trove of a largely unknown collection of costume – everything from the Governor General of Canada's dress uniform to the long blue coats worn by our coachmen 150 years ago. Added to that is a mass of my mother's clothes, some bought from the best-known Paris couture houses, some given to her as hand-me-downs by the late Bunny Mellon, and a few items she had bought at agricultural shows. Then there is my wife's amazing collection of hats, accumulated over the 25 years of our deep involvement with Ascot and especially Royal Ascot. To cap it all are my niece, Stella Tennant's, utterly extraordinary clothes from her long and brilliant career as a supermodel.

We have an excellent selection of my father's clothes, for all occasions, formal and informal, as well as his sweaters which defy description. There are jewels old and new, especially Amanda's ever-growing collection of Andrew Grima, mostly from the 1970s with some modern additions.

And there are uniforms, tweed by the kilometre, shoes, gloves, wedding dresses, children's clothes, black tie, white tie, bow tie, veils, bowlers, top hats, caps, capes and drainpipes. The list is endless, the visual impact staggering.

Bringing all these strands together, this book will tell many stories… of social history, design and of course the way fashion changes, how it is made and who makes it.

Laura persuaded Hamish Bowles to curate and Patrick Kinmonth to design our 2017 exhibition of the same name, and there cannot be a more informed and creative team anywhere in the world to work with on such an exciting project.

I am delighted to thank all those who have contributed chapters to this Rizzoli publication, the ideal publishing house for such a work and a team that has been constantly helpful and continually imaginative.

My biggest thanks go to Laura, without whose inspiration this exhibition and thus the book would never have seen the light of day.

Stoker Devonshire

1 *(page 4)* Deborah Devonshire's 'Carmel' evening dress, Christian Dior Haute Couture, Spring/Summer 1953, laid on a bed in a guest bedroom at Chatsworth.

2 *(opposite)* Rack of state livery jackets, Haldane, Pugh & Co, early 1900s.

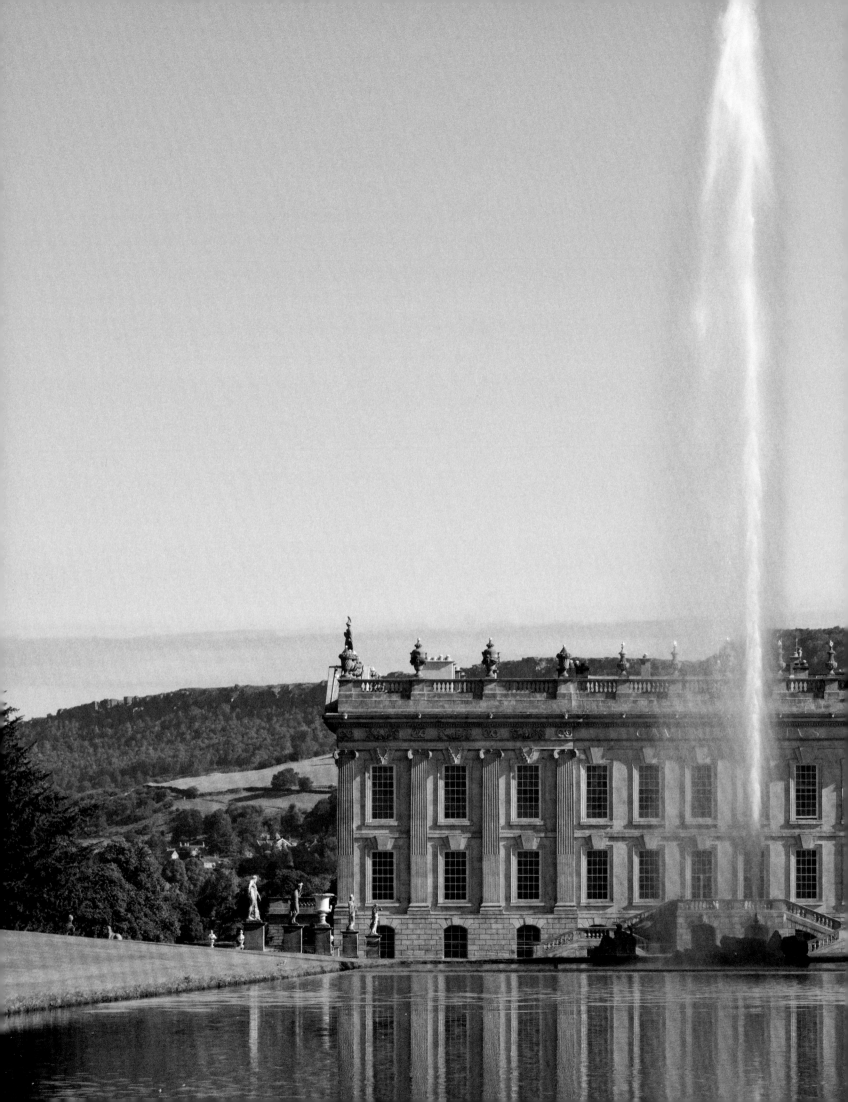

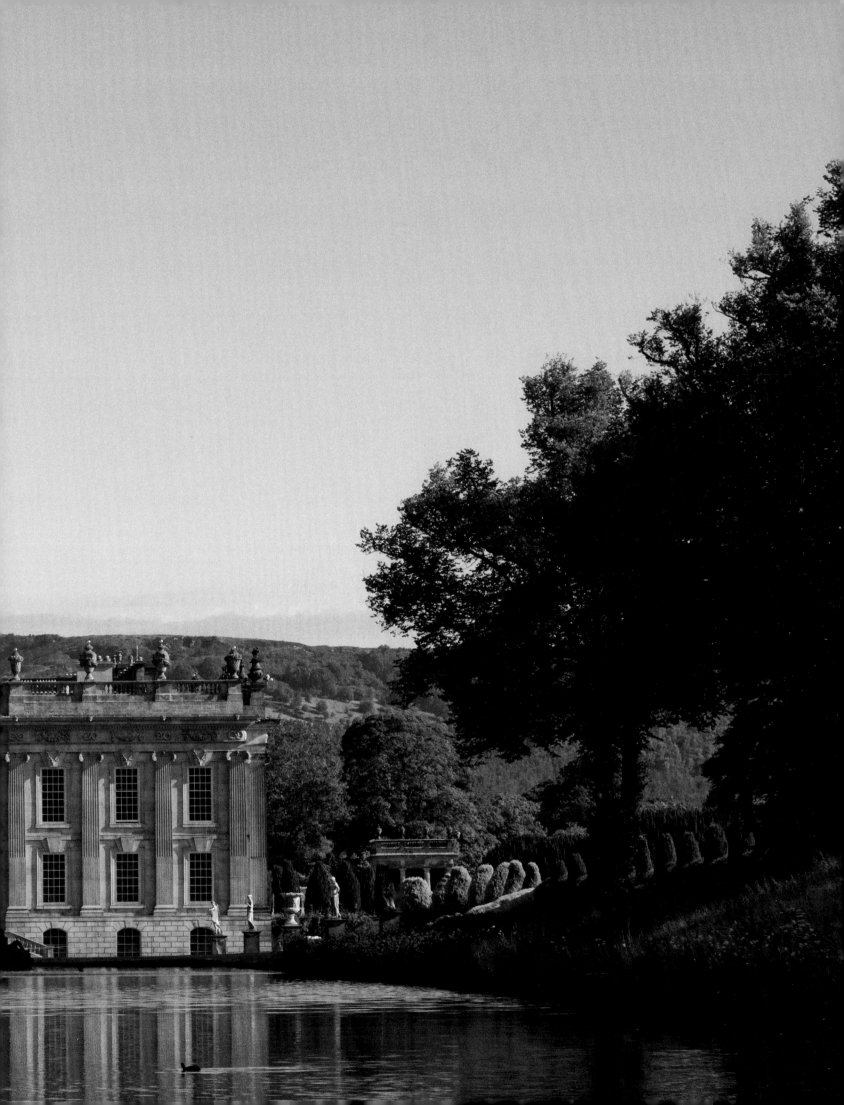

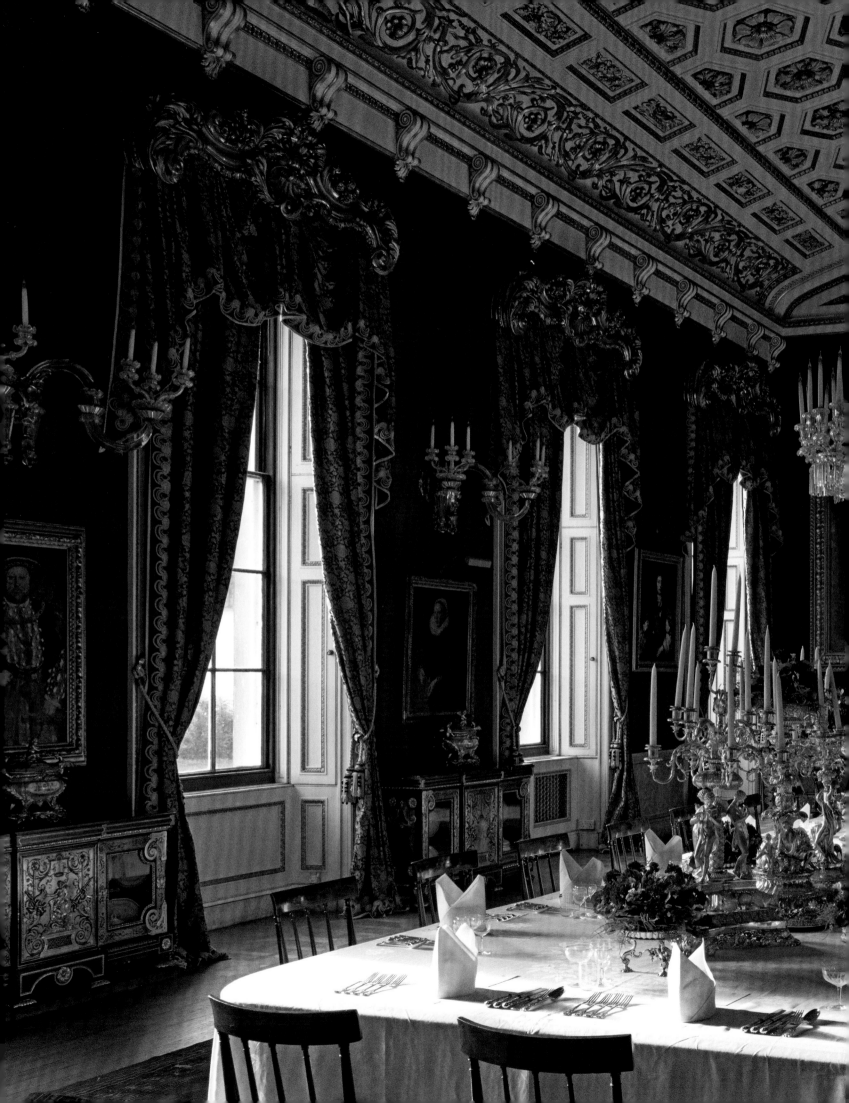

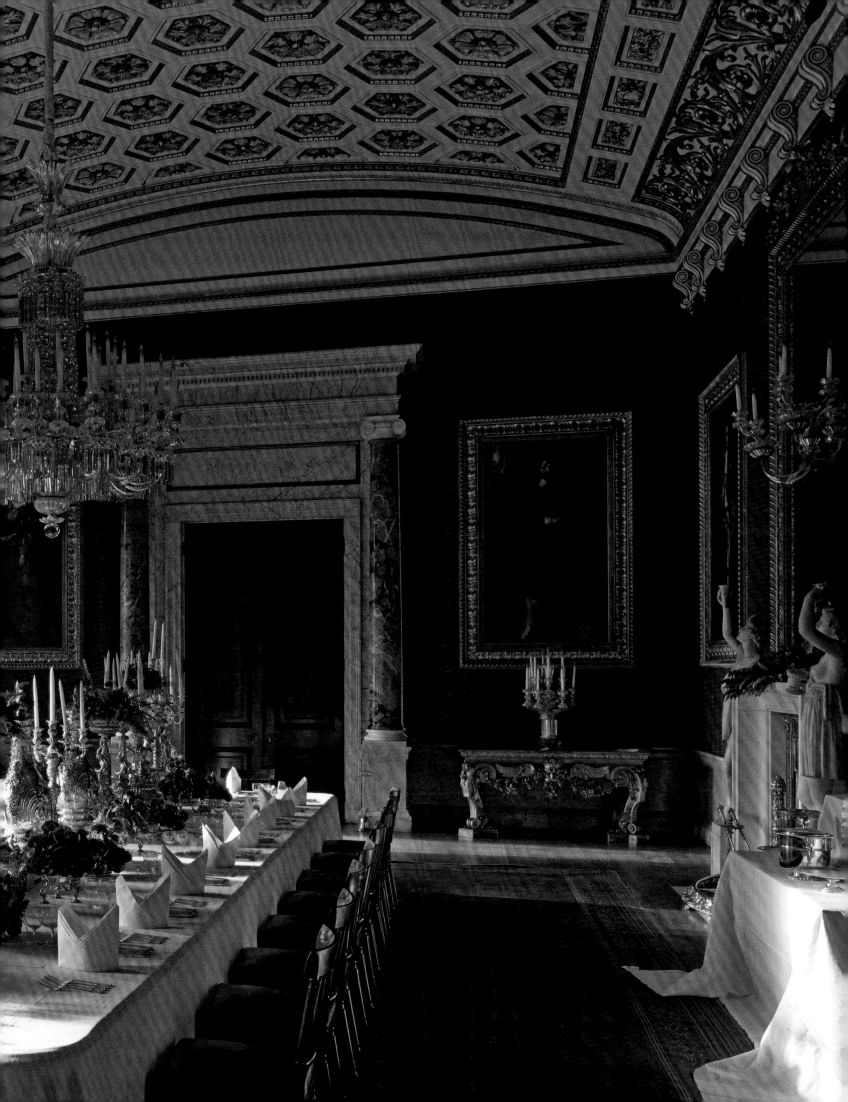

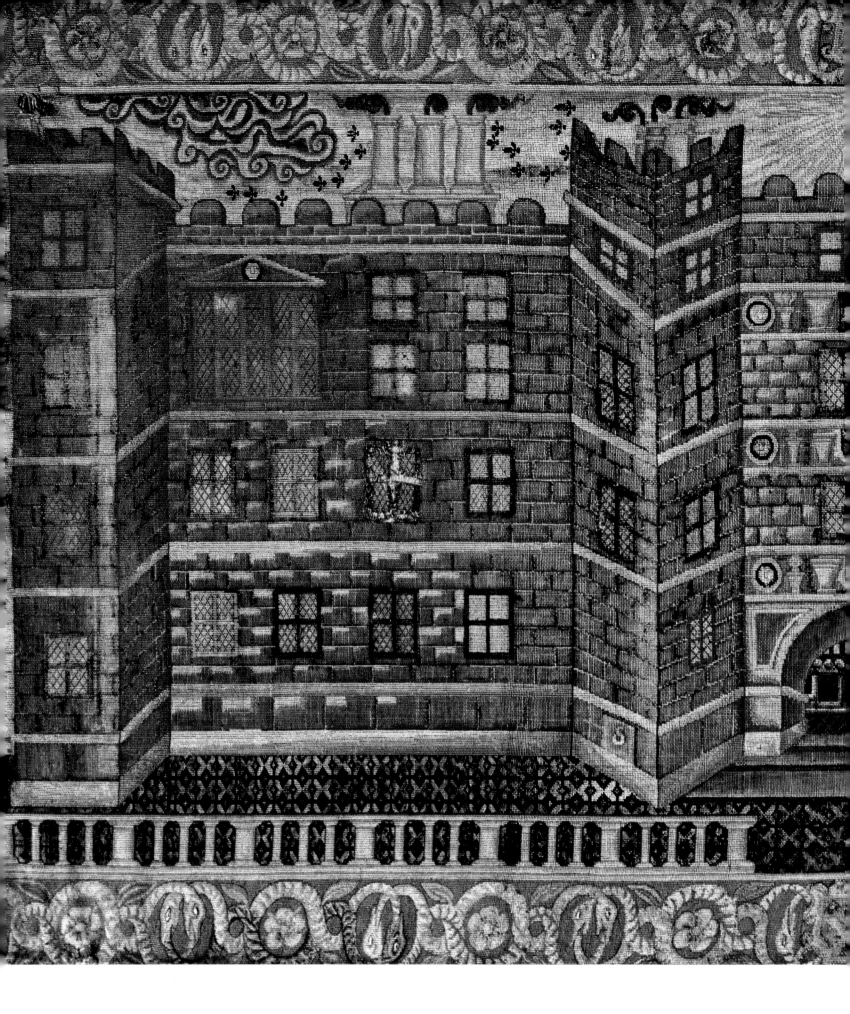

14

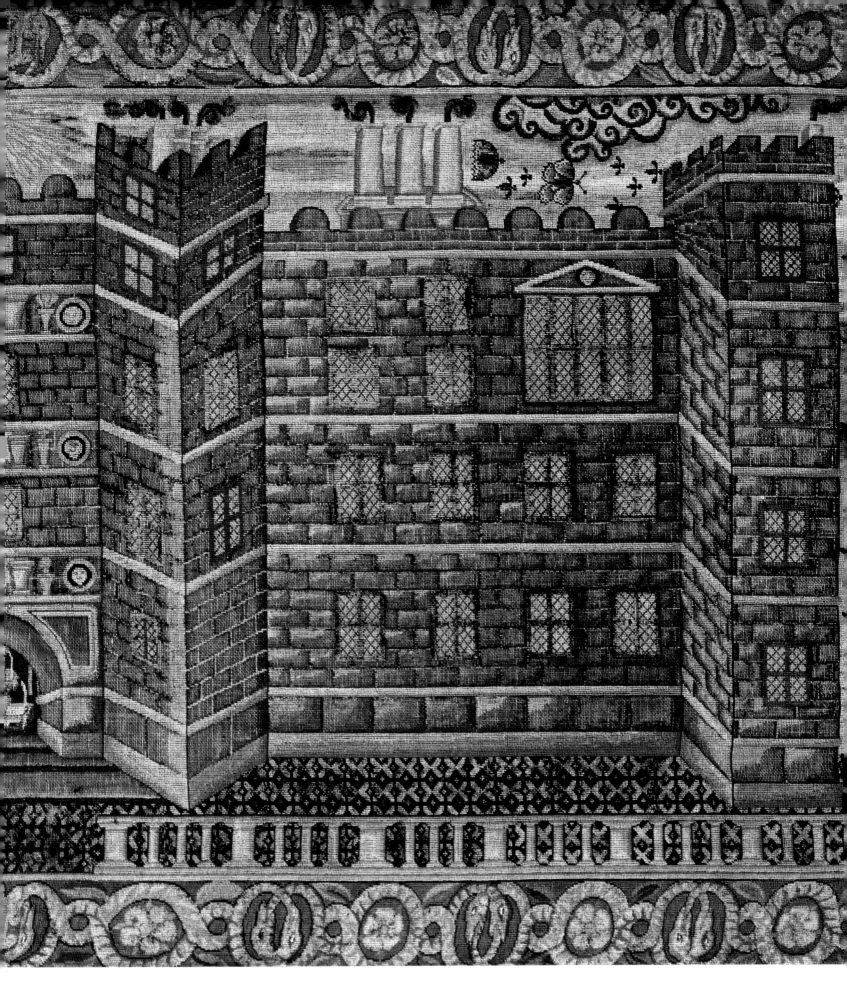

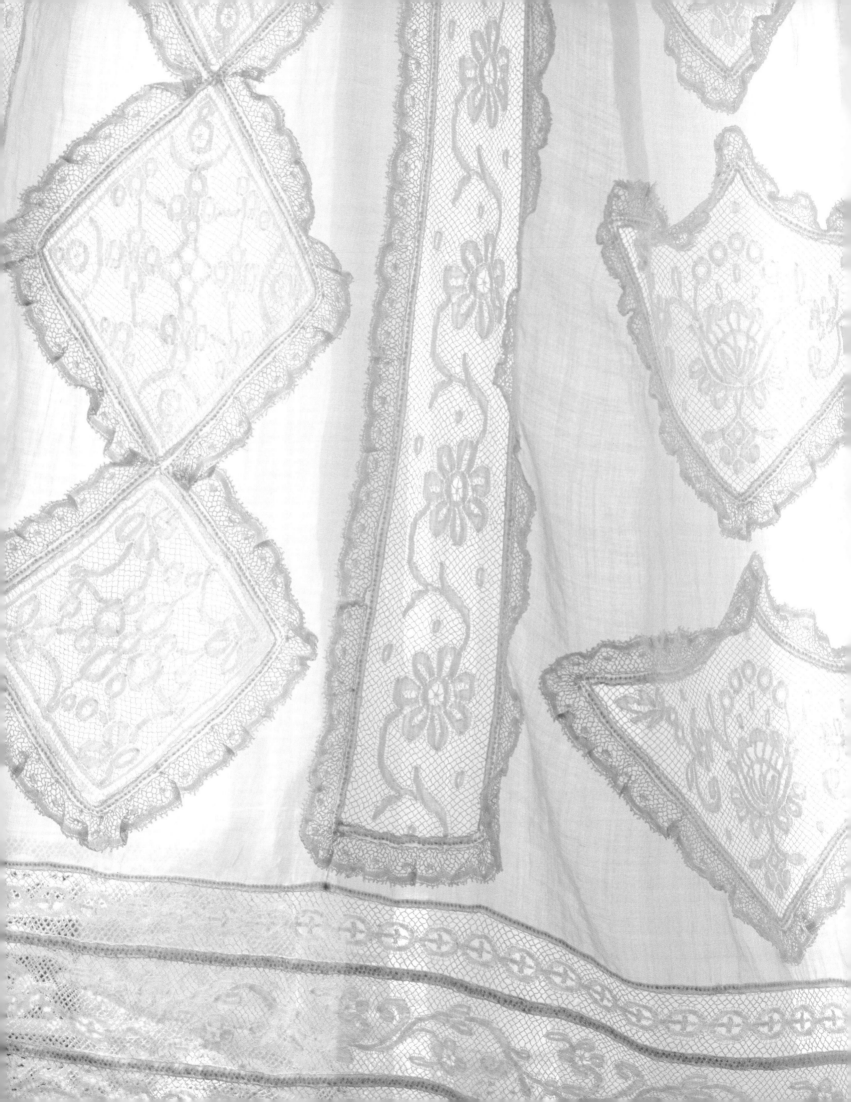

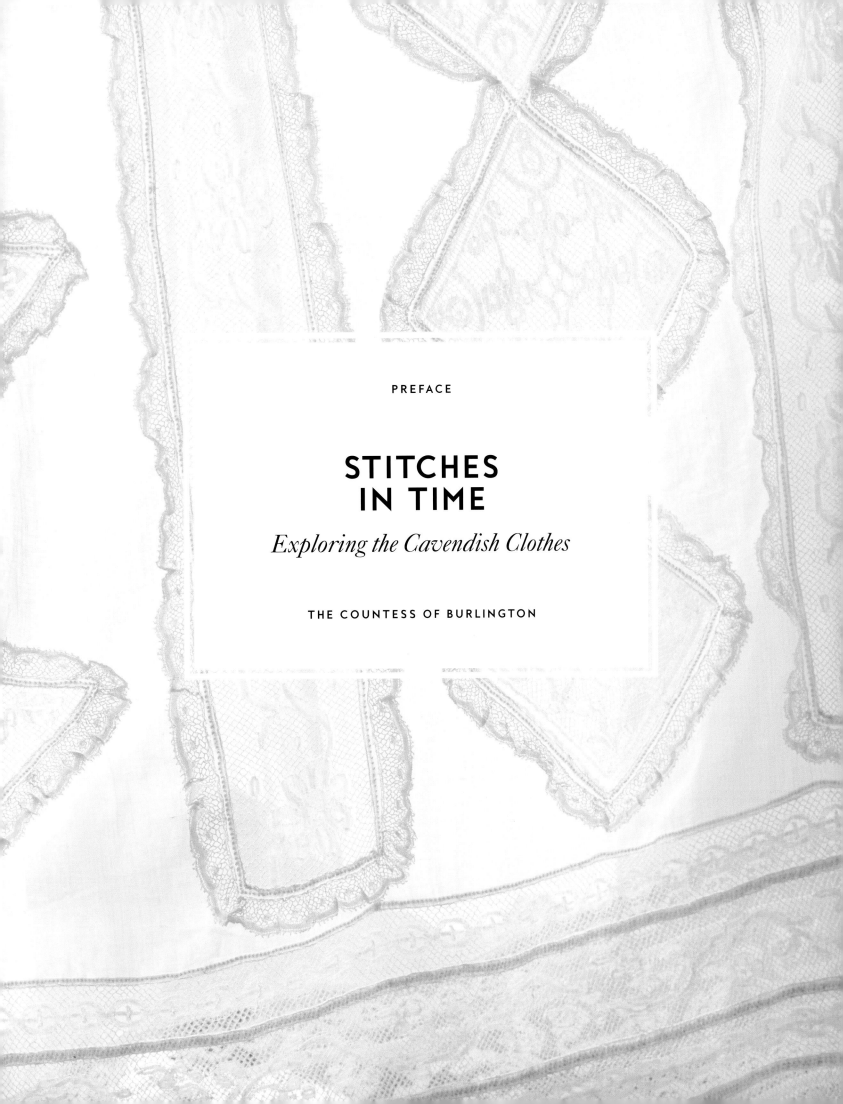

STITCHES
IN TIME

Exploring the Cavendish Clothes

THE COUNTESS OF BURLINGTON

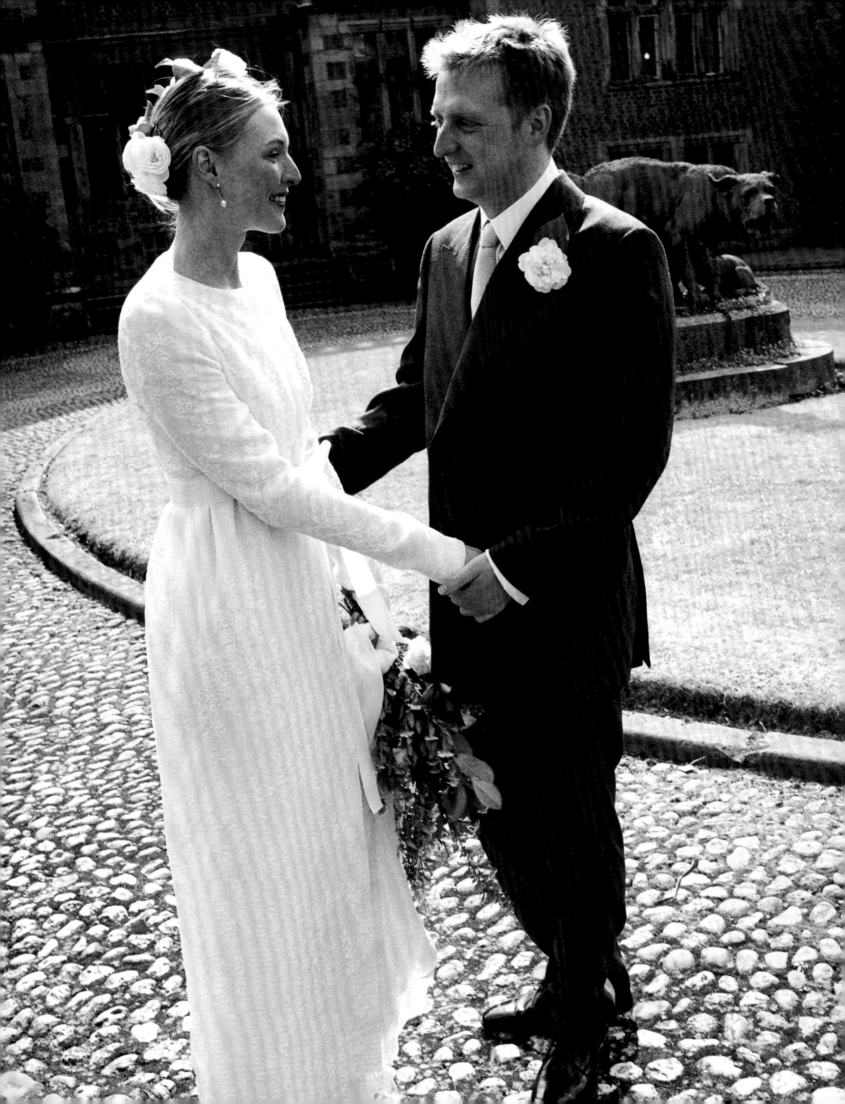

I t will be hard for me to forget that first moment when I opened a box of christening gowns (figs. 4-5) in the textile department at Chatsworth. It was 2009 and William and I (fig. 3) had been married a couple of years, and every few weeks we would come up to Derbyshire to spend the weekend with my parents-in-law. At this point they had lived at Chatsworth for just over three years and we all spent much of these days exploring. My mother-in-law encouraged these trips of discovery, and after our son James was born she suggested that we go to the textile department and look for a christening gown. A large cardboard box was brought down that contained the gown but also underskirts, caps and bonnets, and even capes to wear over gowns. The whole box had been carefully packed with layers of tissue and we saw 30 muslin beauties before we got to the bottom. The room was stacked to the ceiling with other boxes and we opened several more on that day that contained livery (fig. 2), coronation robes (figs. 42, 45), a Jean-Philippe Worth dress (fig. 94), even Adele Astaire's Aran cardigan.

I think it is worth mentioning that I have been interested in fashion since I was a small girl. I'm sure my grandmother was responsible for this; she was a 6-foot clothes-lover very much in the style of Barbara Cartland. I found her exceedingly glamorous, mainly because she wore peach silk bed jackets and a lot of jewellery at 7.30am, which was the time that my brother and I were allowed into her room for morning tea. She was an accomplished dressmaker and gave me sewing lessons from an early age. Looking back on it, I think her greatest quality must have been patience, because she would let me sit in her workroom for hours on end; we would each have a project on the go and hers would be constantly interrupted as I got my bobbin stuck or ran out of thread again. Work commenced straight after breakfast and continued until it became too dark to see what we were doing properly… we took it all terribly seriously.

I continued to sew as a teenager. I painted my bedroom black and for inspiration I pasted the walls with John Galliano asymmetric tailoring from the pages of *Vogue*. The old nursery became a workroom and my parents funded an almost endless supply of fabric and haberdashery.

At 15 my mother suggested that I take an apprenticeship in London with an Austrian couturier called Inge Sprawson. I started work that summer and I think it was a supreme act of kindness on Inge's part that she paid me. My primary role, apart from the obvious tea-making, ran to fumigating the dresses, especially those that had been made by Mr Ray, her star tailor, his speciality being boned corsetry, which he struggled with whilst smoking 40 cigarettes a day. I learned how to do a lot of the basics of sewing, such as making French seams, cutting a skirt without a pattern and sewing a button on with a shank. Over the years that followed I worked for a number of designers, I modelled (figs. 7, 14, 150, 153), I styled for *Harper's Bazaar* and finally I became a fashion buyer. I suppose with this background it was quite normal that I was so excited about the boxes in the textile department.

I wanted to continue exploring the archive at Chatsworth and asked my parents-in-law if I could invite Hamish Bowles to Chatsworth to look through the boxes with me. Hamish is currently the International Editor at Large of American *Vogue* and is a passionate collector of contemporary clothing and historical costume.

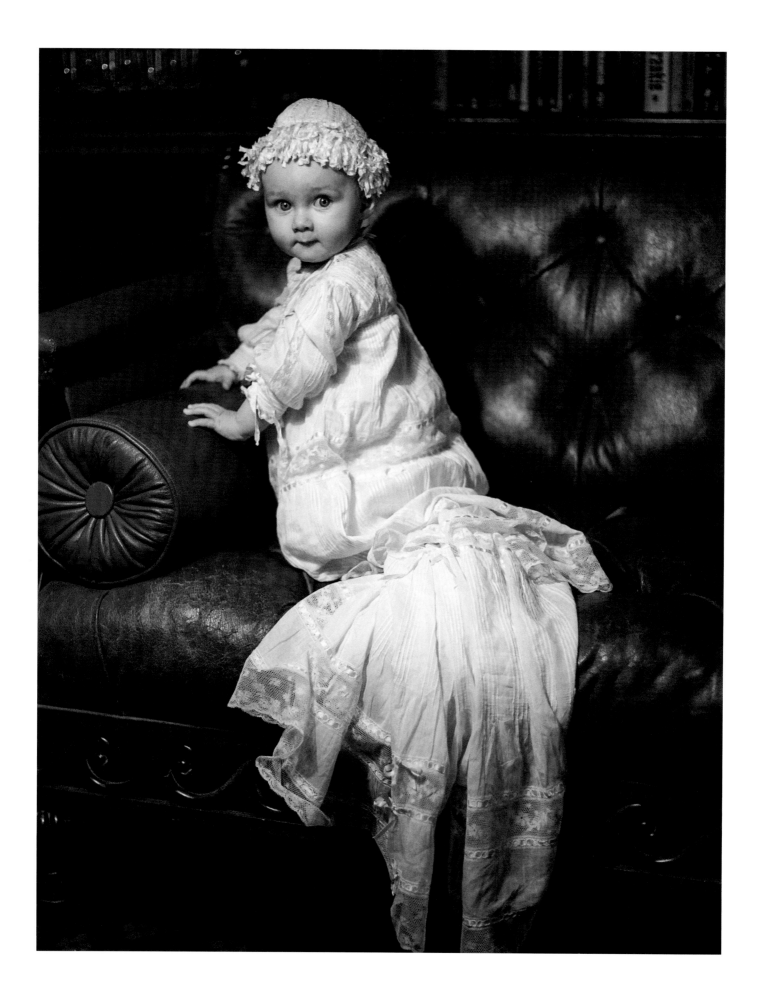

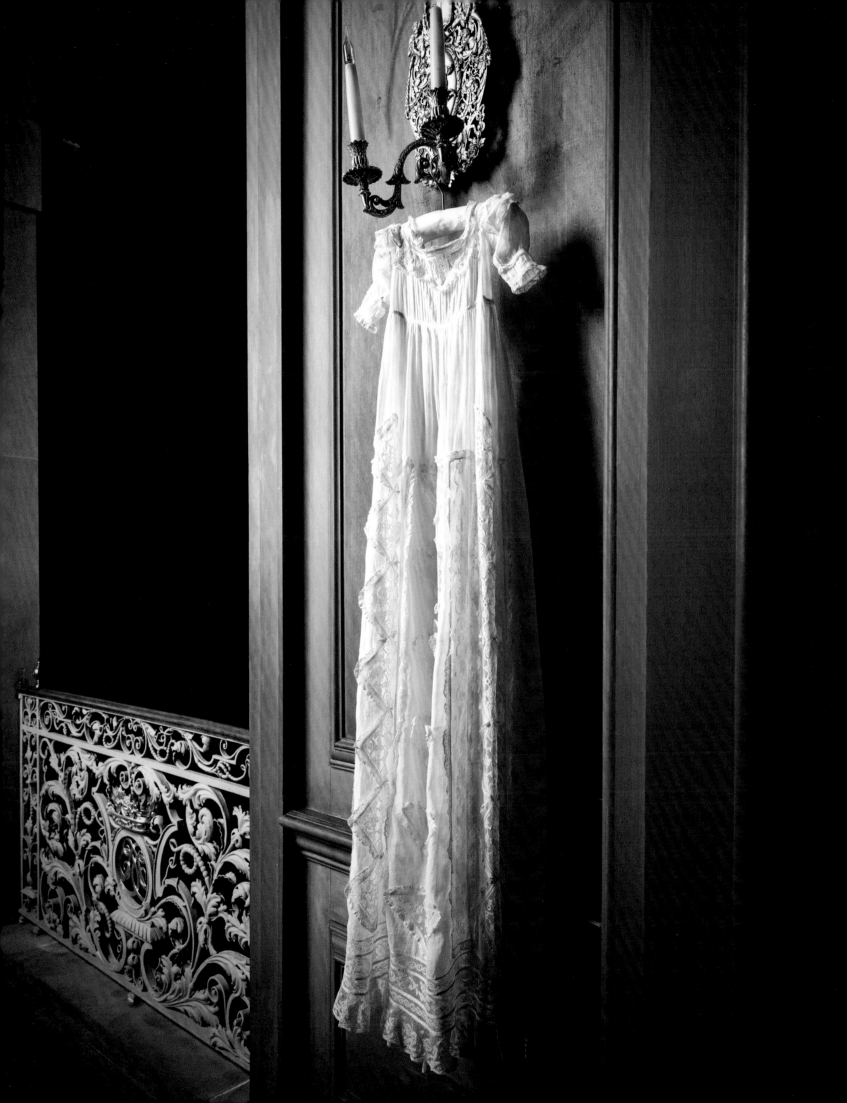

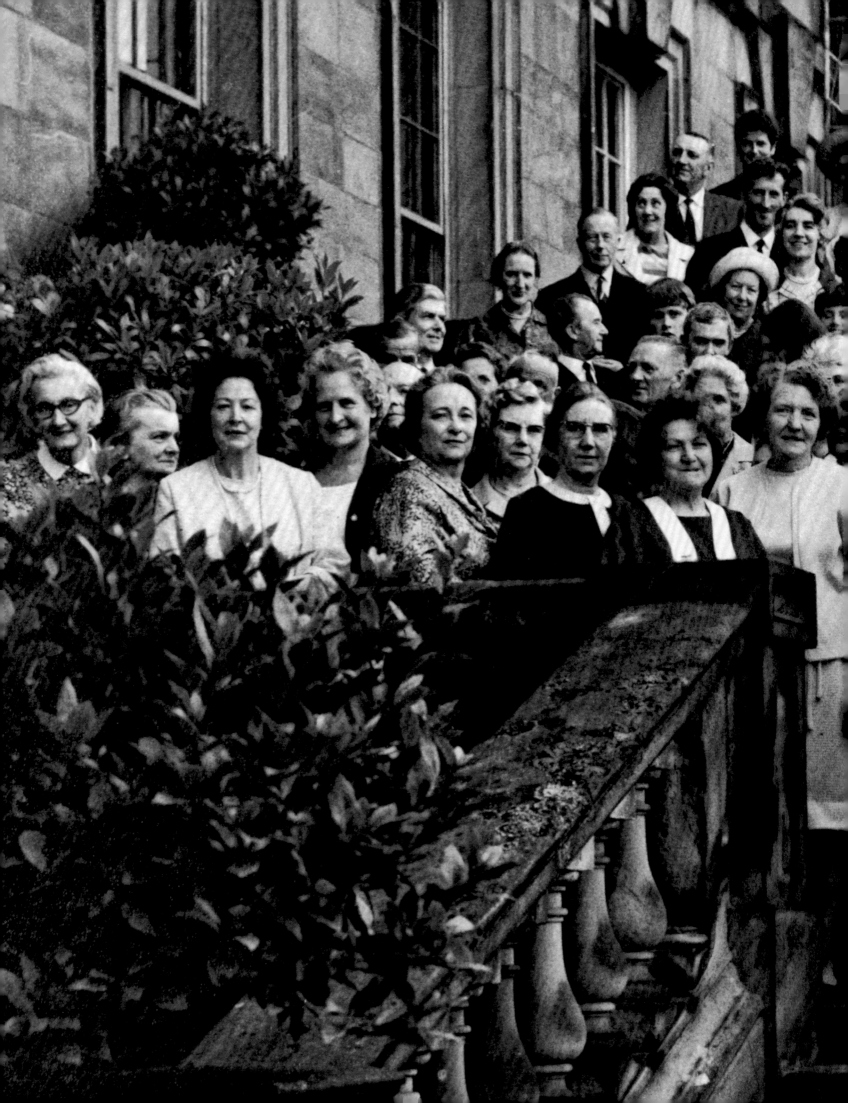

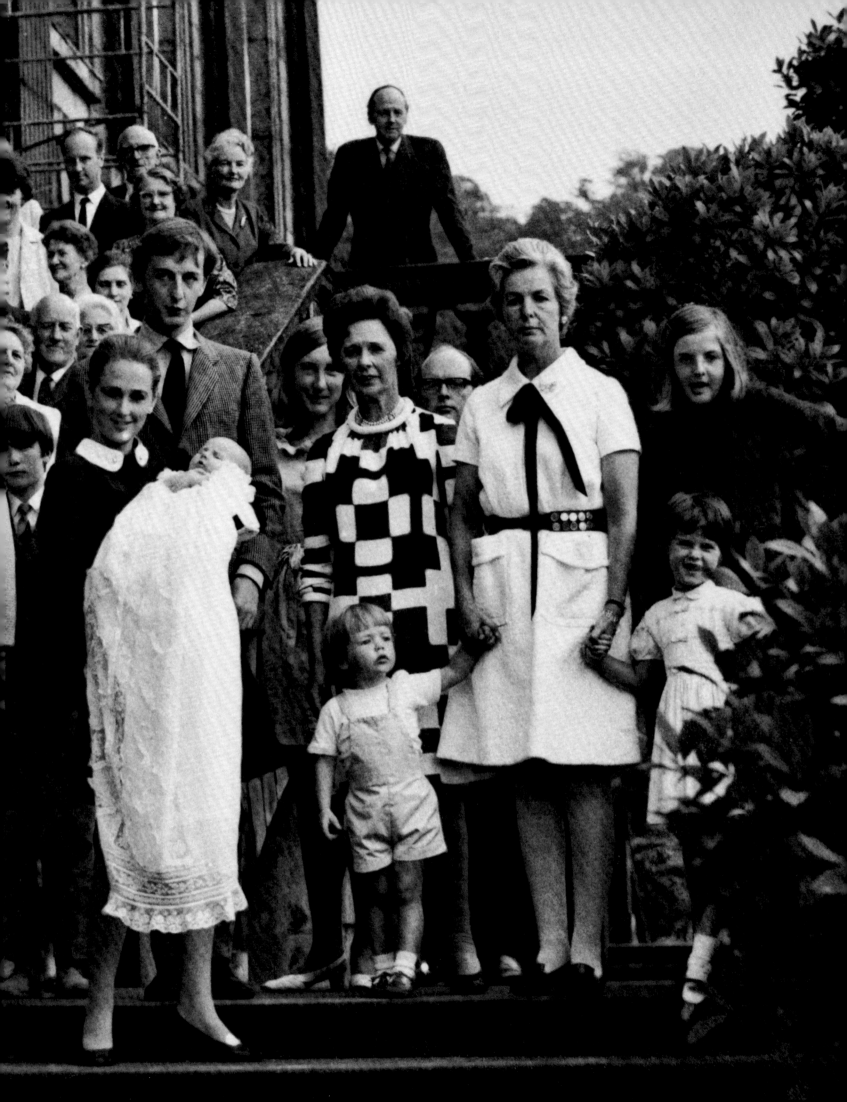

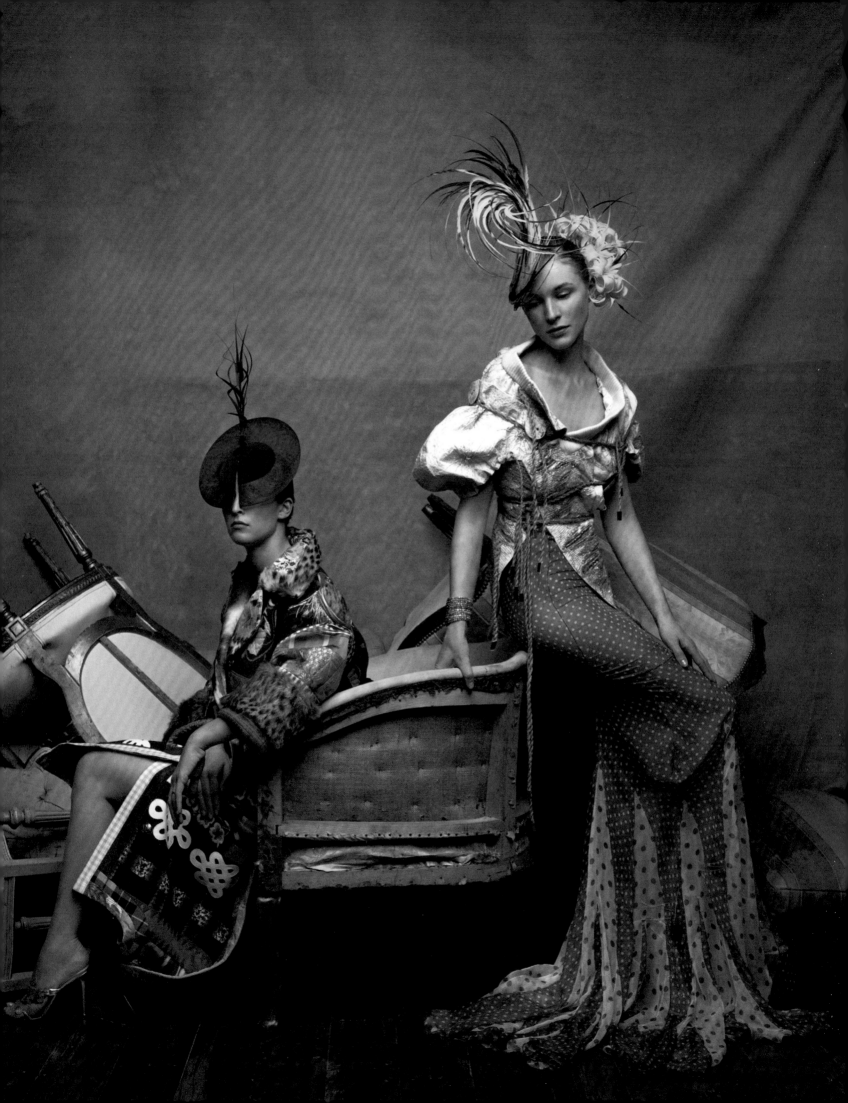

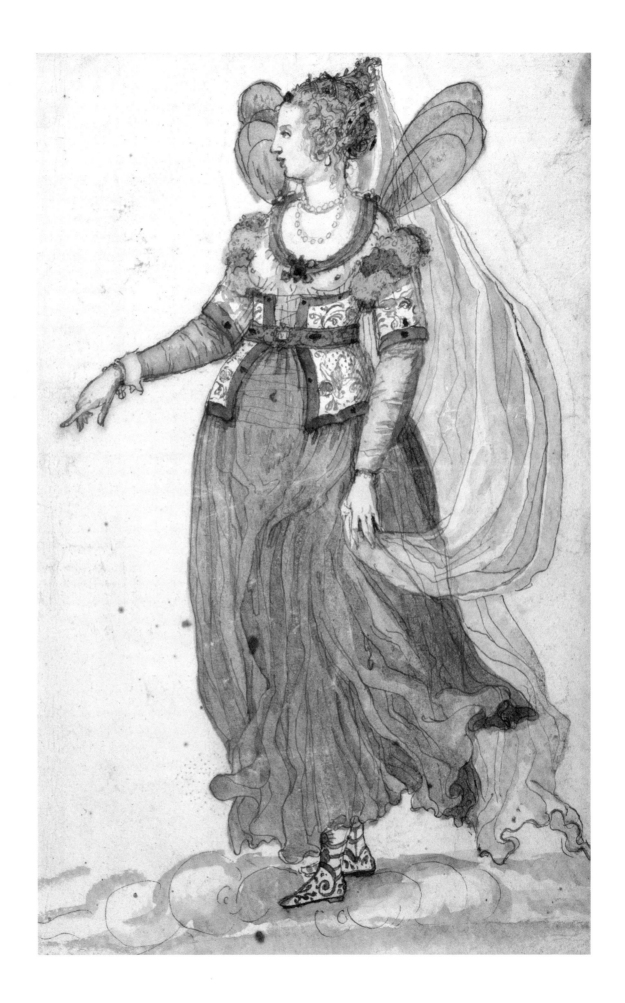

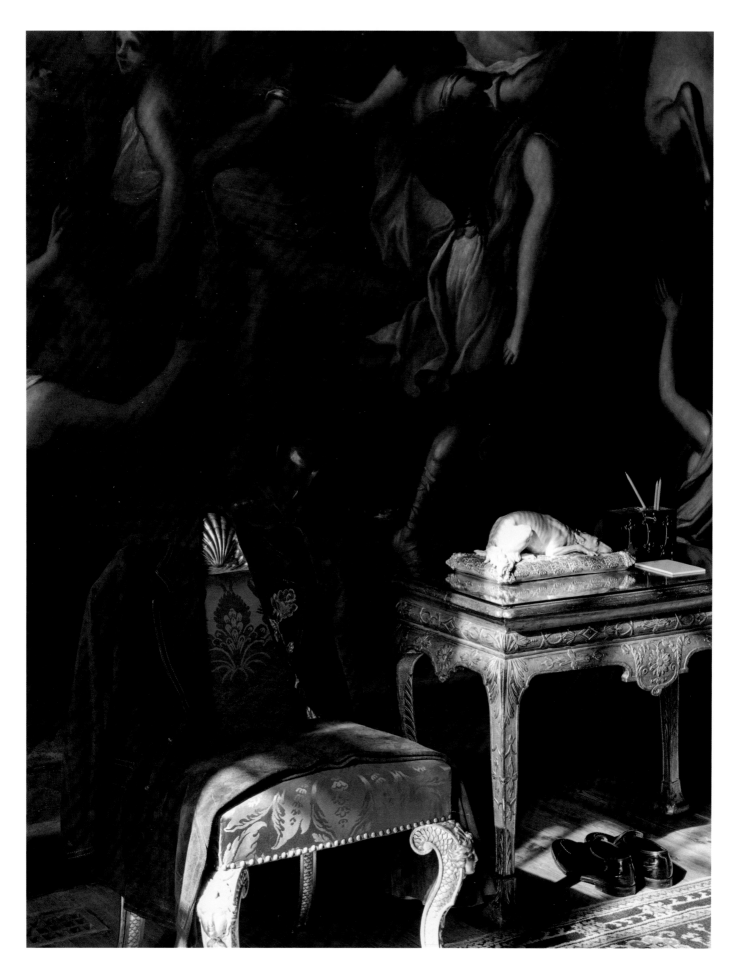

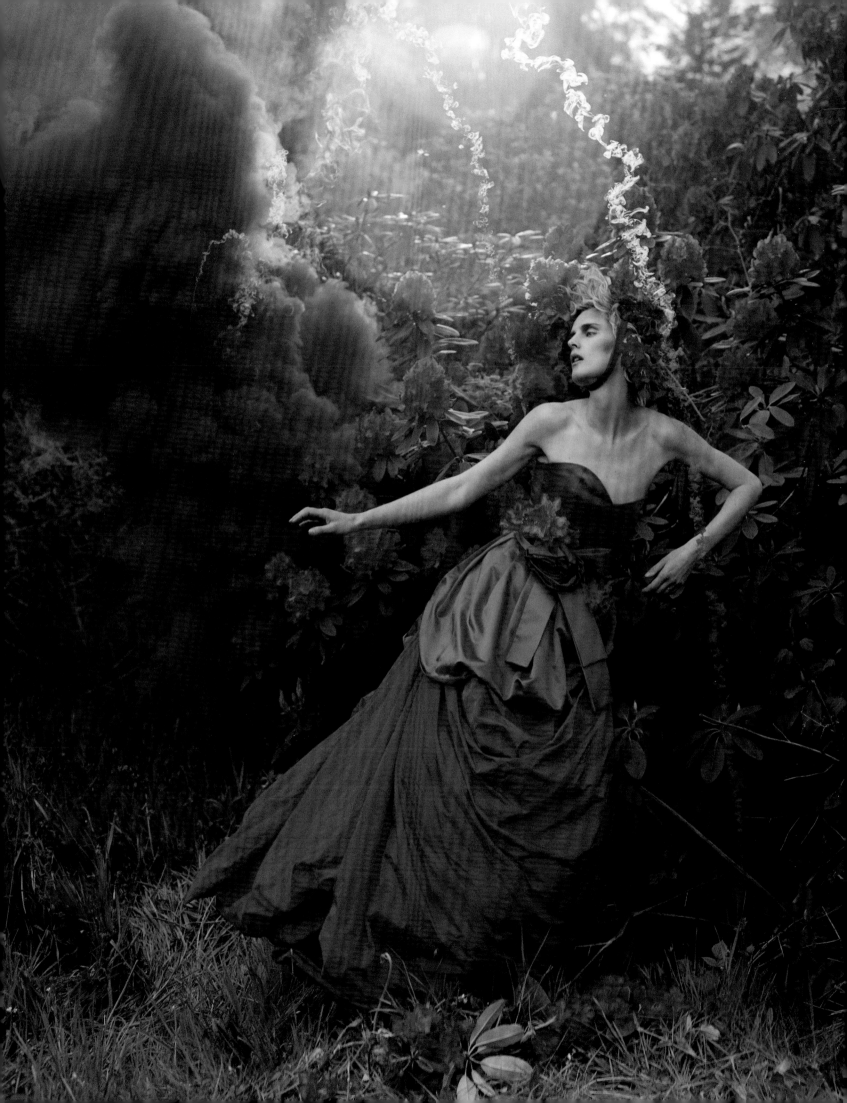

Hamish and I had first met more than ten years before on a fashion shoot when he was an editor at *Harpers & Queen*. I was the model and the clothes included a Botticelli print Vivienne Westwood corset. My hair was put up in a huge bouffant style and a large silk head scarf had been fixed over the huge hair and tied tightly under my chin in the style of Princess Margaret, but with considerable volume. This took a number of hours and a team of four to perfect. When I was ready, Cindy Palmano, the photographer, asked me to perch on a stool, which I did precariously for all of about three minutes and then passed out cold. Hamish was very kind and concerned and brought me sweet tea and didn't mention that my hair was now malformed. I liked him enormously for this.

I wrote to Hamish, and shortly afterwards he arrived at Chatsworth, weary from the Paris shows, and we made quite sure we gave him no time to recover. My parents-in-law showed him the house and garden and then we started rummaging through the cupboards. We went to the photographic archive and found images of Duchess Louise at the Devonshire House Ball (fig. 92) and Deborah Devonshire at the races (fig. 11). Other women in the pictures included those who had married into the family: Adele Astaire (figs. 13, 15), sister and dance partner of Fred, photographed in the garden at Lismore Castle (fig. 53); and Kick Kennedy, sister of JFK, who married Billy Hartington in May 1944, holding a chicken in her army uniform (fig. 12). From the vaults the curators brought up Inigo Jones costume designs from the early seventeenth century (fig. 8) and from the library eighteenth-century books of fancy dress illustrations… Hamish's eyes widened. We went to visit Debo's house and pored over pictures of her Mitford sisters with all their glamour and sass (figs. 108-109). We also found Givenchy in the cupboards and Elvis-embroidered handbags under the bed.

I begged my mother-in-law to show us some of her clothes. She said that she didn't have anything we would be interested in and then proceeded to open a cupboard that contained Bellville et Cie (fig. 20), Troubadour, Catherine Walker, Franka, Biba and an impressive quantity of hats from her days of hosting the Ascot Authority box at Ascot Racecourse (fig. 143). Even William's father produced some suitably dandyish evening suits from Blades and embroidered shirts from Mr Fish. The dressing-up box was opened and out came an array of 1980s ball gowns and a Thea Porter.

By the end of the weekend a plan was formed… Chatsworth would host a fashion exhibition. Hamish felt the person to work with him on the design of this eclectic assortment was his friend Patrick Kinmonth. Pinning Patrick down is no mean feat, as he directs opera and ballet, decorates interiors and stages exhibitions all at the same time. Several imploring emails later and, when I had almost given up, he arrived and it was well worth the wait. A steady flow of ideas continually emanates from him and his collaborator, Antonio Monfreda, as they draw on a deep knowledge of history, art, interiors and costume. Over the last few years I have looked forward to their visits, and the extraordinary energy and commitment they brought with them. The brilliant and organised Denna Garrett was assigned to give the project some backbone and, along with the wonderful team at Chatsworth, we realised we had an exhibition on our hands. A project of this ambition requires a special sort of partner and Antonio had the foresight to introduce us to Gucci, who not only understood what we wanted to achieve, but helped us reach new audiences.

Our first job was to really get a handle on what we had. I was dispatched to Scotland to see what could be contributed by William's cousin Stella Tennant (fig. 10). We spent

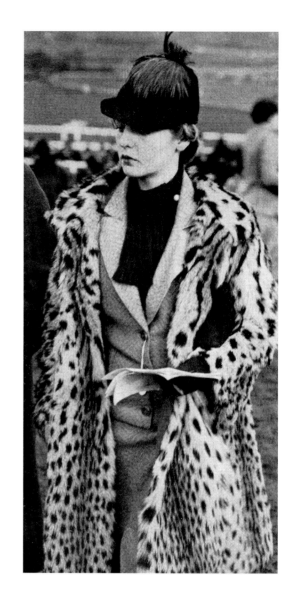

11 *(above)* Deborah Devonshire at Cheltenham Races, 1938.

12 *(opposite, top to bottom)* Kick Kennedy in her American Red Cross uniform, 1943.

13 Adele Astaire and harvesters, circa 1940.

14 *(following pages, left to right)* Walter Chin, Countess of Burlington wearing a suit by Krizia. Originally published in Italian *Vogue*, July 1993.

15 Adele Astaire wearing a costume given to her as a Christmas present by the Duke and Duchess of Devonshire, late 1970s.

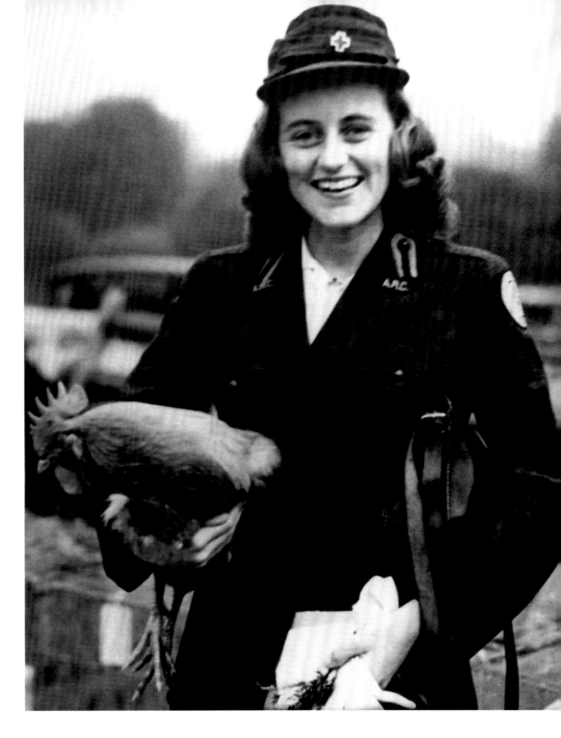

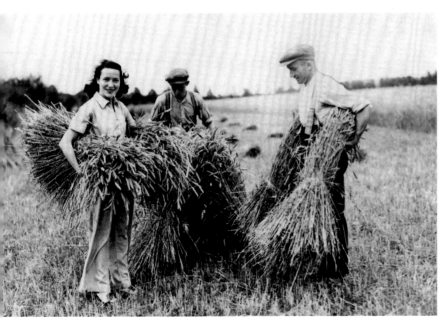

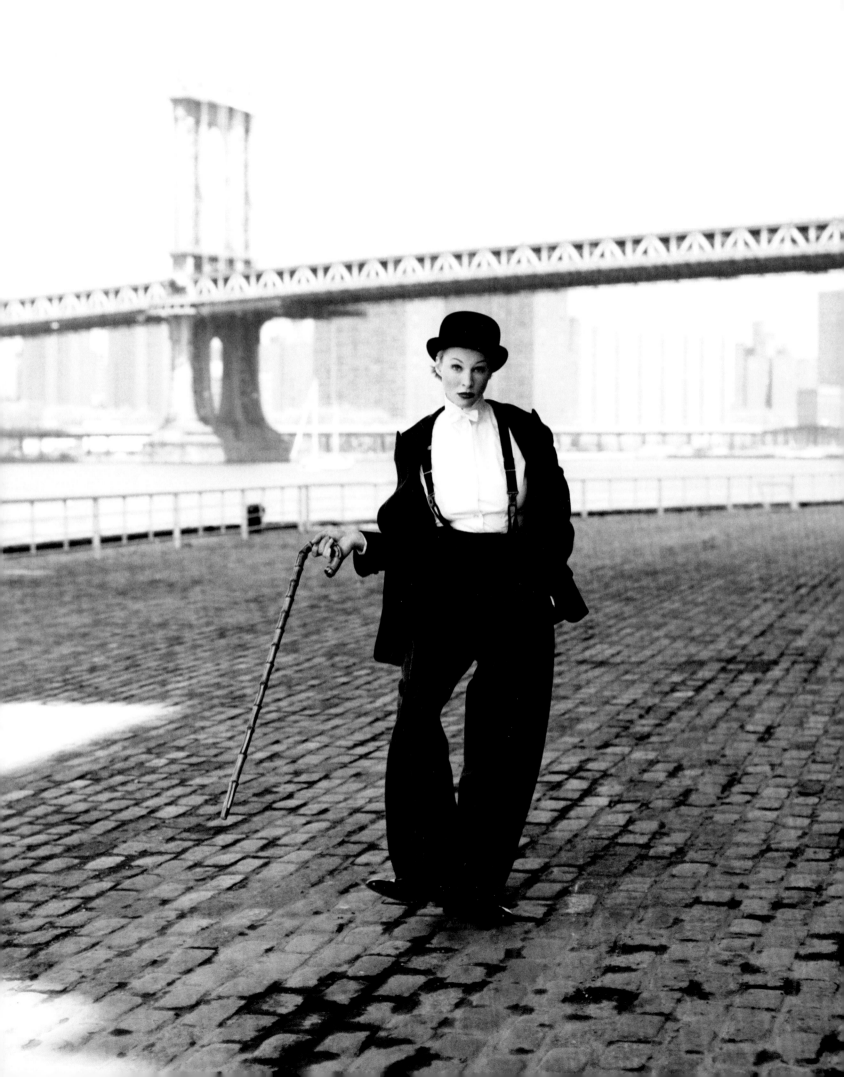

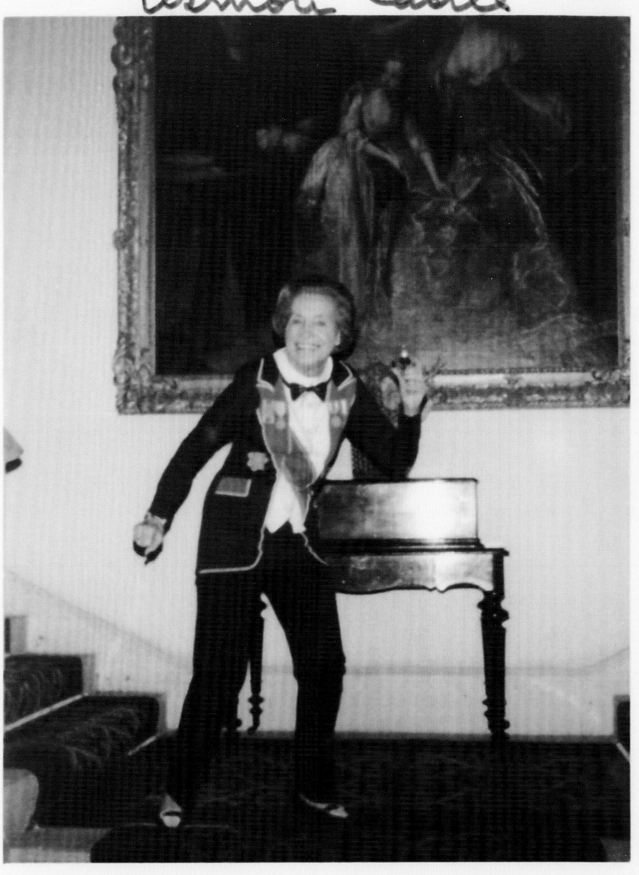

a day going through her clothes and reliving the 1990s. She produced Alexander McQueen dresses (fig. 139), her payment for walking in his show, and some important pieces by Martin Margiela and Helmut Lang. There was also an assortment of bubble gum pink Chanel suits she had put on one side for 'when I grow up and have the vicar for tea'.

We set a date for all the clothes to be accumulated with their boxes in the theatre at Chatsworth (fig. 17). Item-by-item we went through our hoard; unfortunately it turned out to be the hottest day of the year. We'd been at it in 39 degrees for a couple of hours, going carefully through the rails, when Hamish started almost skipping across the room with a pink satin gown in his hands (fig. 1). He knew immediately it was a 1953 design by Christian Dior with a missing label (fig. 121), I can't say that I would have given it a second glance. I suppose this is the fashion equivalent of a Rembrandt in the attic.

Another important find was suggested to me a few weeks beforehand. Charlotte Mosley had asked me if I wanted to go with her and have lunch with Hubert de Givenchy. I leaped at the chance. He had made my mother-in-law's wedding dress (figs. 57-58) and, as a friend of William's grandmother Deborah Devonshire (fig. 120), had visited Chatsworth before. At lunch I was rather nervous and star-struck and I quickly became embarrassed at how bad my French was, nevertheless he was very courteous and spoke English to me, and at the end of the lunch he said to me: 'Your husband's grandfather had the most amazing green tapestry slippers that had been reworked with leather, and they would look wonderful in a vitrine.' This did seem rather like looking for a needle in a haystack but you can imagine my excitement when we opened the box that contained the slippers, exactly as he had described. They had been cleverly archived alongside his Converse trainers used for walking holidays. They are now captured in the book next to the 11th Duke's pyjamas (fig. 18).

We haven't stopped finding treasure in the course of this show. Stella mislaid her wedding dress eighteen years ago and we had little chance of having it remade, as it was a complex combination of tulle and a vest designed by Helmut Lang (fig. 60). A month before this essay was due to go to press, it was found, wrapped in tissue, stored in the same box as her mother's wedding dress and long forgotten. I hope you get as much pleasure seeing these things as we have had discovering them.

I hope that, through the following pages, we have managed to convey the sheer breadth and depth of Chatsworth's collection and give you a glimpse into the ever-evolving relationship between the Devonshire family and fashion. I would like to take this opportunity to thank my parents-in-law who have supported me through the process of creating this book and exhibition. Without their enthusiasm and encouragement I certainly would never have had the opportunity or confidence to make both a reality. They have always made me feel that they were completely behind the project, which is very typical of them.

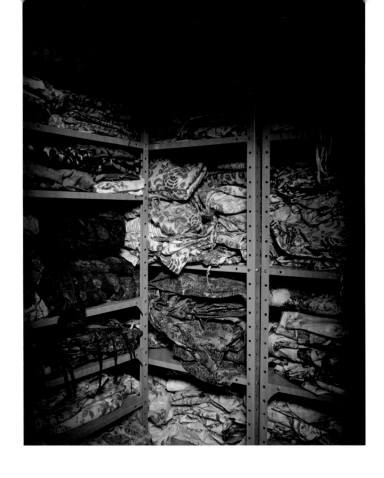

16 *(above)* A storage room filled with piles of chintz case covers, early 1800s-1990s.

17 *(opposite)* Denna Garrett preparing objects for the *House Style* exhibition in the Theatre at Chatsworth, 2015.

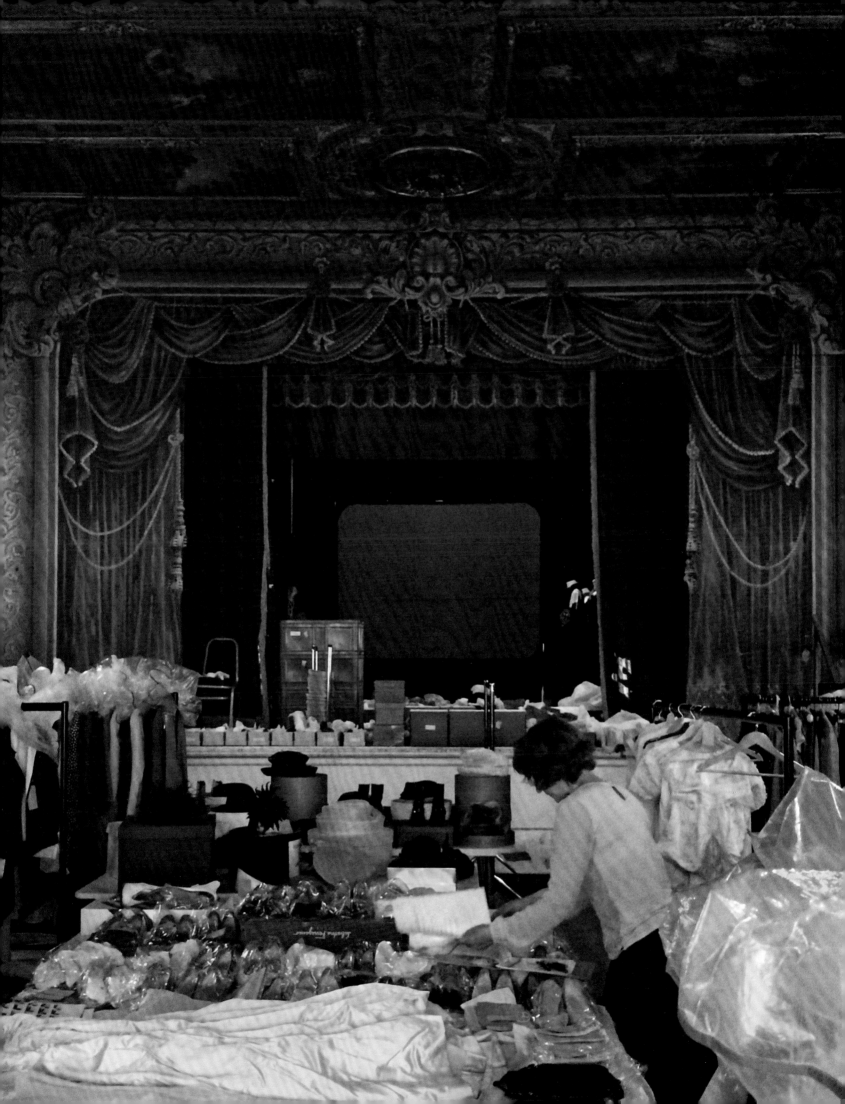

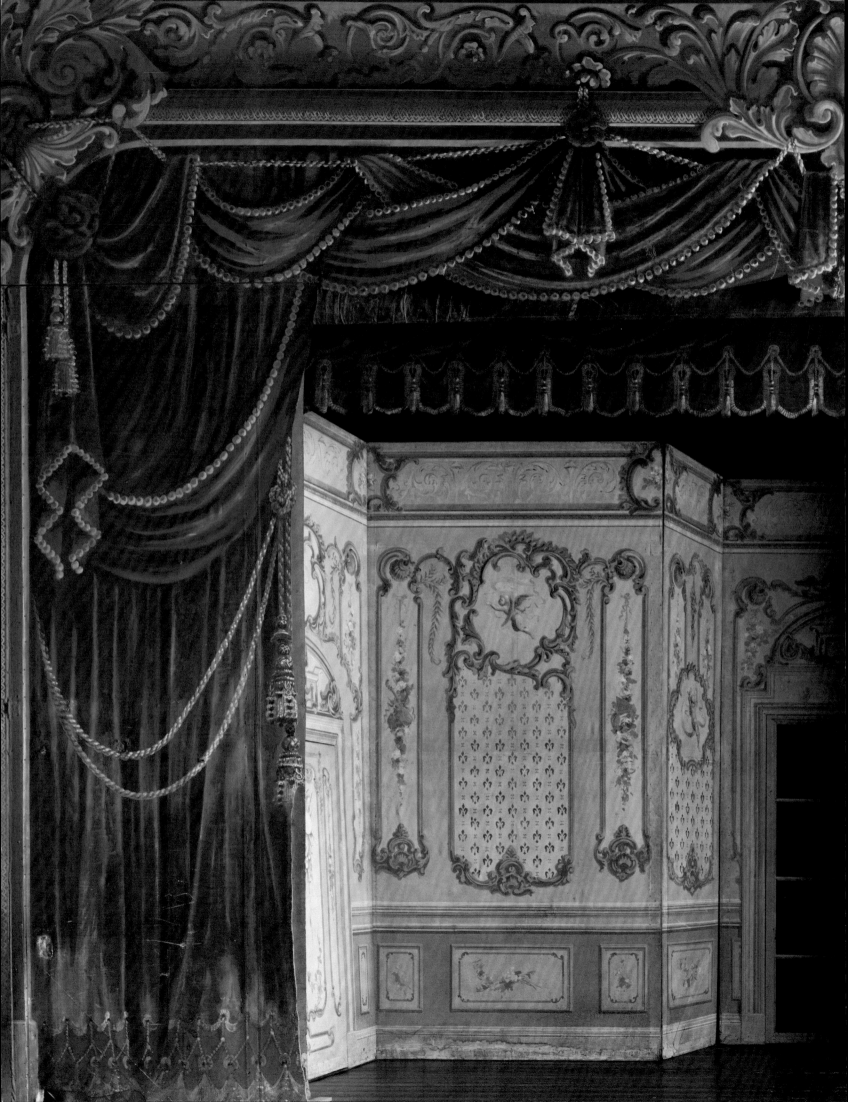

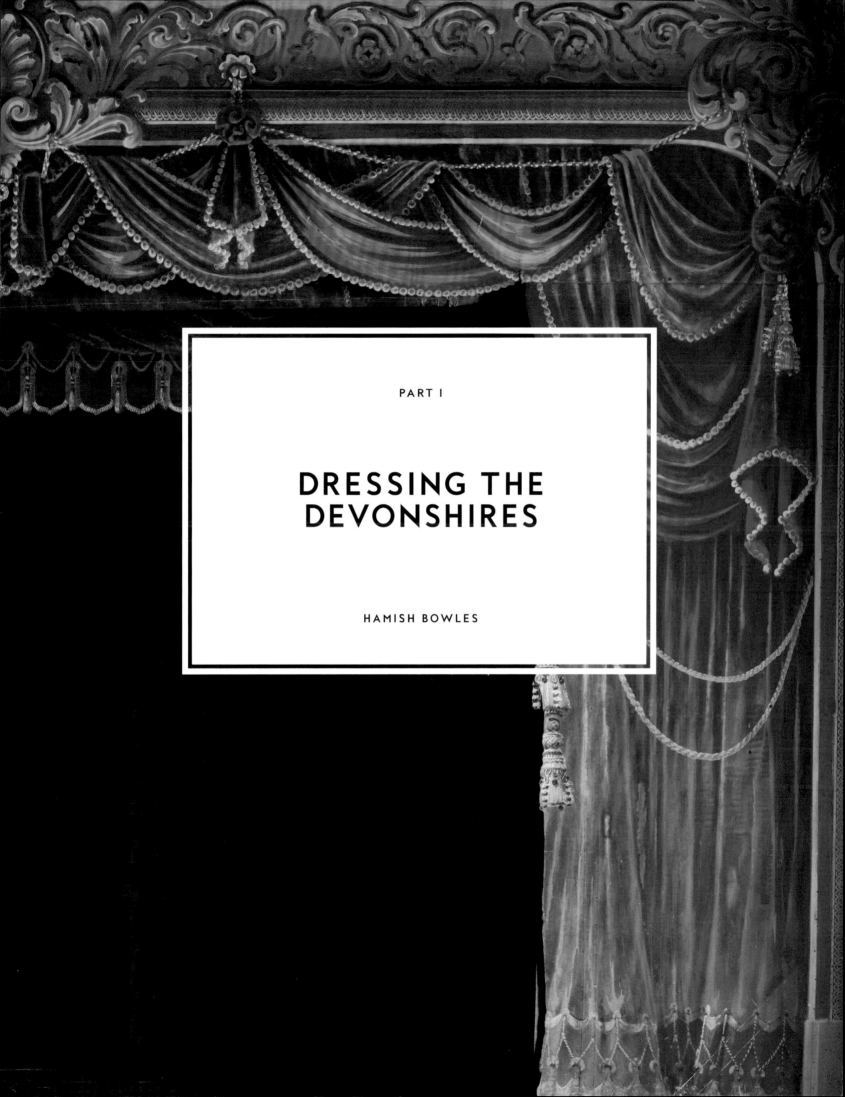

PART I

DRESSING THE DEVONSHIRES

HAMISH BOWLES

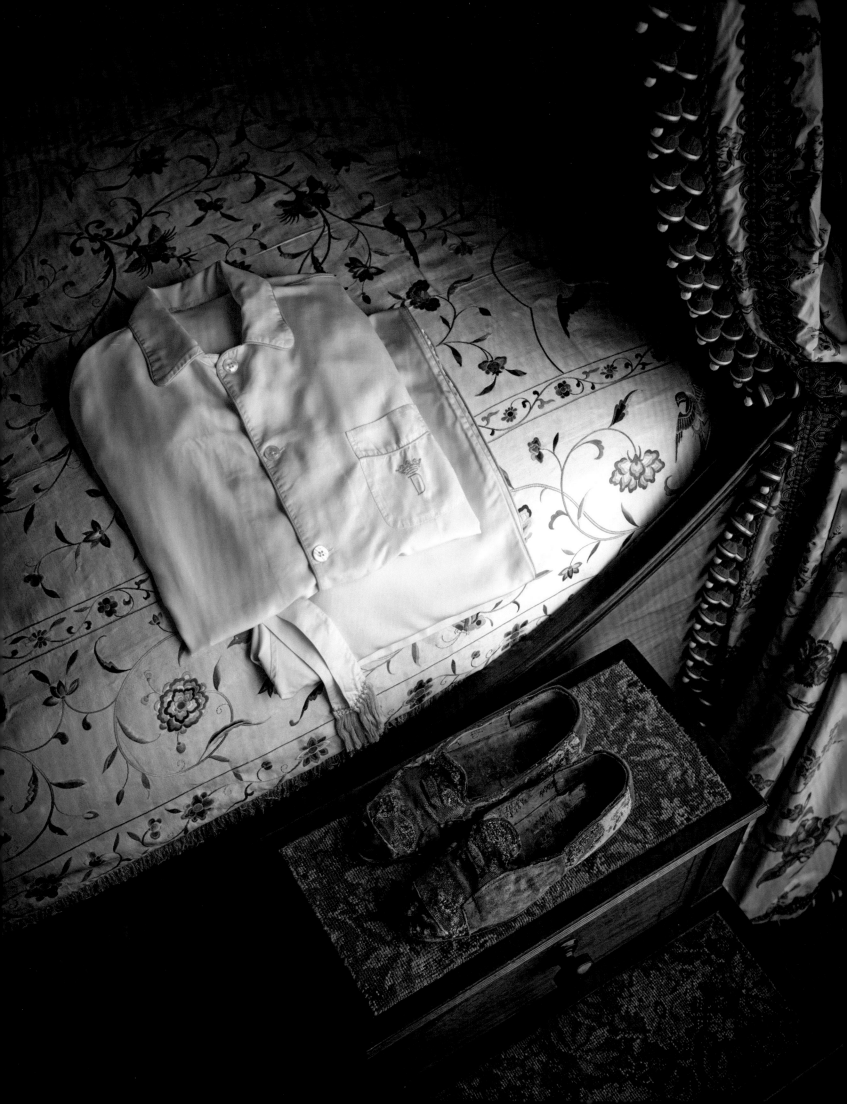

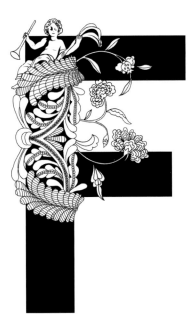

rom Bess of Hardwick (figs. 19, 126) to the present Countess of Burlington (fig. 3), from the swaggering 1st Duke of Devonshire (figs. 70, 74) to the threadbare 10th (fig. 62), in gilded hall and on windswept moor, the Cavendish family has embraced fashion through the centuries with varying degrees of enthusiasm or wariness, economy or profligacy, pragmatism or fantasy. Whatever their approach, however, the family's idiosyncratic members have always used clothing as a vivid expression of their very different personalities and interests.

As I have discovered during my own adventures at Chatsworth, rifling through its closets and muniment rooms, its dressing-up boxes, and its towers of doughty tin travelling trunks, the house brims with the most eclectic and endlessly surprising sartorial treasures that bear witness to the many and varied lives that have been lived there – indoors and out, above and below stairs.

There are pieces from the House of Worth (fig. 94) and from Marks & Spencer; from Ede & Ravenscroft and Vetements' Demna Gvasalia (fig. 154); from the lace-makers of Venice, Mechelen and Brussels, to the workrooms of Franka (fig. 143) and Givenchy (fig. 120) and Dior (figs. 1, 121), and of Helmut Lang (fig. 60), Alexander McQueen (fig. 139) and Philip Treacy (fig. 116). In preserving these textile arts, the Devonshires have painted a vivid picture for posterity of evolving generational tastes. And in Chatsworth itself all the players have had a theatre of *nonpareil* beauty for which to dress the part.

Chatsworth, as Deborah 'Debo' Devonshire noted, is crowded with 'paintings, sculptures, miniatures, incunabula, books, plates, gold and silver objects, furniture, textiles, tapestries, china, pottery, drawings, *objets de vertu*, jewels, bronzes, antique gems, letters, firearms, diaries, estate records, carpets, prints, minerals, household necessities and oddments of all kinds, dates and descriptions… gathered under the 1¼ acres of roof.' Visitors, she added, 'see the formal tip of the iceberg… they totter out into the fresh air exhausted after three furlongs of red carpet, a 101 stairs up and 62 down.'

'It's a rummy old place', the lugubrious Victorian 8th Duke (fig. 64) told one startled visitor, but it is the sentiments of the 6th 'Bachelor' Duke (fig. 22), that great embellisher of the estate's treasures inside and out, that echo more powerfully through the centuries. 'My happiness at Chatsworth is quite different from anywhere else', he wrote, 'I like nothing in the world so much. No, nothing ½ so much.'

The Bachelor Duke, and indeed the Cavendish family, owe their beatitude to a remarkable forebear, the formidable Bess of Hardwick. Bess became the wealthiest and most powerful woman in Elizabethan England after the monarch herself, and one who understood as keenly as her queen the significance and symbolism of architecture, dress and design.

Born Elizabeth Hardwick to minor Derbyshire gentry, she outlived three wealthy husbands before securing the hand of the wily George Talbot, the 6th Earl of Shrewsbury, Earl Marshal of England, and the country's wealthiest nobleman, at what was then for her the far from tender age of 41. The staunchly protestant Bess had wisely supported

18 *(opposite)* The 11th Duke's silk pyjamas by Turnbull & Asser, alongside his oft-worn and much repaired slippers by John Lobb.

19 *(following pages, left to right)* Follower of Hans Eworth, *Elizabeth Hardwick ('Bess of Hardwick'), Countess of Shrewsbury,* circa 1560-1569.

20 The Duchess of Devonshire's evening gown by Bellville et Cie, 1969.

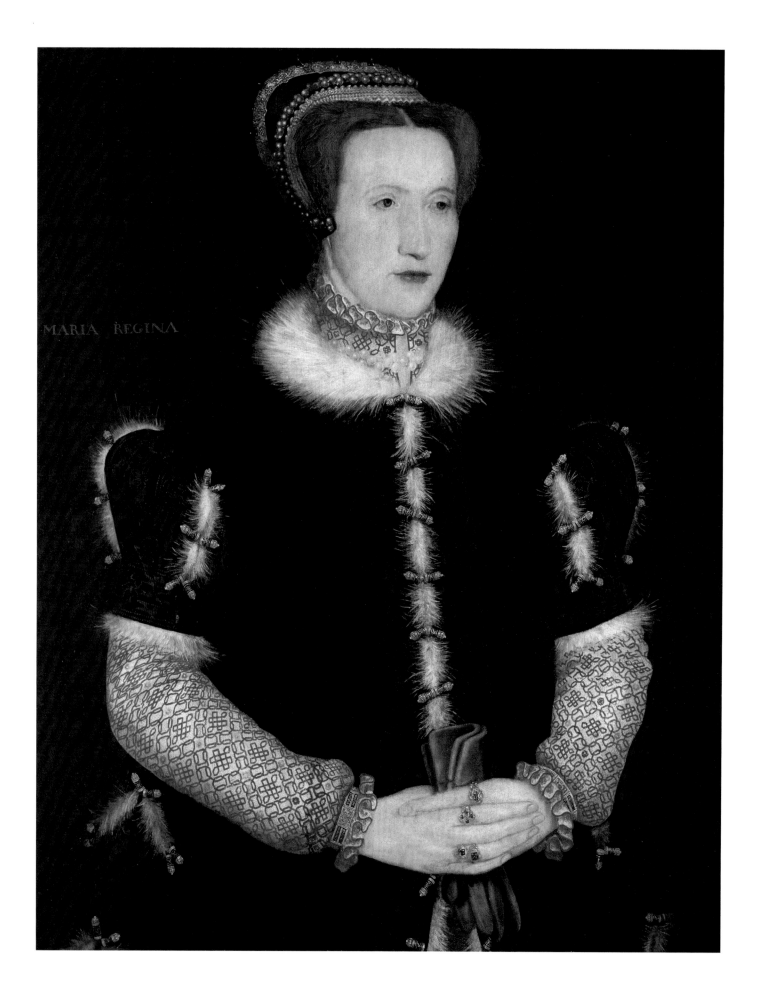

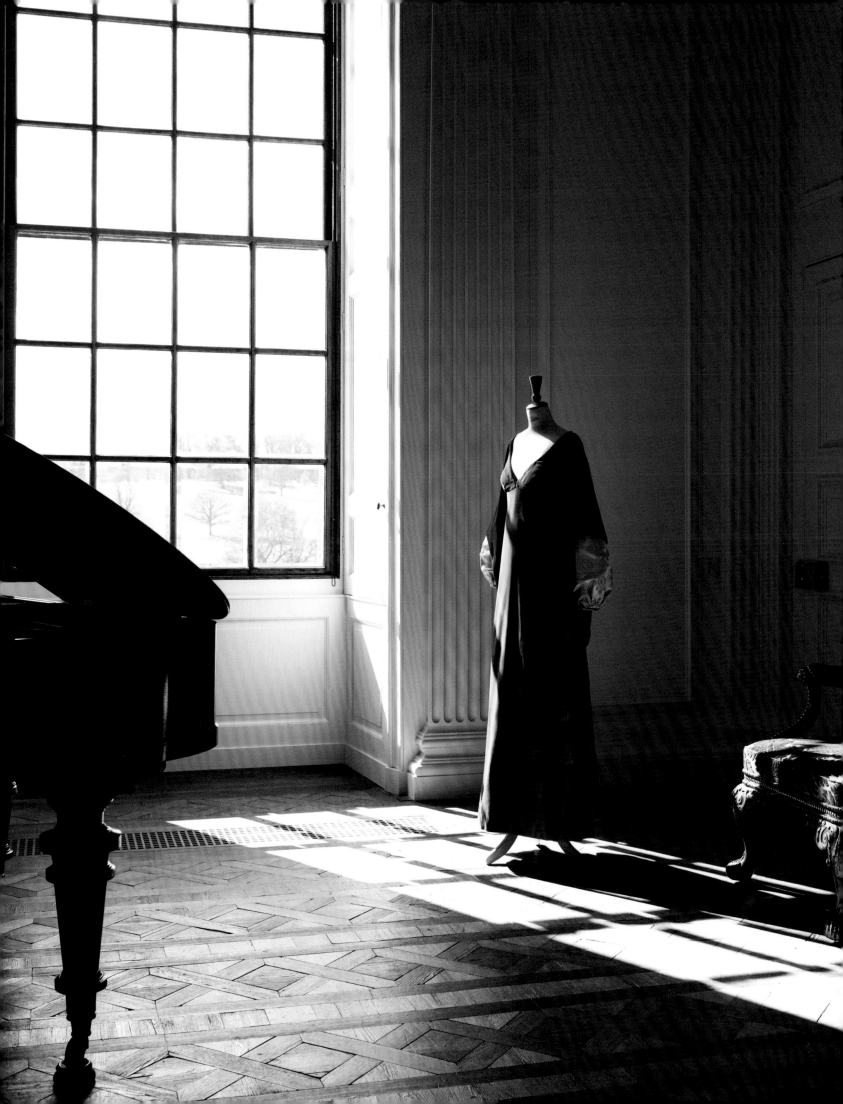

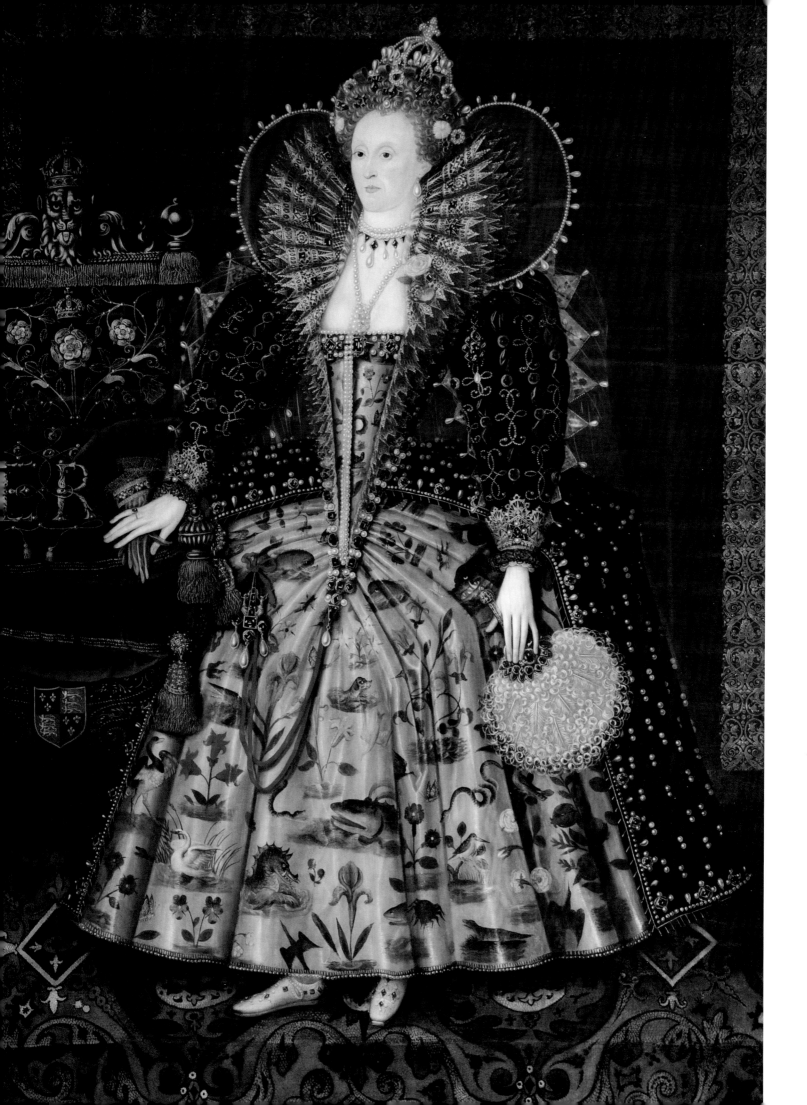

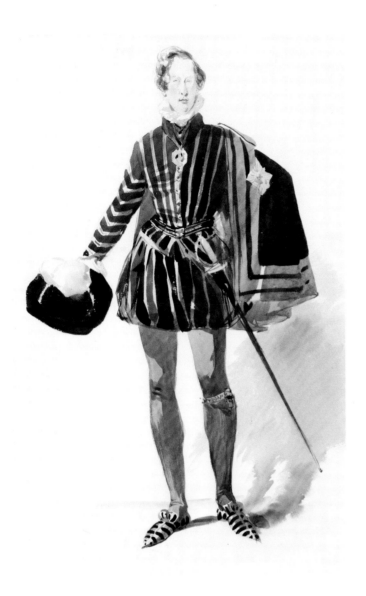

Princess Elizabeth, although her position under the Catholic Queen Mary had been decidedly precarious. Queen Mary died in 1558, however, and Elizabeth ascended, rewarding Bess for her fealty by appointing her to lady-in-waiting. Soon after Bess's fourth marriage, Elizabeth I gave her Earl the dubious honour of serving as the custodian of hapless Mary, Queen of Scots. Mary whiled away the endless hours of her luxurious captivity plotting sundry unsuccessful escape stratagems whilst working superb embroideries with Bess, who had been taught the needle-working arts as a child. Together they produced the celebrated Oxburgh Hangings and many more wonders besides. In these textile adventures they were assisted by their attendant ladies, the male and female members of Bess's staff who had been taught to sew, and occasionally the professional male embroiderer recorded in accounts by the single and appropriate name, Angell.

Bess would soon have some splendid canvases upon which to display the prodigious examples of her handiwork. As the now powerful Countess of Shrewsbury, she set about aggrandizing the existing house atop a hill at Hardwick, Derbyshire (inherited from her second husband). She apparently soon thought better of these interventions, however, leaving that house abandoned and instead hiring the architect Robert Smythson to build her a country palace from scratch a few hundred yards away. Smythson, who also worked on the great Elizabethan trophy houses Longleat and Wollaton Hall, drew on Italian Renaissance, the Loire Valley and Flemish models to create an H-shaped building that is a triumph of the glazier's costly art ('Hardwick Hall, more glass than wall'), and Bess proudly proclaimed her status from the rooftops – quite literally – in a pierced stone-work balustrade frieze that rises above the flat roofs of Hardwick's six square towers and incorporates her 'E S' monogram (for Elizabeth Shrewsbury) surmounted by a coronet, silhouetted against the ever-mutating Derbyshire skies for all to see. (The motif is repeated in a retainer's silver badge in the Devonshire Collection.)

But Bess's architectural ambitions did not end here. She had persuaded her second husband, Sir William Cavendish, one of King Henry VIII's official pillagers of the monasteries, to divest himself of some property and invest instead in 8000 more acres in her own untamed birth county of Derbyshire.

A day's journey by carriage from Hardwick lay the estate of Chatsworth, nestled picturesquely in the Derbyshire Dales above the River Derwent. Under Bess's direction a second Elizabethan palace rose here from the raw landscape of rocky tors and unforgiving moors, in time to be transformed by human ingenuity, vision and labour into an Arcadian vision. Bess proudly recorded her estate's splendours in an elaborately worked embroidery panel of her own devising.

21 *(opposite)* British School, *Queen Elizabeth I*, 1592–1599.

22 *(above)* C Smyth, *William Spencer Cavendish, the 6th Duke of Devonshire in the costume of an Elizabethan nobleman, circa 1600*, worn at the Bal Costumé at Buckingham Palace, 12 May 1842.

As the Countess of Shrewsbury, Bess required an extensive panoply of clothes and jewellery, and her account books are dense with entries relating to the purchase of adornments. 'Bess was born to shop it seems', notes her biographer Mary S Lovell, 'although she spent wisely and insisted on good value', sentiments echoed by Debo, who dressed at agricultural fairs, Marks & Spencer and the Paris haute couture shows declaring that, 'Nothing in between seems to be much good. Properly made clothes should last to the end', she added, 'So forgotten French works of art come out of the back of the cupboard (mixed with Barbours and Derri boots), still beautiful and always comfortable, which is my idea of what clothes should be.'

The Duchess of Devonshire (née Amanda Heywood-Lonsdale), has also preserved many of her own beloved clothes, and a positive flotilla of hats, in wardrobe rooms that are maintained with the scrupulous attention to detail and precision to be found in her stable's tack rooms (fig. 145). These are filled with clothes that bear witness to her various lives – debutante, hipster girl-about-town (fig. 147), hippie de luxe (fig. 140), mother, *égérie* of Royal Ascot (fig. 143), hostess to royalty (fig. 49), enlivener of village fetes and agricultural fairs, winner of gundog competitions (fig. 67), rider and huntswoman (fig. 66) and patron of contemporary artists and artisans.

Bess repaid her monarch's priceless favour with the gift of clothing. No monarch has understood the power and potential of dress as keenly as Elizabeth I. The circa 1599 portrait of the Queen at Hardwick Hall, from the workshop of Nicholas Hilliard (fig. 21), was a New Year's Day gift from Bess to her monarch, and the magnificent gown in which she is depicted was also a tribute from her grateful subject. The superlative embroidery on this costume's stomacher and farthingale skirts, cut short in patriotic and saucy defiance of Spanish custom, and worked with fantastical sea creatures and symbolic fruits and flowers (these latter copied from John Gerard's recently published *The Herball or General Historie of Plants*, a book that is naturally to be found in the Chatsworth library), was once alluringly attributed to Bess herself, but more probably commissioned from John Parr, the Queen's favoured embroiderer. The portrait and the dress were the inspirations for a mock Elizabethan ensemble in Dame Vivienne Westwood's Autumn/Winter 1997-1998 collection.

Bess cherished her embroideries and clothing, as both her expenditures and her will make clear: 'Have speciall care and regard to' p'serve the same from all manner of wett, mothe and other hurte or spoyle thereofe', she wrote firmly in her testament, 'and to leave them so preserved to contynewe at the sayed several houses as foresayed for the better furnishng them therewithall.'

Today, thanks in no small part to Duchess Evelyn (figs. 34, 41), the conservation-minded wife of the 9th Duke, this *nonpareil* collection of embroidered textiles remains

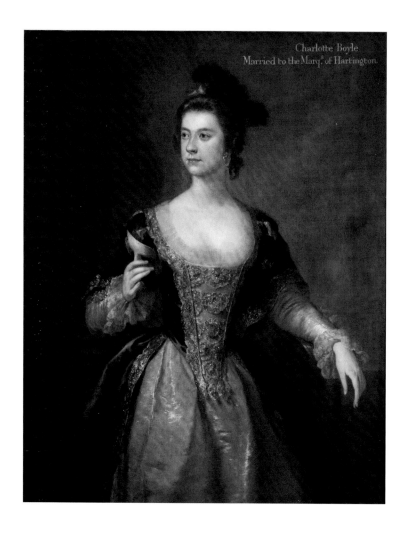

23 *(above)* George Knapton, *Lady Charlotte Boyle, Baroness Clifford and Marchioness of Hartington,* 1748-1756.

24 *(opposite)* Lucian Freud, *Head of a Woman (Portrait of Lady Anne Tree),* circa 1950.

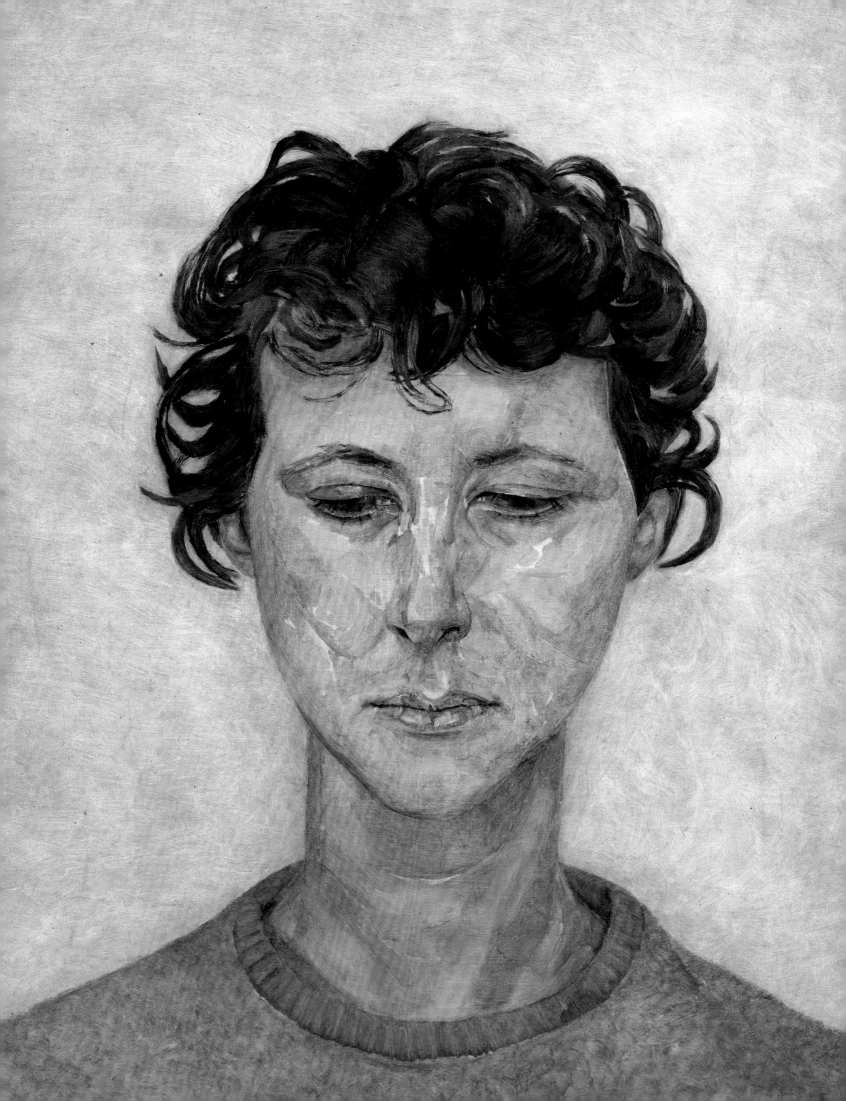

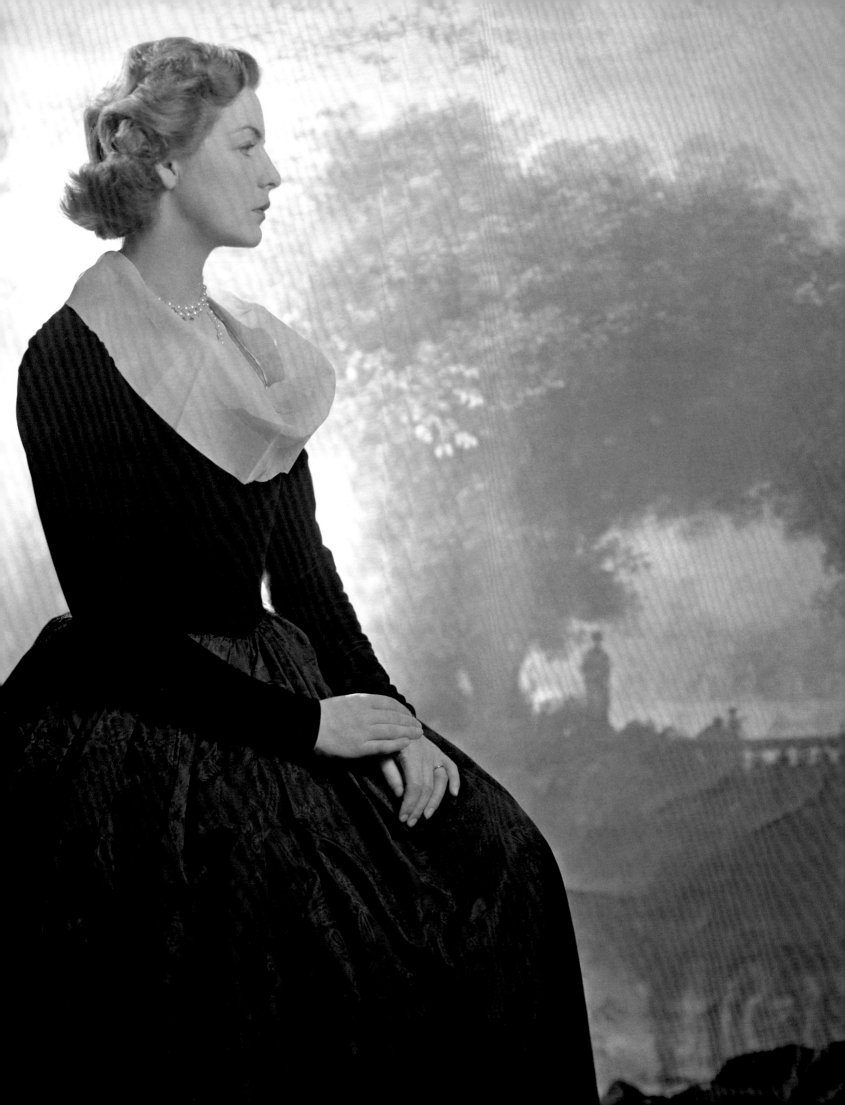

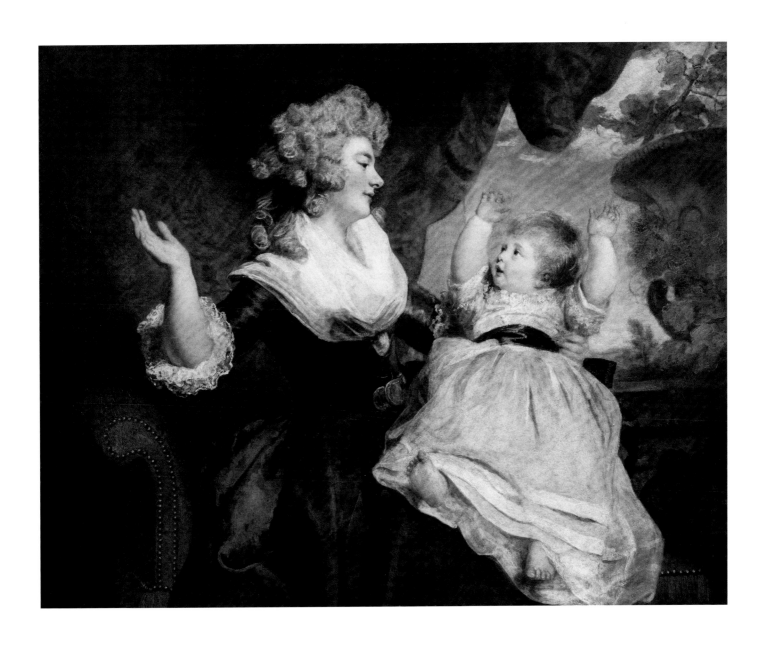

25 *(opposite)* Cecil Beaton, Deborah
Devonshire, 1949.

26 *(above)* Sir Joshua Reynolds,
*Duchess Georgiana with Her
Infant Daughter, Lady Georgiana
Cavendish, Later Countess of
Carlisle,* circa 1759.

astonishingly intact. Much of it was gifted to the nation in 1959, along with Hardwick Hall itself, in lieu, in part, of death duties. By the time of the 10th Duke's death in 1950, Prime Minister Clement Atlee's government had imposed crippling death duties at 80 percent – taxes that took 17 years to pay off.

At Chatsworth, Duchess Evelyn had some precious tapestries washed in the tumbling waters of Paxton's Cascade. A century later, the Mortlake tapestries (depicting scenes from the life of Christ, after cartoons by Raphael) have recently emerged from a state-of-the-art conservation and cleaning program. Maintaining the fabric of Chatsworth is an ongoing and ceaseless project.

Bess bequeathed Chatsworth to her eldest son, Henry Cavendish, but his brother William, 1st Earl of Devonshire, soon bought it from him – for £10,000. William's great-grandson and namesake, the 4th Earl of Devonshire, Francophile in tastes alone, remodelled Chatsworth after Mansart's Château de Marly, where Louis XIV retreated from the formality and much-peopled pomp of Versailles. The Earl's French passions did not, however, extend to that country's religion, and he was an instrumental figure in deposing England's Catholic King James II in favour of the Protestant King William III and his Queen co-regent, Mary II. When the monarchs were duly installed after the Glorious Revolution of 1688, the Earl was rewarded with an elevation to become the 1st Duke of Devonshire, a title now in its twelfth generation's flowering.

In 2004 Peregrine 'Stoker' Cavendish (fig. 72) succeeded to the title, becoming the 12th Duke of Devonshire, and he and Amanda have embarked on an ambitious program of renovation to rationalize the sometimes quirkily haphazard arrangements of the State Rooms, and to integrate the house's storied treasures with their own dynamic collections of contemporary art and ceramics – as generations have done before them. This is a house, after all, that can boast a Painted Hall (fig. 42) with murals by Louis Laguerre from 1687-1694, with scenes from the life of Julius Caesar (in overt homage to William III), and a mural of giant cyclamens on a guest bathroom's wall painted by Lucian Freud when he came to stay in 1959 (fig. 152).

These latest twenty-first-century home improvements alone involved a kilometre of hand-stitching for the window draperies and bed hangings (fig. 1). The familial interest in fine textiles continues at Chatsworth to this day. The Duchess of Devonshire embroidered

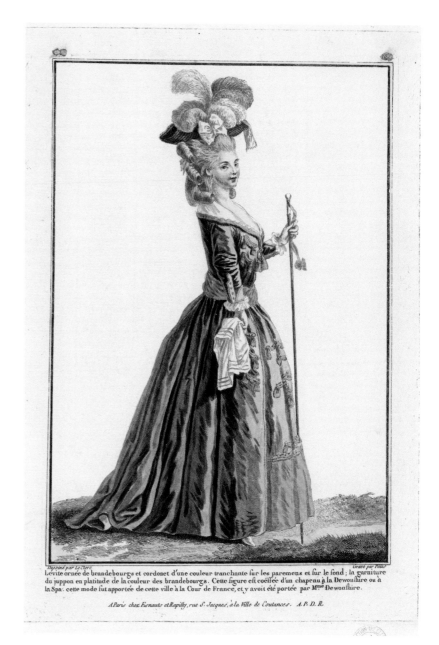

27 *(above)* Pierre-Thomas LeClerc, *Lévite ornée de brandebourgs*, Galerie des Modes et Costumes Français, 1779.

28 *(opposite)* 'Shepherdess' fancy dress costume by Russell & Allen, worn by Duchess Evelyn in India, 1889.

29 *(following pages, left to right)* Duchess Louise's silk and lace bag with gold work embroidery, 1890s, on a George III giltwood chair by François Hervé, late eighteenth century.

30 John Lucas, *Blanche, Countess of Burlington* (2nd creation), 1840.

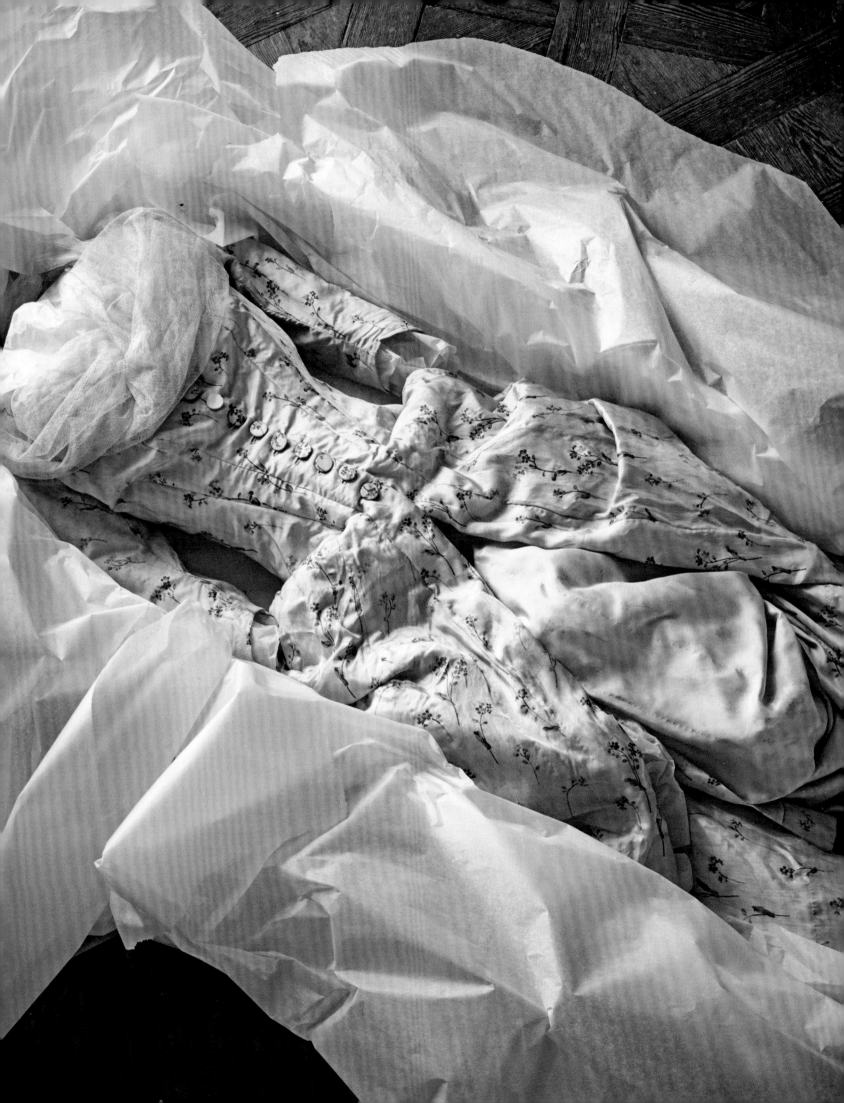

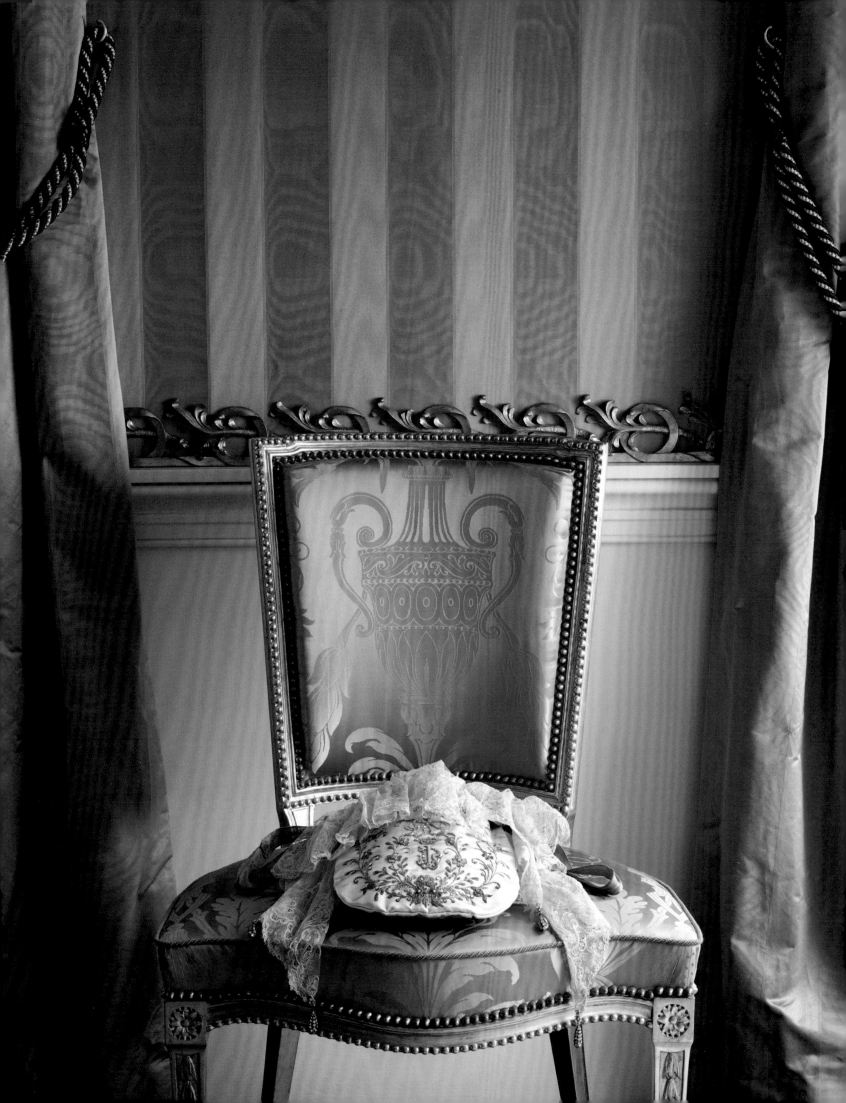

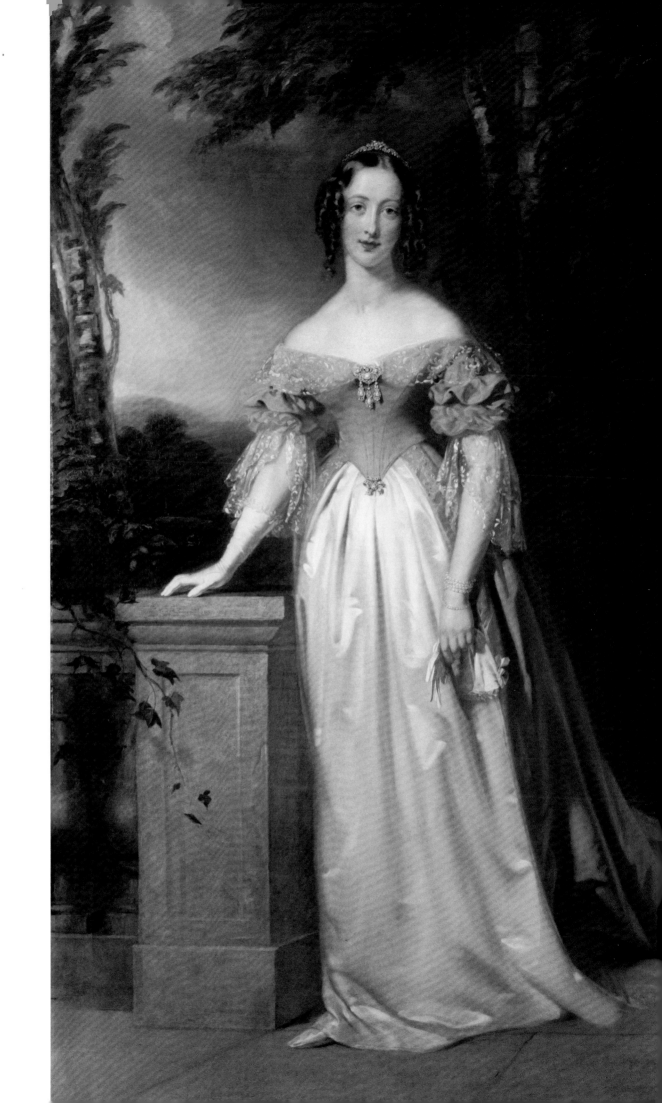

a Thomas Hope footstool in the Wellington Bedroom – so named because the victorious Duke spent the night there in 1843 when the young Queen Victoria came to stay – herself, carefully matching its High Empire scheme of arsenic green and silver damask. The Countess of Burlington, in turn, was taught to sew by her glamorous grandmother, Ann Roundell, who engendered in her a passion for fashion that would flourish in Laura Burlington's future lives as a model, a muse to the designer Roland Mouret and a fashion editor. When Jacob van der Beugel was commissioned in 2009 to create the *North Sketch Gallery Sequence*, a ceramics installation including representations of family members' DNA, each was asked for a subject that had special significance for them; Lady Burlington chose a stitch pattern that her grandmother had taught her as a child. In the twentieth century Duchess Evelyn not only conserved the textiles at Hardwick Hall, but contributed embroideries of her own working. Such was Evelyn's love of Hardwick that it became her 'dower house', and she continued to live there, until her death in 1960.

The Duke's intriguing aunt, Lady Anne Tree (fig. 24), meanwhile, a self confessed 'Victorian do-gooder', put her own passion for needlework to philanthropic use. Lady Anne was a prison visitor for many years and she lobbied the Home Office for over 20 years in an attempt to change the rules so that prisoners could earn money by working while they were incarcerated. 'Sewing', she averred, 'not only provides a small nest egg to ease prisoners' lives on release, it also has a spiritual quality… It is meditative, a way of thinking, of taking stock.' In 1997 her efforts were rewarded and she established Fine Cell Work, a scheme in which prisoners are taught needlepoint skills and produce items whose profits devolve to them. The majority of these newly minted embroiderers, like Angell before them, were men. 'If you feel this is poofy, don't bother us', Lady Anne thundered at any who dared to object, 'because we don't want to train you.'

Chatsworth's custodians have enjoyed an unusual engagement with the modern art of their day, but they have also been surrounded by inspiring material to nurture their historicist instincts. The 4th Duke exponentially added to the treasures and real estate holdings of his family by the deft expedient of marriage – to Charlotte Boyle, heiress to the breathtaking collections of her father, the 'Architect' 3rd Earl of Burlington, dubbed 'the Apollo of the Arts', a follower of Andrea Palladio, Inigo Jones and William Kent.

The lovely but short-lived Charlotte Boyle herself was depicted by George Knapton (circa 1750) brandishing a silvery half mask and dressed in masquerade costume of black

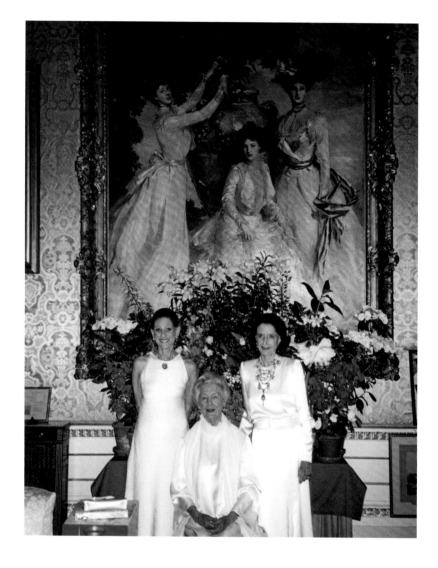

31 *(above)* Annette de la Renta, Deborah Devonshire and Jayne Wrightsman, July 1995, standing in front of *The Acheson Sisters* by John Singer Sargent, 1902.

32 *(opposite)* Robert Fairer, Stella Tennant, Erin O'Conner and Nadejda Savcova backstage at John Galliano for Christian Dior Haute Couture's Autumn/Winter 2005 presentation.

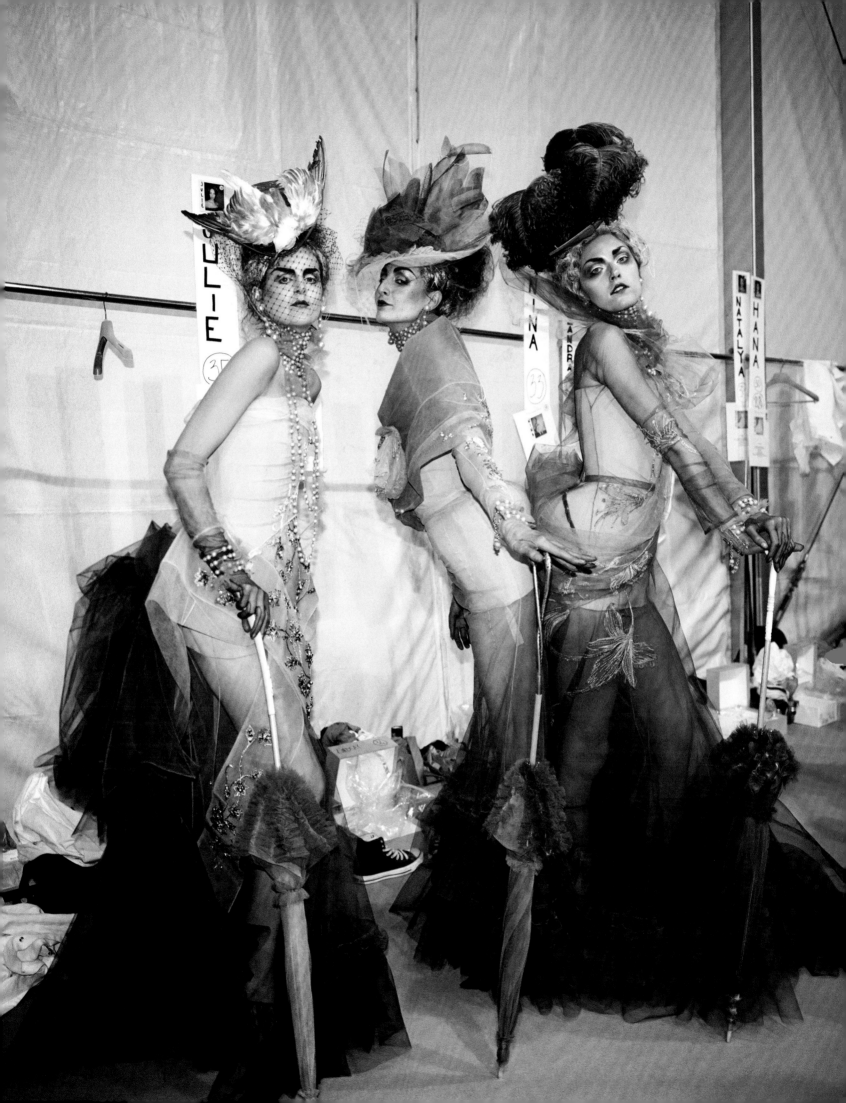

TATLER

VOL. 258   No. 3,348   LONDON JUNE 1968   Price Five Shillings

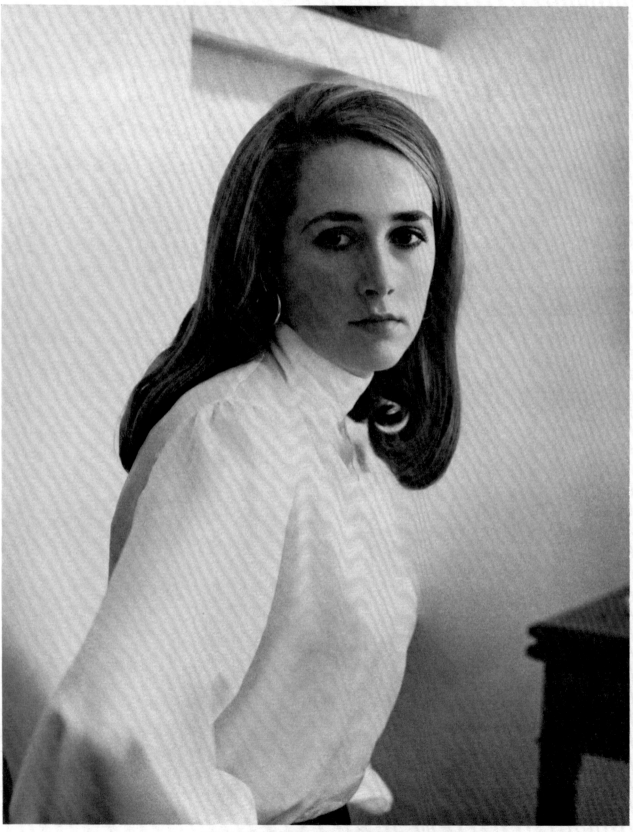

THE MARCHIONESS OF HARTINGTON

Lady Hartington is the wife of the Duke of Devonshire's heir. She was formerly Miss Amanda Heywood-Lonsdale, the only daughter of the late Cmdr. Edward Heywood-Lonsdale, R.N. and of Mrs. Heywood-Lonsdale.

The Hartingtons married last year and live in London and Derbyshire.

Portrait by Barry Swaebe

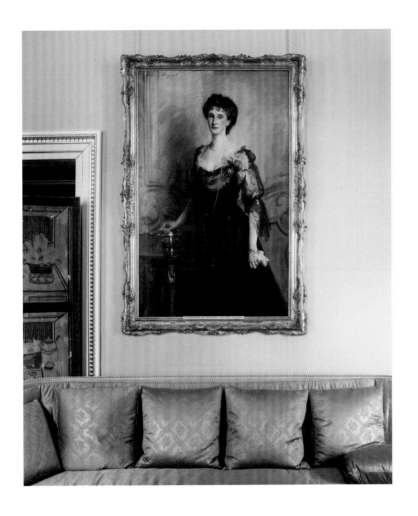

satin and silver tissue and lace, with an ostrich-feathered cap – an ensemble that was fondly presumed at the time to suggest the clothing worn in the age of Rubens (fig. 23).

The 6th Duke of Devonshire was the model of a Romantic-era aristocrat, with refined tastes in contemporary art and culture, an interest in scholarly as well as fashionable life, and a passion for the theatre, dressing up and historicism. Inspired by a visit to the Château de Fontainebleau, for instance, the Duke installed stamped leather panels in the State Music Room and State Bedchamber, and on a whim he acquired at auction some thoroughly un-Chatsworthian carved sixteenth-century panelling from a German monastery and had it installed in the low-ceiling Oak Room, which now provides a faintly tenebrous ante room to the Chapel. At Lismore Castle, meanwhile, he worked with the architect William Atkinson, and subsequently with Joseph Paxton and the artist-designers Crace and Pugin to create a bewitching High Gothic fantasia of towers and turrets in one of the loveliest settings in Ireland, on a bluff above the Blackwater River.

The Duke carried the royal orb at the coronation of his friend George IV, his Mock Tudor revival costume part of the elaborate *mise-en-scène* designed for that aesthetic monarch (who managed to spend an astounding £24,000 on his own coronation robes, just short of £1 million in today's currency). The 6th Duke was further able to indulge his Tudorbethan fancies when Queen Victoria and Prince Albert held a Plantagenet Ball for 2,000 guests at Buckingham Palace in 1842. The artist James Robinson Planché was responsible for the costumes of the Royal Household; Prince Albert was dressed as Edward III, Queen Victoria as his consort Philippa of Hainault. Guests outside the royal household could be costumed as they wished and the 6th Duke chose to appear as Elizabeth I's favourite Robert Dudley, the Earl of Leicester, (who visited Chatsworth in 1577 and stayed in a bedroom subsequently converted by the 6th Duke in the 1830s). Dressed in a short crimson cape, pinned with the Garter star that George IV had given him, he cut a convincing figure, despite his windswept, defiantly early Victorian coiffure (fig. 22).

When the Duke's nephew Earl Granville was appointed to head the British delegation to the coronation of Tsar Alexander II in 1856, the Duke was inspired to commission for his wife, Lady Granville, a magnificent parure in the neo-Renaissance 'Holbein' style from the London jeweller C F Hancock, (designer of the Victoria Cross), using many of the antique intaglios and cameos that had been assembled by the 2nd Duke in the early eighteenth century. Existing family jewels were cannibalized to provide the diamonds required to give this parure – with its stomacher, coronet, diadem, comb, necklace, bracelet and bandeau – the requisite sparkle (figs. 127-128). They didn't sparkle in the parure for too long. The formidable 'Double Duchess' Louise, widow of the Duke of Manchester,

33 *(opposite)* The Duchess of Devonshire on the cover of *Tatler*, June 1968.

34 *(above)* John Singer Sargent, *Duchess Evelyn*, 1902.

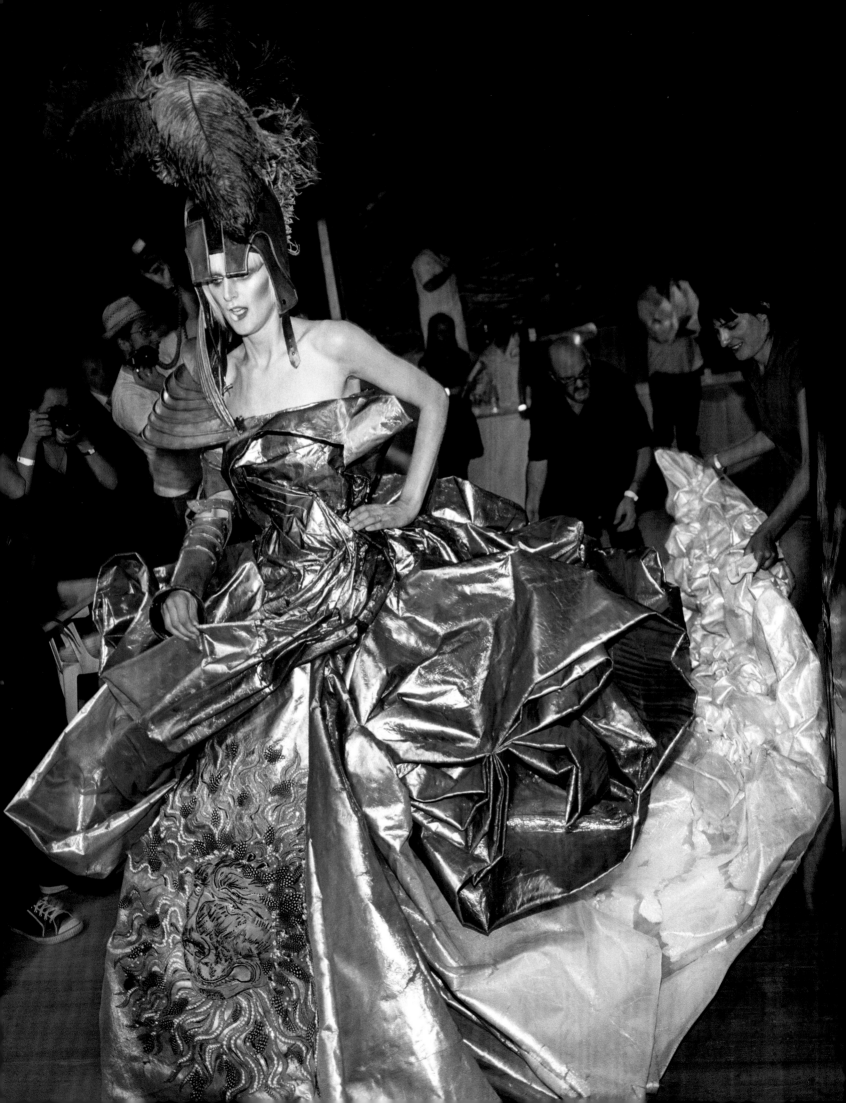

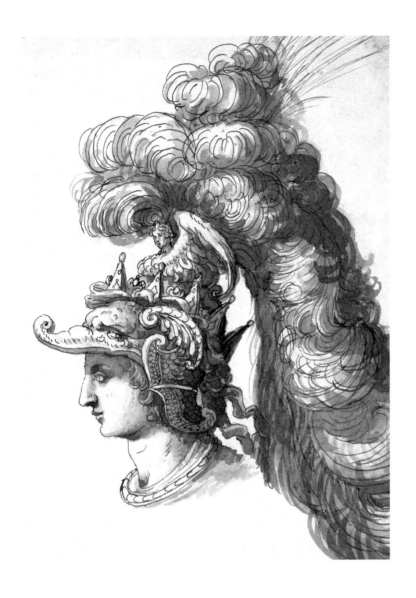

wife of the 8th Duke, and celebrated Whig hostess, intent on creating a magnificent tiara for herself, picked them all out, and while she was at it had *all* the diamonds in her husband's Garter star removed as well.

In her new palm-leaf and lotus-motif diadem, commissioned from the jeweller A E Skinner (fig. 124), however, Duchess Louise was suitably bedazzling. 'She set everything on fire', observed Benjamin Disraeli, 'even the neighbouring Thames.' Duchess Louise's splendid satin evening bag, frothy with lace and crusted with embroidery, is a sparkling memorial to her opulent tastes (fig. 29).

Lady Blanche Cavendish, the 6th Duke's beloved niece and wife of the future 7th Duke, shared her uncle's Romantic tastes in dressing. When she dressed as Flora for charades at Chatsworth in 1831, she was decked with garlands that were made by Joseph Paxton himself. She was depicted by the artist Henry Howard in Tudor costume à la Anne Boleyn (in a portrait at Castle Howard), and in a posthumous portrait by John Lucas (fig. 30) in the lavender and white satin dress that she wore to Queen Victoria and Prince Albert's 1840 wedding, a gown intended to suggest Restoration costume. (The tulle-trimmed gloves that she holds were recently identified in Chatsworth's textiles collection.)

Amanda has also embraced the Mediaeval and Tudor-bethan romanticism of the late 1960s and the early 1970s, with evocative designs from Troubadour and Bellville et Cie. It was Belinda Bellville's appropriately sixteenth-century looking dress of brown velvet and ivory brocade (fig. 20) that she wore in 1969 to the opening of the exhibition of *Old Master Drawings from Chatsworth* at the National Gallery of Art in Washington, DC. This influence continued into the 1980s with an Elizabethan-inspired ball gown made by the Duchess's favourite couturier, the Yugoslavian-born Franka.

Although Debo also wore some clothes of frankly Tudor inspiration, including some stately velvet and watered silk ball gowns made by Hubert de Givenchy (fig. 120), her tastes generally ran more to the eighteenth century, and looked to the rich visual legacy of the 6th Duke's mother, the beautiful and flamboyant Duchess Georgiana (fig. 82). As Kimberly Chrisman-Campbell notes in her chapter, Georgiana was the unchallenged leader of style in Georgian England, dubbed 'the glass and model of fashion' by the press, whose influence reached even to the court of her great friend Queen Marie Antoinette. (Not every duchess has been so warmly received in the capital of fashion. Duchess Mary, in Paris in 1947 with the Duchess of Rutland, went to see the much vaunted collection of the new designer Christian Dior, but in their shabby wartime tweed coats they were denied admittance by the disdainful saleswoman.) Georgi-

35 *(opposite)* Robert Fairer, Stella Tennant in an evening dress by John Galliano for Christian Dior Haute Couture, Autumn/Winter 2006.

36 *(above)* Inigo Jones, *Design for a Helmet from the Court Masque, Prince Henry's Barriers or Tilts,* 1610.

ana, a famously reckless gambler, ran up bills at Rose Bertin, the French queen's brilliant dressmaker, (whom she patronized even as the French Revolution was waging), that remained unpaid at the time of her death. Georgiana's husband, the 5th Duke, dressed à la mode himself in his youth. As a 20-year-old Grand Tourist in 1768 he sat for Anton von Maron in a suit of startling lapis-blue velvet and an ermine-lined strawberry pink cloak intended to evoke the age of Van Dyck, and soon after Georgiana met him he appeared at a masquerade dressed in a blue and gold suit à la française, with white leather shoes topped with blue and gold roses. To Georgiana's dismay, however, this vein of frivolity soon withered on the vine.

Immortalised by the great swagger portraitists Gainsborough (fig. 82), Reynolds (fig. 84), Downman (fig. 87) and Cosway (fig. 91), among many others, and more or less affectionately lampooned by the caricaturists Rowlandson (fig. 86) and Gillray, Duchess Georgiana has proved an enduring inspiration to the Cavendish ladies. When Lady Evelyn Petty-Fitzmaurice married the future 9th Duke in 1892 her bridesmaids wore ensembles à la Georgiana, with fichus and 'white Gainsborough hats trimmed with feathers and caught up at the sides with pink roses' – a style that Georgiana introduced to the French court. (As a young woman in India, where her father, the 5th Marquess of Landsdowne, was the Viceroy, Duchess Evelyn wore an eighteenth-century-inspired shepherdess costume (fig. 28) for a theatrical performance or costume ball, its curvaceous buttoned bodice showcasing her 52-cm, or 20.5-inch, waist.)

The 11th Duke of Devonshire's sister, the embroidering Lady Anne, wore an Edward Molyneux gown for her 1949 wedding to the gossipy Michael Tree (dubbed 'Radio Belgravia' by his friends), loosely inspired by the one worn by Duchess Georgiana in Reynolds's delightful 1786 portrait with her daughter Lady Georgiana Cavendish (fig. 26); Debo subsequently sat for Cecil Beaton wearing a dress even more literally drawn from this source (fig. 25).

In 1951 the 11th Duke (Andrew) and Debo were invited to the celebrated ball given by the mysterious Mexican silver mining millionaire Carlos de Beistegui to inaugurate his newly restored Palazzo Labia in Venice. There were 18 *entrées* organized in the manner of the 8th Duke and Duchess Louise's 1897 Devonshire House costume ball. The legendary beauty Lady Diana Cooper led this series of highly elaborate tableaux, impersonating Cleopatra as imagined by Tiepolo in the palazzo's fresco. The ferocious hostess Daisy Fellowes (fig. 38) arrived as *America, 1750*, and Salvador Dalí and Christian Dior concocted a tableau of 14-foot-tall Giants.

Andrew and Debo wore eighteenth-century dress, Debo's costume (fig. 88) inspired by John Downman's 1787 portrait of Georgiana (fig. 87), but also evoking her own 1941

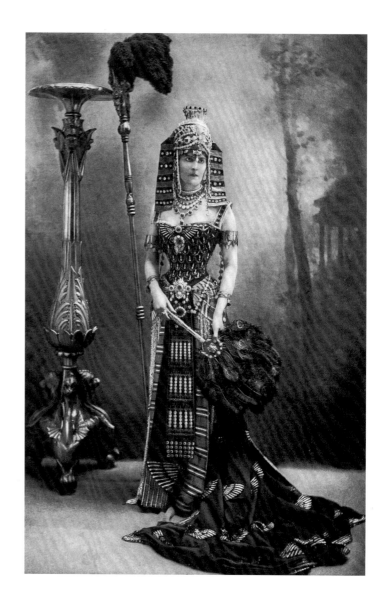

37 *(above)* John Thomson, photogravure by Walker & Boutall, Mrs Arthur Paget as Cleopatra, wearing a dress by Jean-Philippe Worth for the House of Worth, at the Devonshire House Ball, photogravure 1897, published 1899.

38 *(opposite)* Cecil Beaton, Daisy Fellowes at the Beistegui Ball, Venice, 1951.

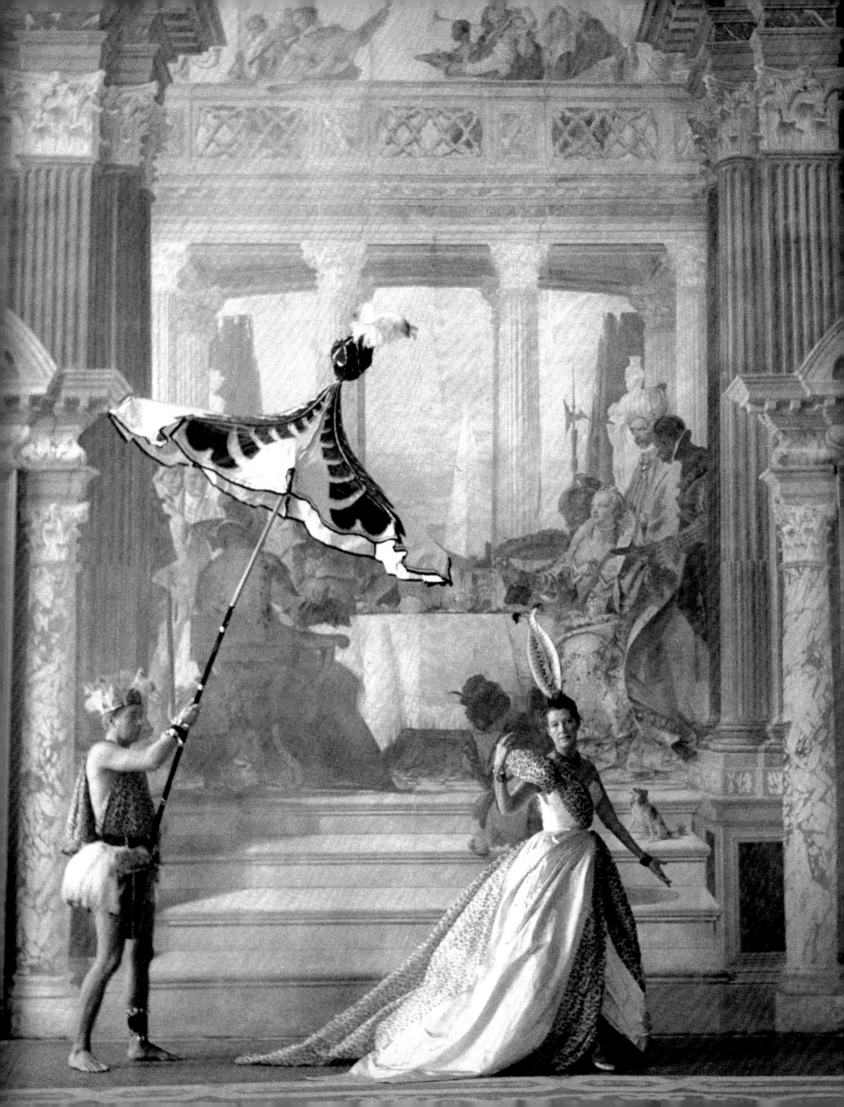

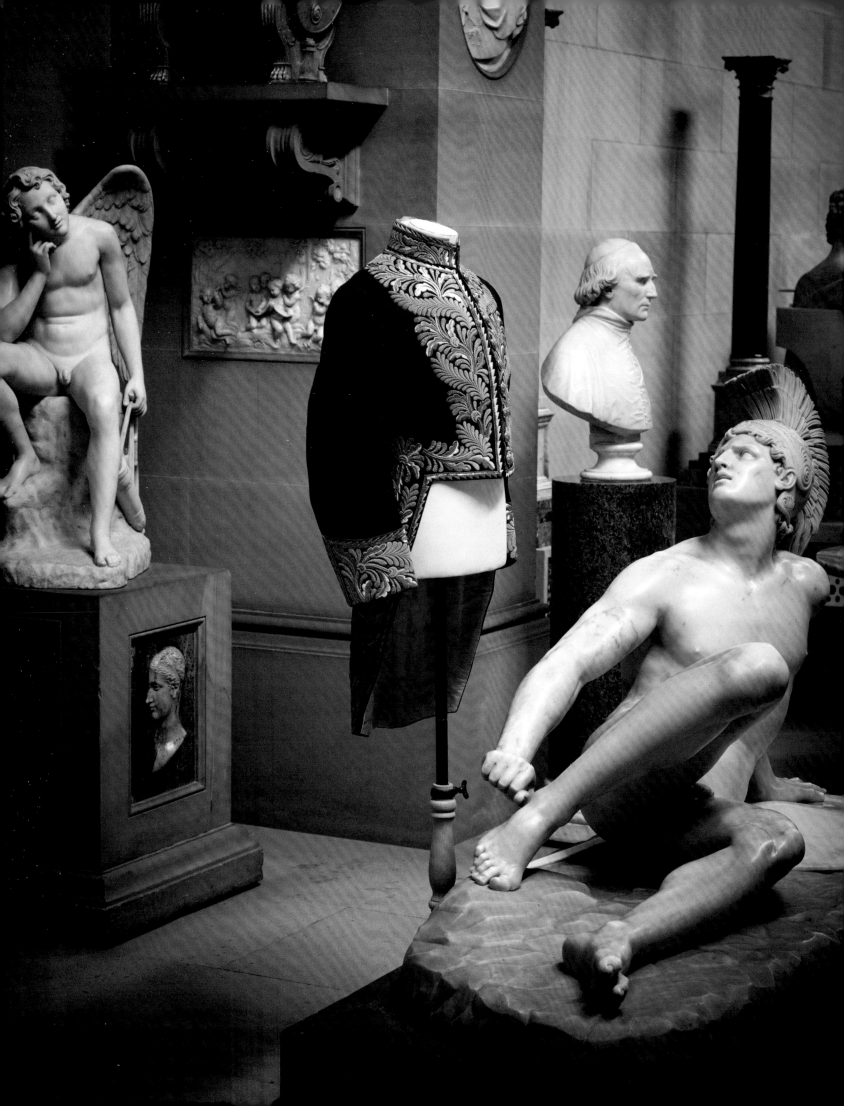

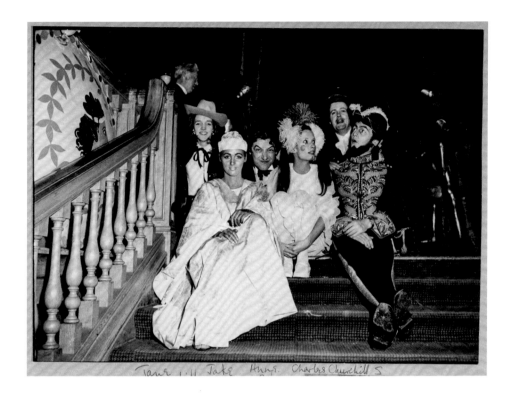

wedding dress (fig. 113), made by Victor Stiebel from 80 yards of silk tulle and a last gasp of extravagance before wartime rationing kicked in.

The Georgiana influence continued into the turn of the twenty-first century, when Debo's friend Oscar de la Renta made her a series of Watteau-back dresses in soft blue and green warp-printed silks and paper taffetas (fig. 119), and Amanda chose Ralph Lauren's coatdress of spangled, eighteenth-century-inspired striped and rose-patterned silk for house parties.

As a muse to designers like John Galliano, Karl Lagerfeld, Vivienne Westwood and Alexander McQueen, Stella Tennant has brought their own historical fantasies to life. Nor was she the first family member to flaunt borrowed finery for posterity. Elizabeth Cecil, the wife of the 3rd Earl, had to borrow the sable tippet and jewels worn for her portrait by Van Dyck: ''Tis no great matter for another age to think me richer than I am', she noted.

Stella was dressed by Galliano for his Autumn/Winter 2006 Christian Dior haute couture collection as a fanciful Roman centurion (fig. 35) in a helmet recalling Inigo Jones's designs (fig. 36), whilst in the spring of 1998 she was one of the designer's ghostly belle epoque figures (fig. 32), evoking the Edwardian panache of the three Acheson sisters, Aldra, Mary and Theo (granddaughters of Duchess Louise from her first marriage to the Duke of Manchester), depicted in John Singer Sargent's epic 1902 portrait that now commands a view of the Oak Stairs at Chatsworth (fig. 31). When Amanda sat for the cover of the *Tatler* in 1968, she also wore an Edwardian-style blouse, then the height of nostalgic chic (fig. 33).

Duchess Georgiana sometimes illustrated her lively correspondence with her own delightful sketches indicating the latest fashion trends, or the idiosyncrasies of regional dress that she observed on her many travels. Her son shared these interests, and the 6th Duke's fascinating diaries, letters and scrapbooks are filled with details of fashion and local costume. At the Geneva jewellers Baute et Moynier in 1824, for example, he acquired a pair of bracelets composed of enamelled pictures of women dressed in the costumes of Switzerland's 22 cantons, whilst his scrapbooks from the late 1820s include contemporary fashion plates, as well as thickets of letters from hopeful future duchesses, and theatre playbills, then printed on ivory or bright coloured satin (one of these is depicted in Landseer's 1832 portrait of the Duke in his box at Covent Garden). The 6th Duke bought the large collection of plays and playlists of the great actor John Philip Kemble and at Devonshire House he turned a suite of state rooms into a temporary theatre where, in 1851, he staged a charity production of a play written by Charles Dickens.

39 *(opposite)* The 9th Duke's Royal Household full dress uniform jacket photographed alongside *The Wounded Achilles*, 1825, by Filippo Albacini in the Sculpture Gallery, Chatsworth.

40 *(above)* The Duke and Duchess of Devonshire at Christie's fancy dress ball, 1972. Left to right: Jane Spencer-Churchill, Duchess of Devonshire, Jonathan Morley, Anne Peto, Charles Spencer-Churchill, Duke of Devonshire.

The 8th Duke, or rather his Duchess Louise, revelled in pageantry, transforming Sir Jeffry Wyatville's 1836 ballroom at Chatsworth into a private theatre in 1897 – the year they gave their great costume ball in London. The theatre still preserves its painted proscenium drop curtain and sundry sceneries, designed by the noted William Hemsley, as well as its spotlights and its footlight pillars (fig. 17). As a young man, the 9th Duke belied his somewhat dour reputation by appearing in amateur theatricals and burlesques as a student at Trinity College, Cambridge, to some local acclaim.

The apotheosis of the Devonshires' mania for dressing up was the Devonshire House Ball, given by the 8th Duke and Duchess Louise as the crowning celebration of Queen Victoria's Diamond Jubilee festivities. True to form, Duchess Louise went for it hammer and tongs, commissioning Attilio Comelli, the 'Artist in Chief' at the Royal Opera House, to design her ensemble but entrusting its fashioning to her preferred couture establishment, the famed House of Worth, then newly under the direction of Jean-Philippe Worth, son of the founder, the great Charles Frederick Worth (figs. 92, 94).

Although a noted beauty in her youth, the Duchess cut a formidably Wagnerian figure in later life. 'Rumour had her beautiful', the undeniably lovely Duchess of Marlborough recalled, 'but when I knew her she was a raddled old woman, covering her wrinkles with paint and her pate with a brown wig. Her mouth was a red gash.'

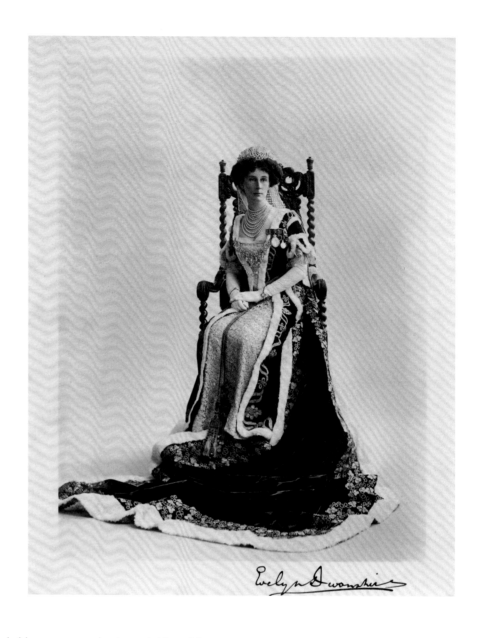

Undaunted, Duchess Louise decided to represent Queen Zenobia, the belligerent third-century Queen of Palmyra, whose fabled beauty was said to eclipse Cleopatra's. In the circumstances, Comelli and Worth worked wonders. Comelli also designed the costumes for some of the Devonshire House staff who were fancifully dressed as fan bearers, trumpeters and shepherdesses. 'Nothing succeeds like excess', wrote the reviewer Harry Lovell in the American newspaper *City Affairs*. It was, the Duchess of Marlborough conceded, 'a fitting climax to a brilliant season.'

Many of the costumes were recycled for the play *The White Heather* at the Drury Lane Theatre, a spectacular piece of Victorian stagecraft that also featured a wedding on a yacht and an underwater fight in which the protagonists wore helmets out of Jules Verne. 'We beheld again the very dresses worn by so many famous men and lovely women',

41 *(above)* Duchess Evelyn dressed as Mistress of the Robes, 1911 coronation.

42 *(opposite)* Mistress of the Robes coronation gown, worn by Duchess Evelyn at the 1911 and 1937 coronations and Duchess Mary at the 1953 coronation.

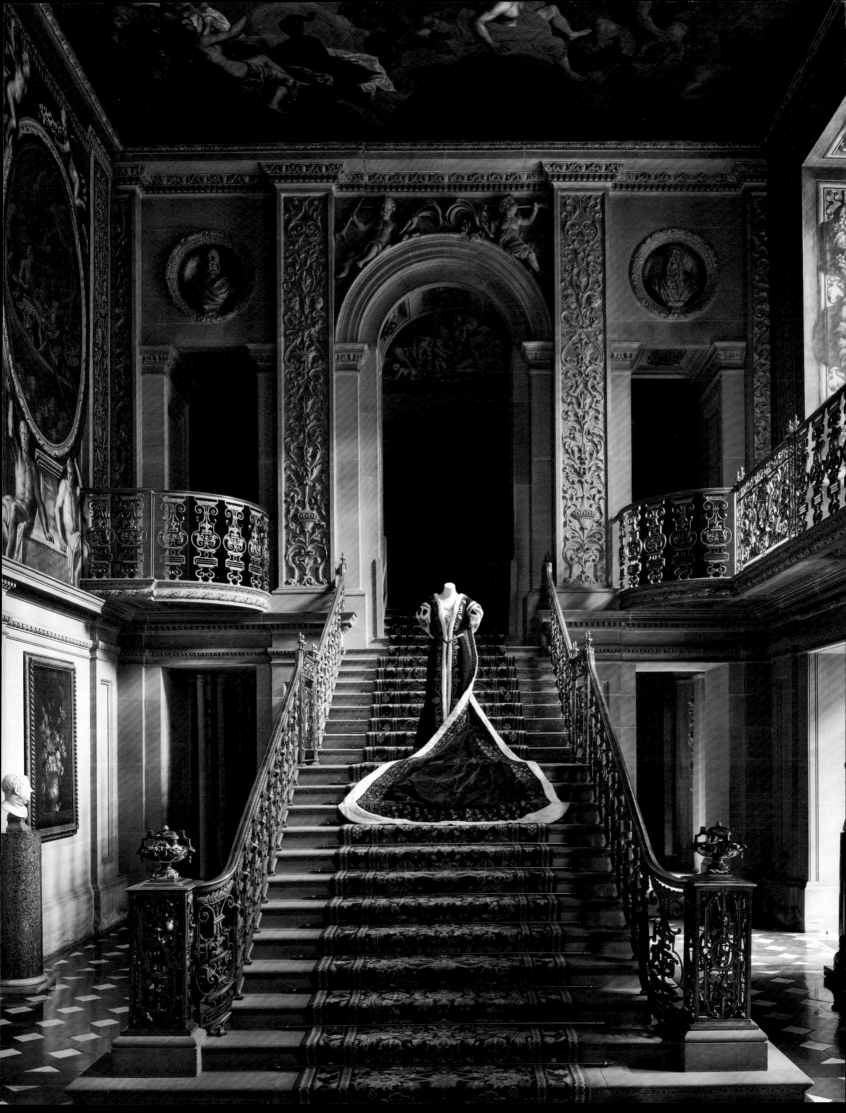

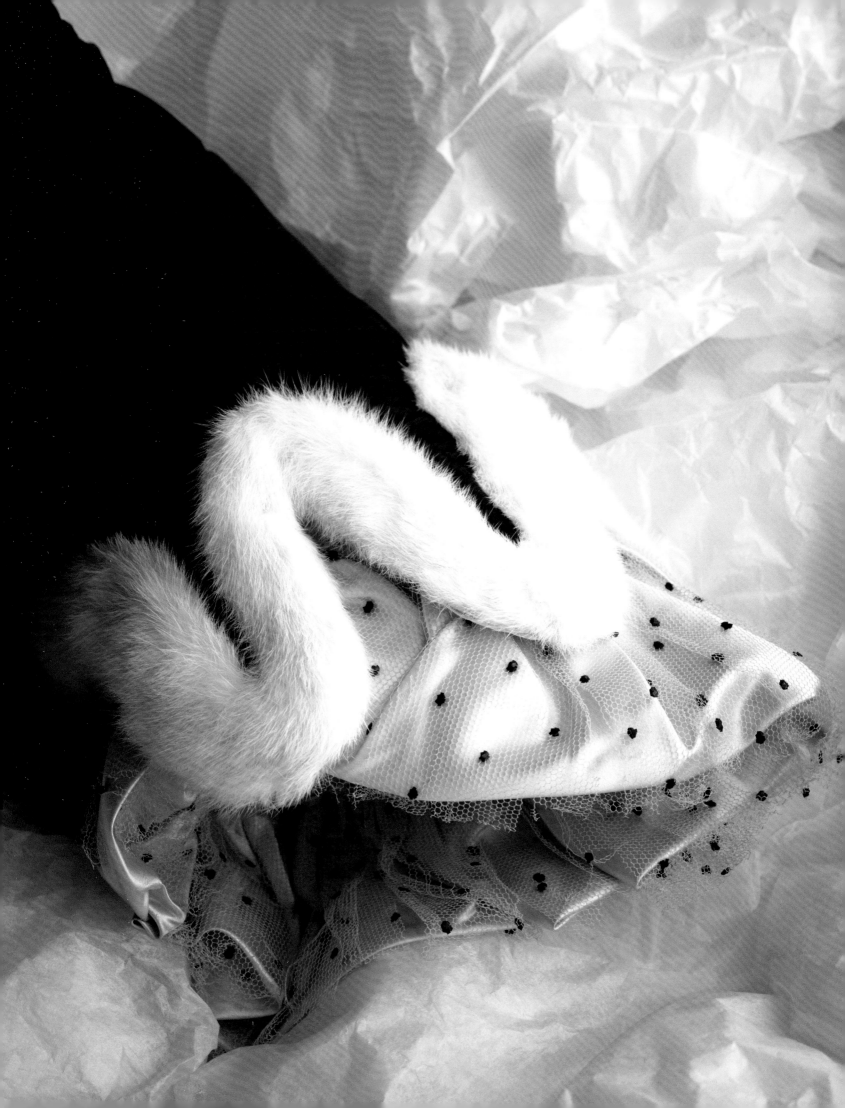

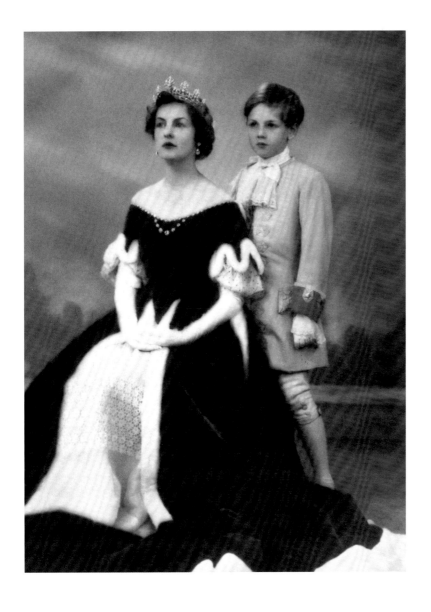

wrote the *Courier's* critic, 'but I'm bound to say that these looked second hand and dowdy; the new dresses were much better.'

Other costumes met even more ignominious ends. Jean-Philippe Worth costumed Mrs Arthur Paget (née Minnie Stevens, daughter of a Bostonian hotelier) to represent Cleopatra (fig. 37). The *Daily Mail* considered her 'lithe, and seductive, a lovely serpent of the old Nile', and she was deemed to have outshone the cultural *saloniste* Lady de Grey who chose the same subject and whose dress was rumoured to have cost £6,000. At the auction of Mrs Paget's effects in 1911, however, her spectacular ensemble fetched a paltry £9.

The Devonshire costumes, meanwhile, were more fortunate in being consigned to the dressing-up box. The 9th Duke's daughter Lady Maud Baillie wore her father's Ambassador costume (fig. 95) for a childhood production of *The Merchant of Venice*, staged at Holker Hall, and Debo wore the Duchess Louise's Zenobia costume to celebrate her 80th birthday, discovering in the process that 'it weighs a ton.' The love of dressing up is shared by Amanda and Stoker, who attended the Christie's Ball in 1972, the duchess in silvery robes given to the 11th Duke by an African chieftain, and the duke dressed – in classic 60s rock star fashion – in a borrowed uniform coat very similar to the 9th Duke's Royal Household full dress uniform jacket (figs. 39-40).

The Chatsworth uniforms and their accoutrements tell their own stories of ceremony and gallantry, and include the splendidly plumed helmet worn by the 9th Duke when he was made 2nd Lieutenant of the Derbyshire Yeomanry in 1890, and the greatcoat made for Billy Hartington, the dashing elder son of the 10th Duke and Duchess Mary, in the Second World War that would claim his life.

The twentieth century saw some other star guest appearances at Chatsworth. In 1932 the hard-drinking Lord Charles Cavendish married the vivacious Adele Astaire (fig. 54), sister of Fred and at one time the more admired half of their dancing partnership – 'a puckish thistledown with the energy of a hurricane', as *Vogue* wrote. Duchess Mary recalled the family's unforgettable first meeting with Adele. 'All gathered, like stone pillars, in the library: the heavy doors opened and there stood this tiny girl, beautifully dressed. We waited for her to approach us, but instead of walking she suddenly began turning cartwheels. Everyone loved it.'

As the chatelaine of Lismore Castle, Adele developed an interest in Irish crafts, and knitted up a storm herself. The Countess of Burlington recently unearthed a 1970s long-sleeved T-shirt of Adele's, trompe l'oeil-printed to look like a man's formal eve-

43 *(opposite)* Sleeve detail of the 1831 Peeress Robe worn by Deborah Devonshire at the 1953 coronation.

44 *(above)* Deborah Devonshire wearing the 1831 Peeress Robe for the 1953 coronation, accompanied by her son the Duke of Devonshire, who was page to Duchess Mary, Mistress of the Robes.

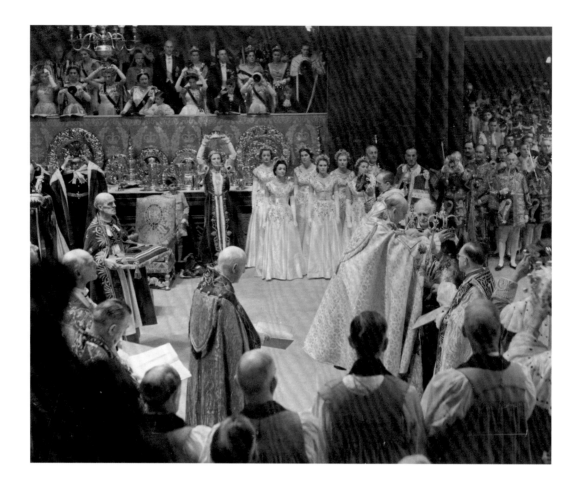

ning suit, complete with a be-medalled sash (fig. 15). It was a gift from Stoker and Amanda, and a witness to Adele's enduringly antic spirit.

Kathleen 'Kick' Kennedy (fig. 12), beloved sister of the future President of the United States, also brought her own joie de vivre into the family when she wed Billy Hartington in 1944. Alas, her happiness was to prove short-lived, for Billy left for combat and was killed four months later by a sniper in Belgium. In her first public appearance as a presumed future Duchess of Devonshire, at the local Bakewell Show, the fairgoers were awed not only by Kick's easy manner, but by her nylon stockings sent from America – an unheard-of luxury.

America provided more than nylons. Soon after the war, the 11th Duke's sister, Lady Elizabeth Cavendish (future Lady in Waiting to Princess Margaret), visited her aunt Adele in Manhattan and wrote to her sister Lady Anne to tell her that the New York girls 'all wear false rubber bosoms. I am buying you a pair. So do be excited – they give you the most wonderful shape.'

In 1932 the chic Adele, newly converted from Catholicism that very morning, was dressed for her wedding in a short beige satin dress 'with touches of orange at the waist and a set of blue fox furs', designed by the recently established Chicago-born Parisian couturier Mainbocher (fig. 59), who was to dress Wallis Simpson for her 1937 marriage to the Duke of Windsor.

Adele was not the only fashion-forward Cavendish bride. Amanda wore Hubert de Givenchy's sleek A-line dress and a floret-embroidered bolero (figs. 57-58) for her 1967 marriage to Stoker, having been introduced to the designer by her stylish godmother, Carmen Esnault-Pelterie. In 1997 Stella Tennant's sister Issy wore a lilac chiffon dress by John Galliano, its translucency daringly underscored by a black thong. For Stella's own marriage to the photographer David Lasnet in 1999, the couple were both dressed by the innovative Austrian-born designer Helmut Lang (fig. 60). Stella's dress was so diaphanous that it was considered lost for fifteen years (and has only recently been discovered by projects coordinator Denna Garrett), having lain in a box underneath

45 *(above)* Duchess Mary, with her coronet aloft paying homage to Queen Elizabeth II at the 1953 coronation.

46 *(opposite)* Coronet worn by the Duchess of Devonshire to coronations.

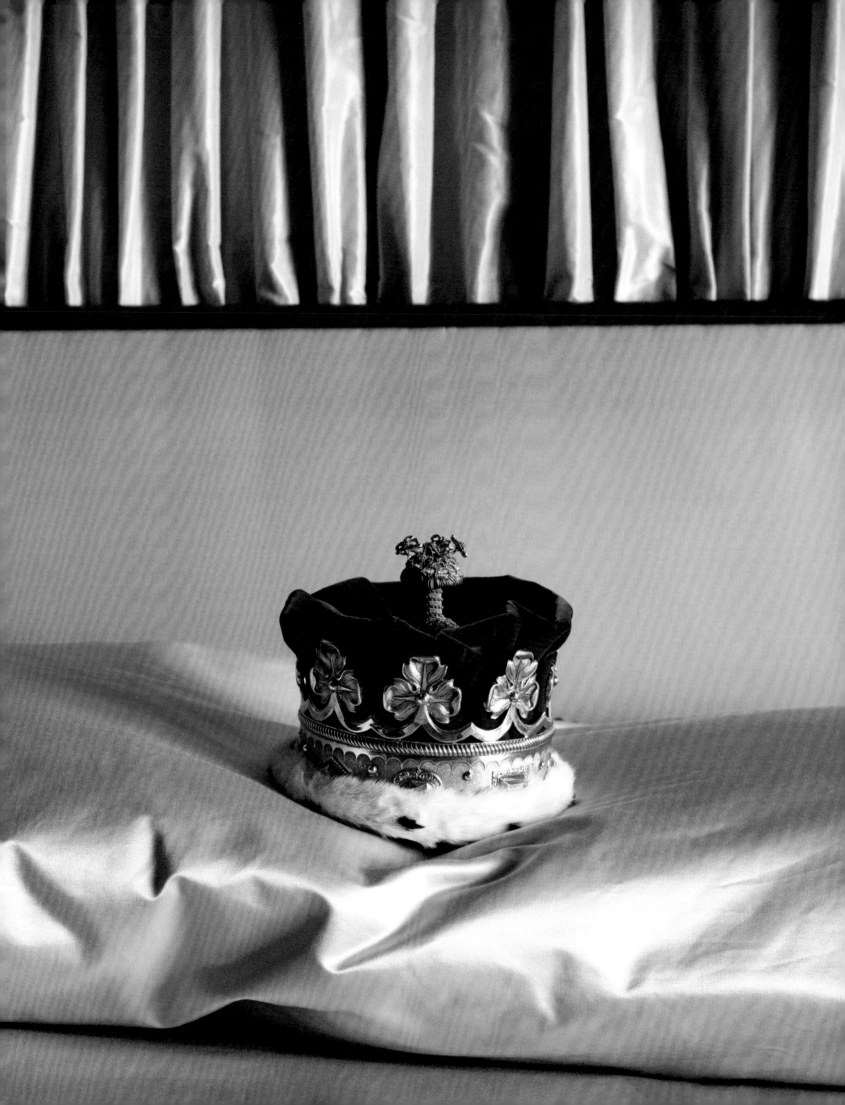

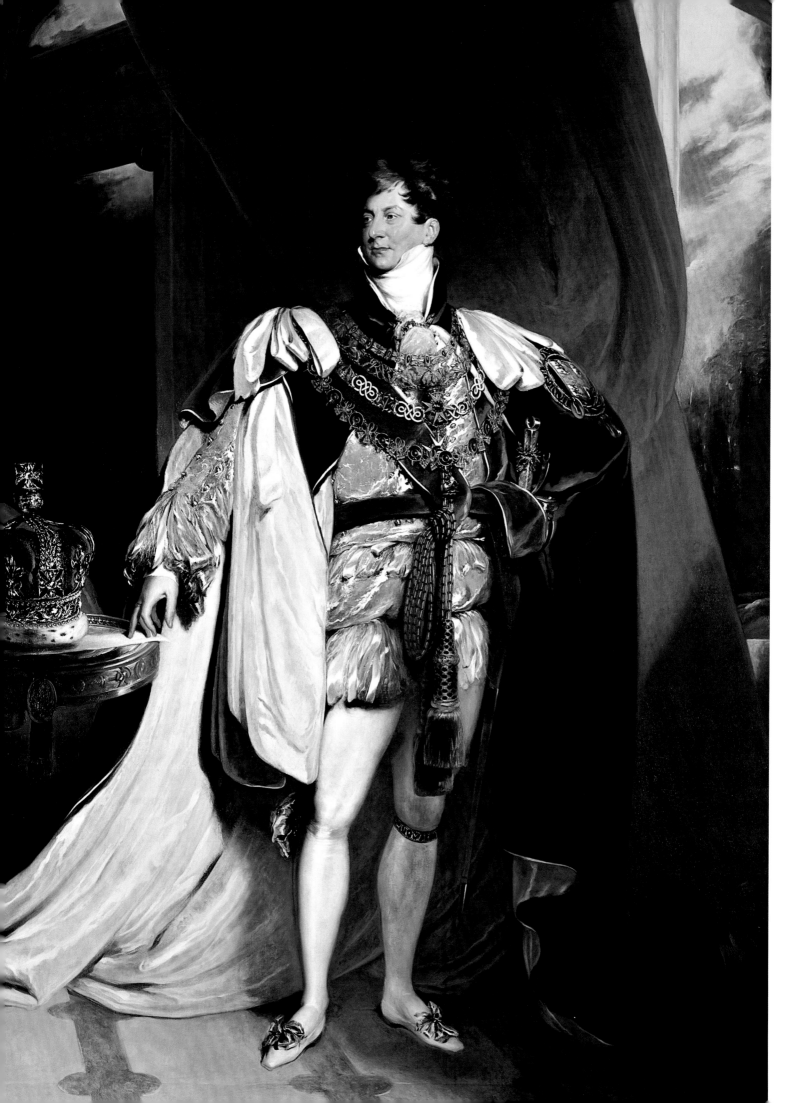

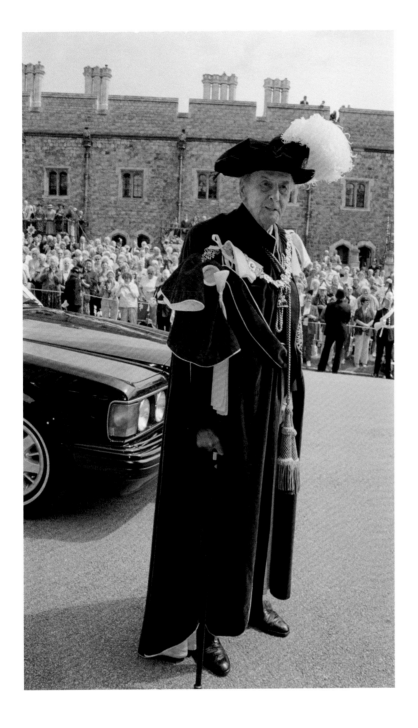

her mother Lady Emma's voluminous wedding dress, unnoticed between sheets of tissue paper as fragile as the dress itself.

The characters of the Duke's daughters Lady Jasmine and Lady Celina, meanwhile, are revealed in their own choices of wedding dress. For her 2003 wedding to Nicky Dunne, Lady Jasmine sleuthed an antique satin wedding dress made on the eve of the First World War at a vintage clothing store. Lady Celina, meanwhile, went to her mother's dressmaker Franka in 1995 for a classical princess-line gown of slubbed silk, its traditionalism gently mitigated by the large buttons down the back, each hand-embroidered with an image from *Winnie the Pooh* (fig. 56).

Some items of children's costume in the collection have been preserved for the most deeply poignant of reasons. In the eighteenth and nineteenth centuries childbirth – and indeed childhood – could be life-threatening conditions. As Georgiana lay pregnant in 1791 with her fourth child, the illegitimate Eliza Courtney (whose father was the politician Charles Grey), she penned heartbreaking letters to her three other children and to her son, the future 6th Duke, written in her own blood, in case she did not survive the birth.

Her niece Lady Blanche Georgiana Howard, (wife of the 7th Duke), lost her beloved infant son William 'Can' Cavendish at the age of three. 'I heard his last sigh', she wrote in her diary, 'I felt his pulse flutter, & all was still.' She kept not only a lock of his hair, but his tiny cherry-red leather shoes, and a little dress that she had made him (boys were traditionally not 'breeched' until the 'age of reason' at seven or so). Lady Blanche's second son, Spencer Compton Cavendish, survived to become the procrastinating 8th Duke of Devonshire who thrice refused Queen Victoria's invitation to become Prime Minister. He did, however, manage the singular feat of falling asleep whilst delivering his maiden speech at the House of Lords.

In the traditional way, christening clothes and some of the finer baby clothes have been passed from generation to generation. The present Lord Burlington was christened (fig. 6) in the Devonshire robe (fig. 5) worn by his great-great-grandfather, as was his daughter Nell Cavendish. Nell's siblings, James and Maud (fig. 4), however, both older at the time of their respective ceremonies, wore the larger Mitford family christening robe.

Even when clothing is as ritualized and hidebound as it is for a royal coronation, the characters of the various players are revealed. Concerning the coronation of King George VI,

47 *(opposite)* Sir Thomas Lawrence, *King George IV*, 1818.

48 *(above)* The 11th Duke of Devonshire at the entrance of St George's Chapel, Windsor Castle, after his investiture as a Knight of the Garter, June 1996.

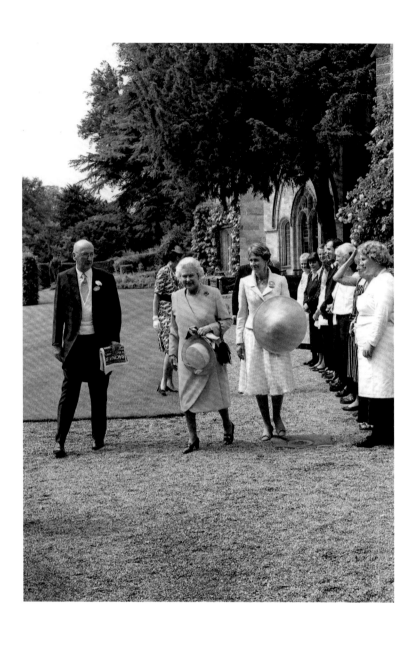

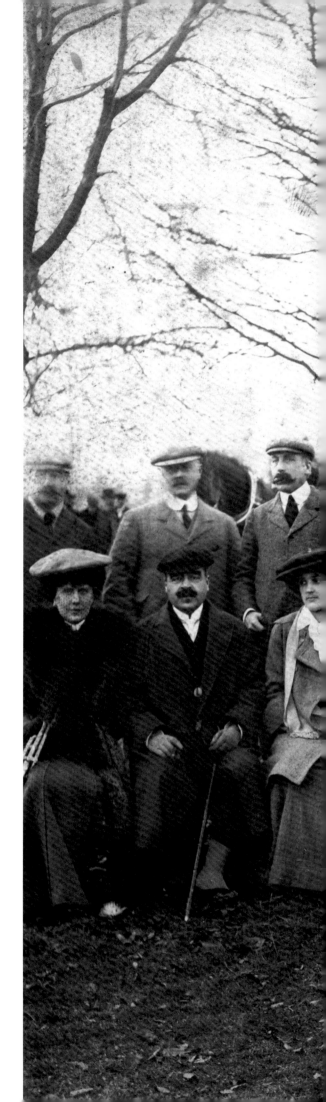

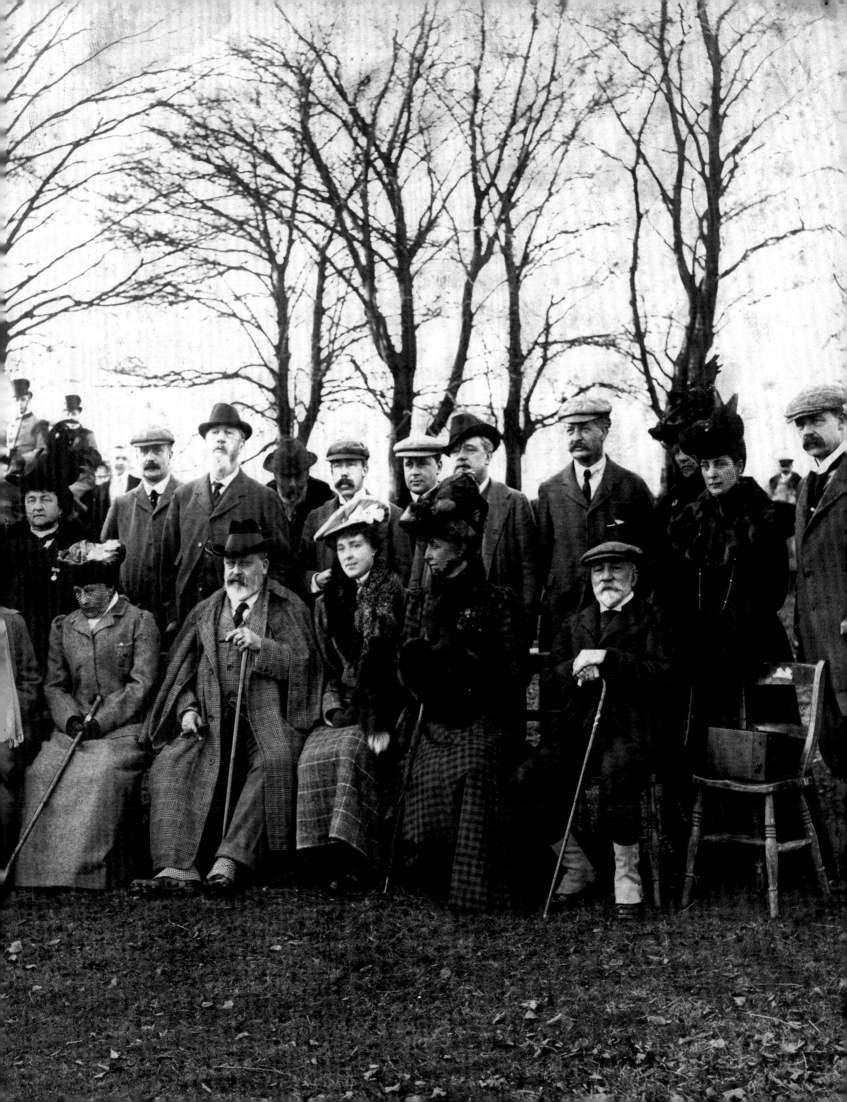

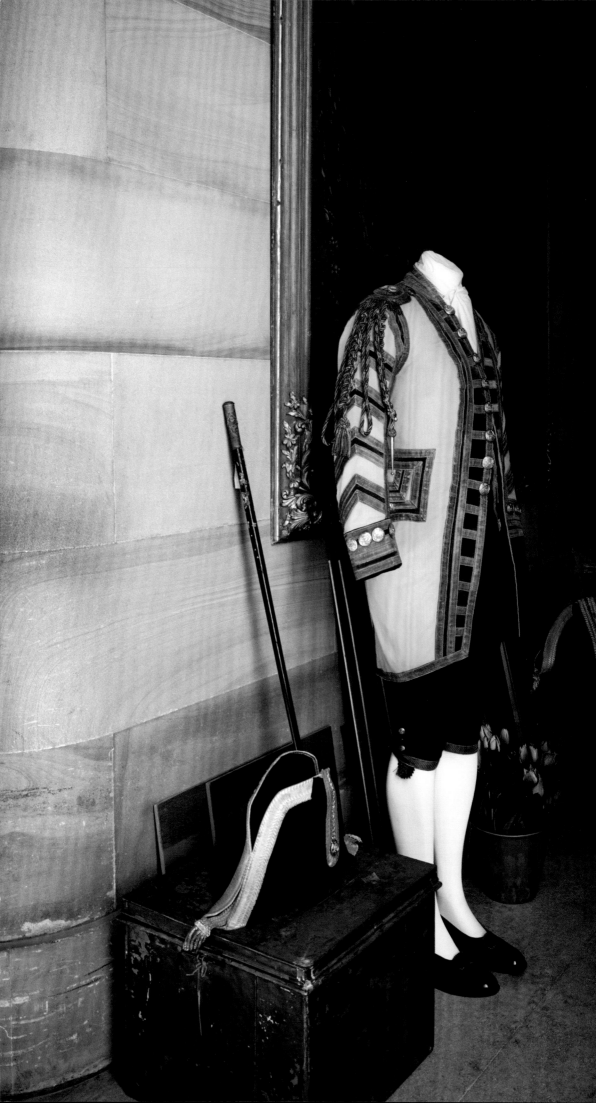

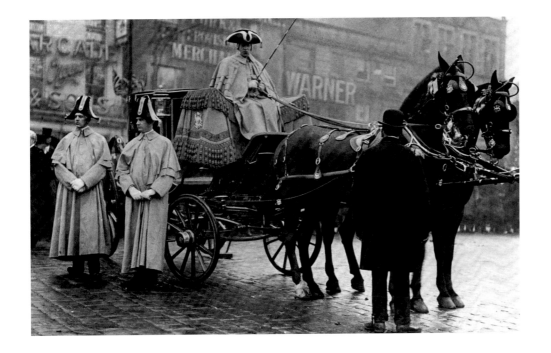

the Earl Marshal wrote to reassure the thrifty Duchess Evelyn, Queen Mary's Mistress of the Robes, that 'any robes may be used again. The dressmakers have gone quite mad over the prices', he added, 'but it is their funeral as many people will have them made by maids.'

For Edward VII's coronation Lady Evelyn's mother (née Lady Maud Hamilton, daughter of the 1st Duke of Abercorn), had provided her with an under-dress of Indian embroidery, but as this had tarnished by the 1911 coronation of King George V and Queen Mary, the duchess laid an extraordinary length of superb seventeenth-century Venetian point lace over cloth of gold to make her gown (fig. 41).

For the coronation of King George VI and Queen Elizabeth (the Queen Mother) in 1938, some of this robe's ermine trims were missing or defective. The duchess dispatched a splendid ermine pillow muff, stole and collar (in which she had been photographed in the Edwardian era), to the furriers Hewitt & Vincent to be cannibalized and fill in the gaps. By the time Elizabeth II's coronation loomed in early 1953, however, even these replacements had become unsatisfactory. Duchess Evelyn, however, had grown more resourceful still, writing to her daughter-in-law, Duchess Mary, 'It strikes me that – if Debo got busy at once – she could breed some white rabbits, which, when young, look just like ermine.'

Debo herself was concerned about what she might wear to Elizabeth's crowning: the economies following those punitive death duties having already firmly kicked in. 'Chatsworth, as always, came to the rescue', she recalled, 'There were a number of tin boxes containing old uniforms and other relics. In the vain hope of finding something for me, we started going through them and, lo and behold, from beneath a ton of tissue paper in the box that had held Moucher's (Mary, Dowager Duchess of Devonshire), appeared a second crimson peeress's robe (figs. 43-44).'

These appear to have been made for the 1831 coronation of William IV, probably for the 5th Duke's niece. 'The velvet is of exceptional quality', noted Debo, 'so soft your fingers hardly know they are touching it, and of such pure, brilliant crimson as to make you blink... but there was a hitch: unlike other peeresses' robes it was cut off the shoulder.' The new Queen's permission was sought and granted for Debo to wear 'this irregular style'. Cecil Beaton, writing on the ceremony for *Vogue*, considered her 'undoubtedly the most beautiful' of all the peeresses present.

Something of the atmosphere of a coronation was vividly captured by Edward Cavendish, the future 10th Duke, who served as the page to his great uncle, the 8th

49 *(preceding pages, left to right)* The Duke and Duchess of Devonshire with Her Majesty The Queen, Bolton Abbey, 2005.

50 The Royal Shooting Party at Chatsworth with King Edward VII and the 8th Duke and Duchess of Devonshire, 1907. (Queen Alexandra stands behind her camera on the chair.)

51 *(opposite)* Head Coachman's state livery ensemble, early 1900s.

52 *(above)* Chatsworth coach and horses in Chesterfield for the Mayor's Sunday, circa 1911.

Duke (Spencer Compton Cavendish), at the coronation of King Edward VII and Queen Alexandra in 1902. Then seven years old, Cavendish dutifully sat down with his tutor to write up his remarkable memories of the day. At home at Devonshire House in the morning his nanny was terrified by the cannon fire, and there was 'a great fuss' about his tie, braces, stockings and sword. At Westminster Abbey the Archbishop of Canterbury asked him if he 'knew subtraction & then he asked me if I had got to Euclid yet!'

During the ceremony itself he remarked:

> I saw the King beautifully & a lot of other grand people. Soon after, all the peers & peeresses put on their coronets & at the same moment a lot of lights were switched on at all the corners & they all sparkled, it was just then I saw a looking glass being passed 'round all the peeresses... Then the King came to his throne & Lord Rothschild lifted me up, I can't explain what it all looked like because it kept changing gold & scarlet & silver, reds, greens & blues. The King's crown looked very strange because it was so plain & not at all dazzling. The Queen's train was all pure white with fleur-de-lys in gold, it looked like a sheet... A lot of Princesses came & everybody had to bow to them, & some had such long trains that people had to hold them up & they had such long trains that someone had to hold theirs, this looked so funny.

After these excitements Master Cavendish was understandably 'so hungry that I ate a bigger luncheon than I had ever had before (mutton, chicken, jelly, biscuits & cakes).'

Characteristically, the coronation page boy ensembles later saw double duty as costumes in the children's plays and for fancy dress – a tradition perhaps initiated by Georgiana's scandalous niece Lady Caroline Lamb, who chose to be dressed in man drag as a page boy in her alluring 1814 portrait by Thomas Philips (fig. 141).

Edward Cavendish may not have noticed another moment of unexpected human comedy at the coronation. Whilst the 6th Duke bore George IV's orb, the 8th Duke was the bearer of King Edward VII's crown at his coronation. Edward Cavendish's great-aunt, Duchess Louise, however, proved a less able guardian of her own coronet. In her eagerness to get to the ladies' room after the lengthy ceremony, she pushed past the guardsmen at the tail end of the royal procession and swiftly came a-cropper, losing her footing and hurling headlong down a flight of steps, where she landed at the feet of the bemused Chancellor of the Exchequer. Quick-witted Margot Asquith retrieved the Duchess's coronet, which had gone rolling along the stalls, and deftly placed it back on her head.

Bess of Hardwick's extensive retinue of 72 house servants had been dressed in Cavendish blue, or 'mallard colour' livery. By the nineteenth century, this colour had been

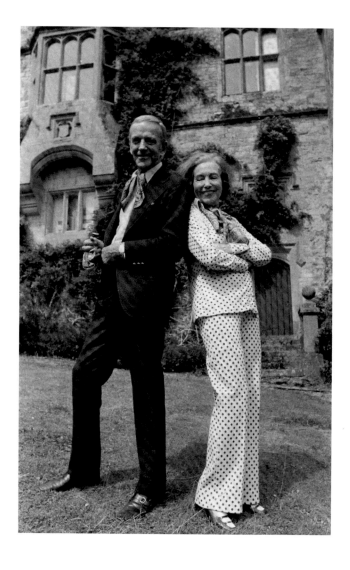

53 *(above)* Fred Astaire and Adele Astaire at Lismore Castle, 1975.

54 *(opposite)* Cecil Beaton, Adele Astaire and Cecil Beaton, New York, 1931.

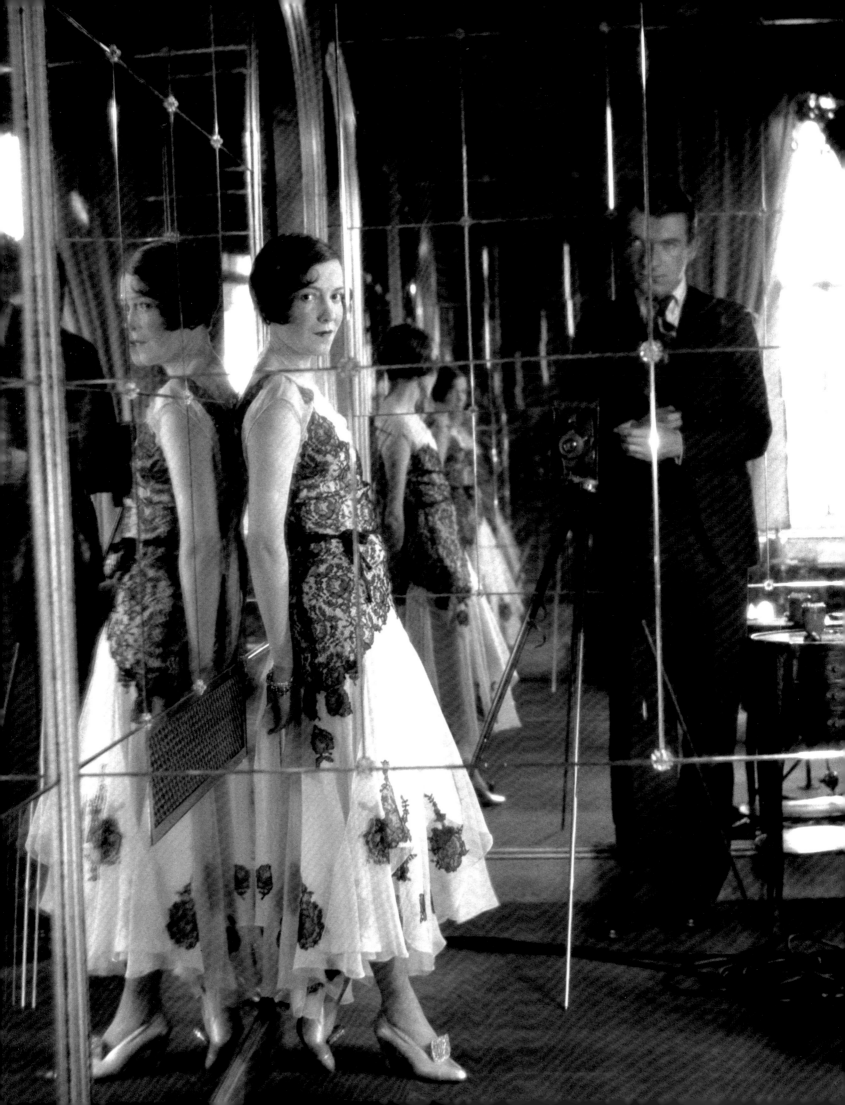

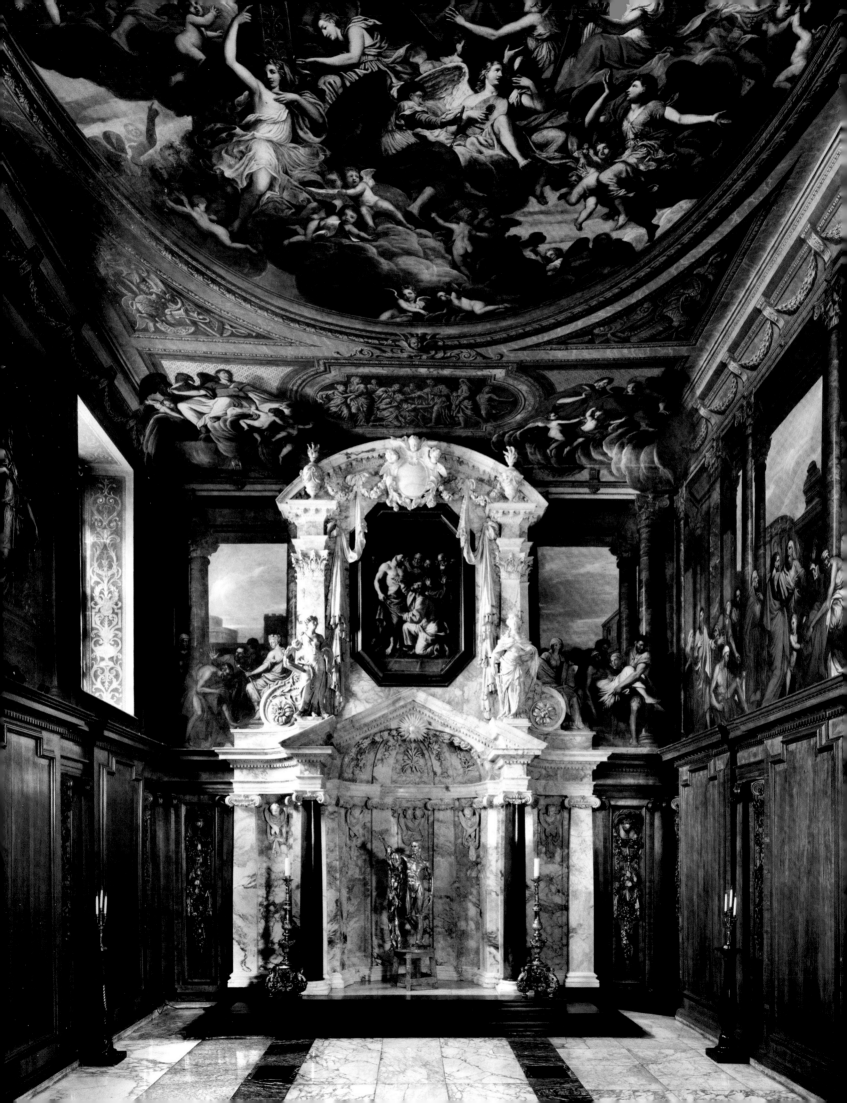

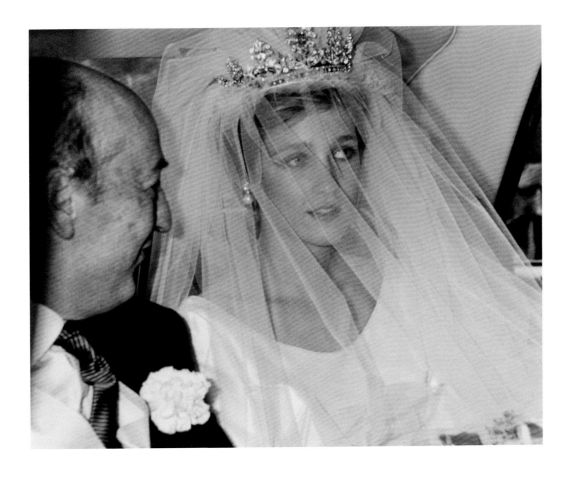

55 *(opposite)* The Chapel at
Chatsworth with a sculpture
by Damien Hirst (b. 1965), *St
Bartholomew, Exquisite Pain*, 2008.
Walls and ceilings by Louis Laguerre,
1688–1693. Painting over the altar,
The Incredulity of St Thomas by
Antonio Verrio, 1692.

56 *(above)* Lady Celina Cavendish
with her father, the Duke of
Devonshire, on her wedding day,
3 June 1995.

57 *(page 76)* The Duchess of Devonshire on her wedding day, 28 June 1967.

58 *(page 77)* Beaded bolero by Hubert
de Givenchy, worn by the Duchess
of Devonshire on her wedding day,
1967.

59 *(page 78)* Lord Charles Cavendish
and Adele Astaire on their wedding
day, 1932.

60 *(page 79)* Mario Testino, wedding of
Stella Tennant and David Lasnet, 1999.

61 *(pages 80-81)* Sixteen of the
9th Duke of Devonshire's 21
grandchildren, Christmas 1931.

62 *(pages 82-83)* The 10th Duke of
Devonshire with his children William,
Andrew, Elizabeth and Anne at
Bolton Abbey, Yorkshire, circa 1938.

sublimated to the trim-
mings of the full dress
liveries, the coats being
made in sharp lemon yel-
low (fig. 2). Most splendid
of all the remaining Chatsworth liveries is the head
coachman's ensemble (fig.
51), glittering with silver
thread braid, and worn
with a blue-coloured coat
made from woollen cloth
so tightly loomed that the
hems of its various short
capes are simply sheared
and left unfinished (fig.
52); after a century and
more there is no hint of
fraying.

The splendid effect was
completed with a long stick,
the purpose of which was
to lift ladies' skirts. Andrew
and Deborah almost didn't
make it to the Coronation of Queen Elizabeth II. To amplify the theatricality of their
arrival at Westminster Abbey, they brought the state coach from Chatsworth, but unfortunately the Derbyshire coachman, though magnificently attired, didn't know London and
soon lost his way. 'There was no way to communicate from inside the coach', Debo recalled,
'so my husband had to scream outside the window, "Left! Right!" The crowd thought it
was the funniest thing they'd ever seen.'

The Most Noble Order of the Garter was founded in 1348 by King Edward III, and
remains the highest order of chivalry in the United Kingdom, frivolous as its origins may
seem. As legend has it, Joan of Kent, the Countess of Salisbury, was in full dancing fig
when one of her garters accidentally fell to her ankle. She was a favourite of the king, who
gallantly stooped to retrieve it for her and restore her imperilled dignity. *'Honi Soit Qui Mal
Y Pense'* he glowered at the disapproving onlookers: 'Shame on him who thinks badly of it.'

Successive monarchs have bestowed each of the 11 deceased Dukes of Devonshire
with the honour, which has been received with mixed feelings through the generations.
'One's impression is that the whole thing is rather ridiculous', wrote the 7th Duke to his
daughter Lady Louise, after having attended the Garter Ceremony. Debo, however, was
characteristically more stirred by the historic pageantry. 'Like a medieval play, clothes,
language & background', she wrote to her sister Diana, 'Disney with Knobs On.'

Andrew was fortunate in having two sets of Garter robes to choose from, one of which
(originally made for the towering 7th Duke), suited his own attenuated figure. For the
ceremonies, he wore the Garter over his suit (fig. 48), but in 1996 was required to wear it

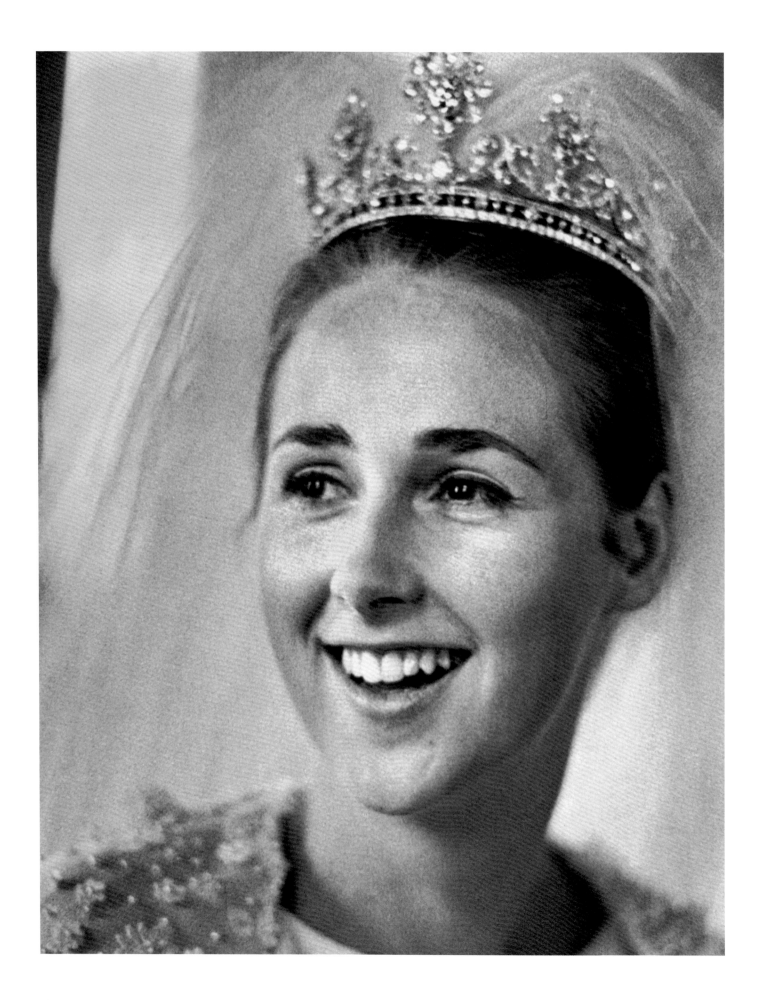

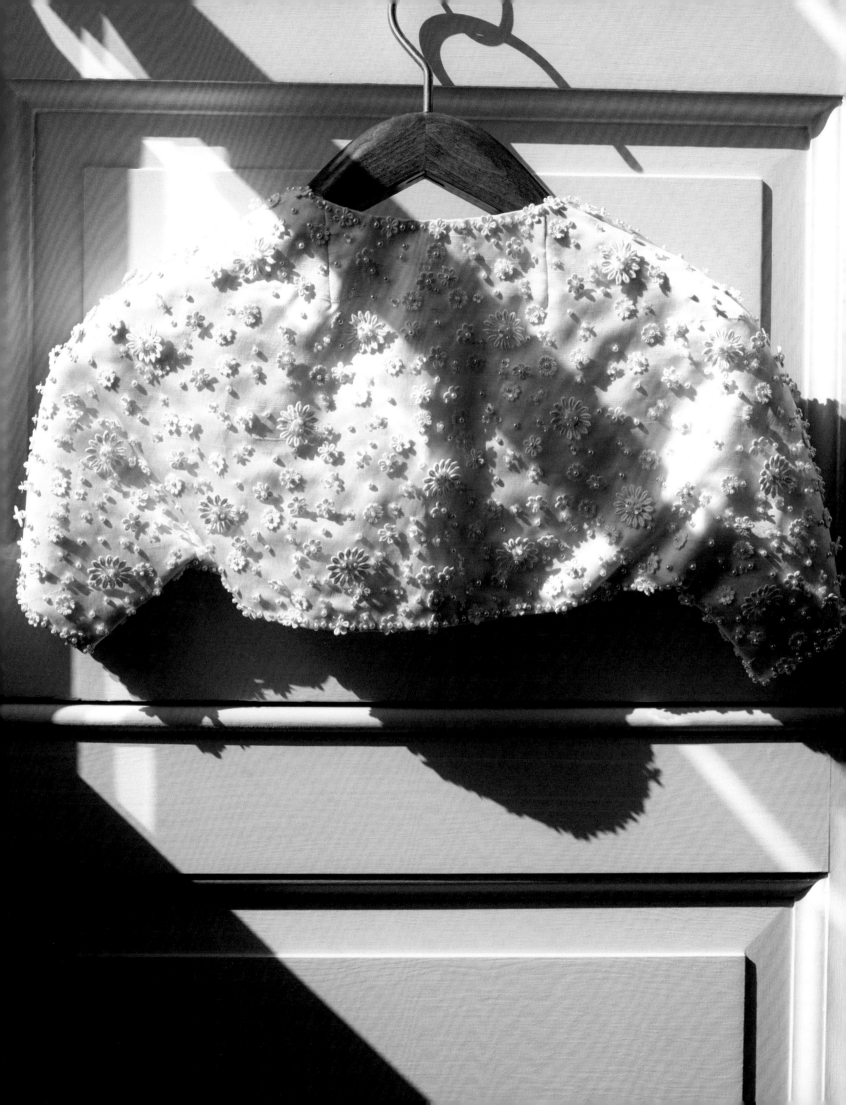

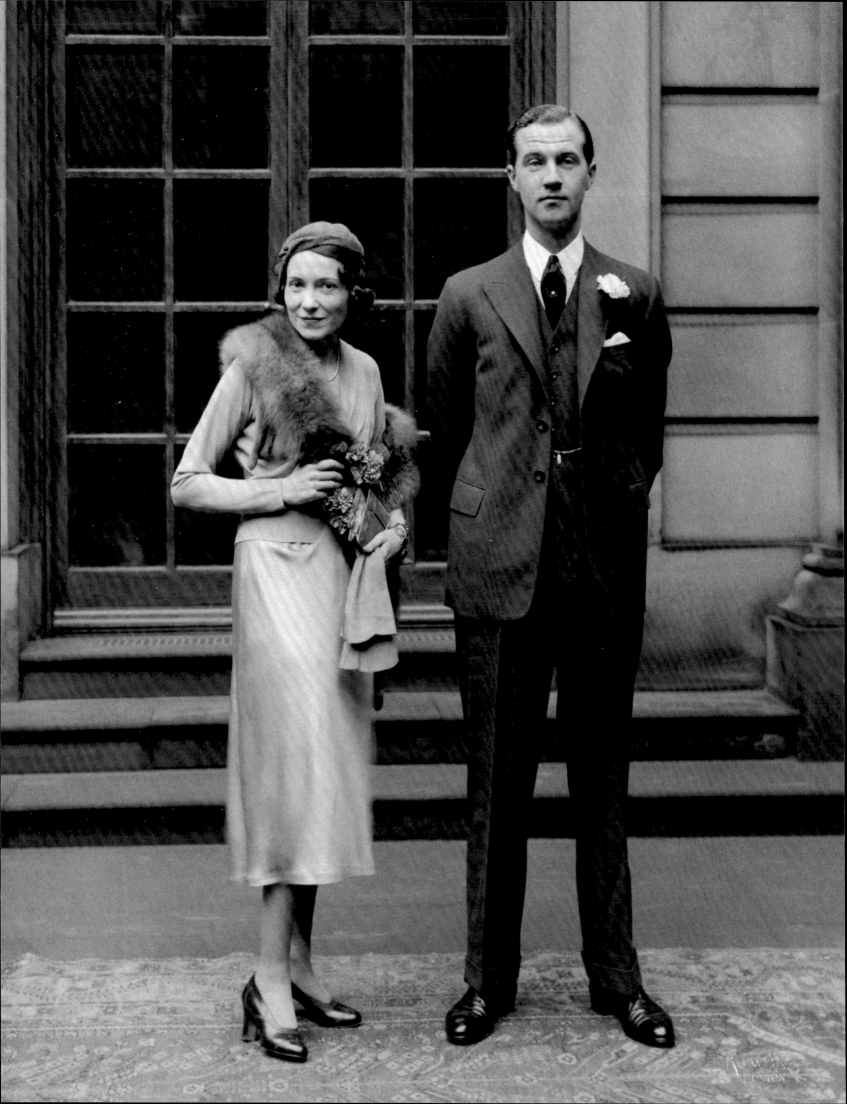

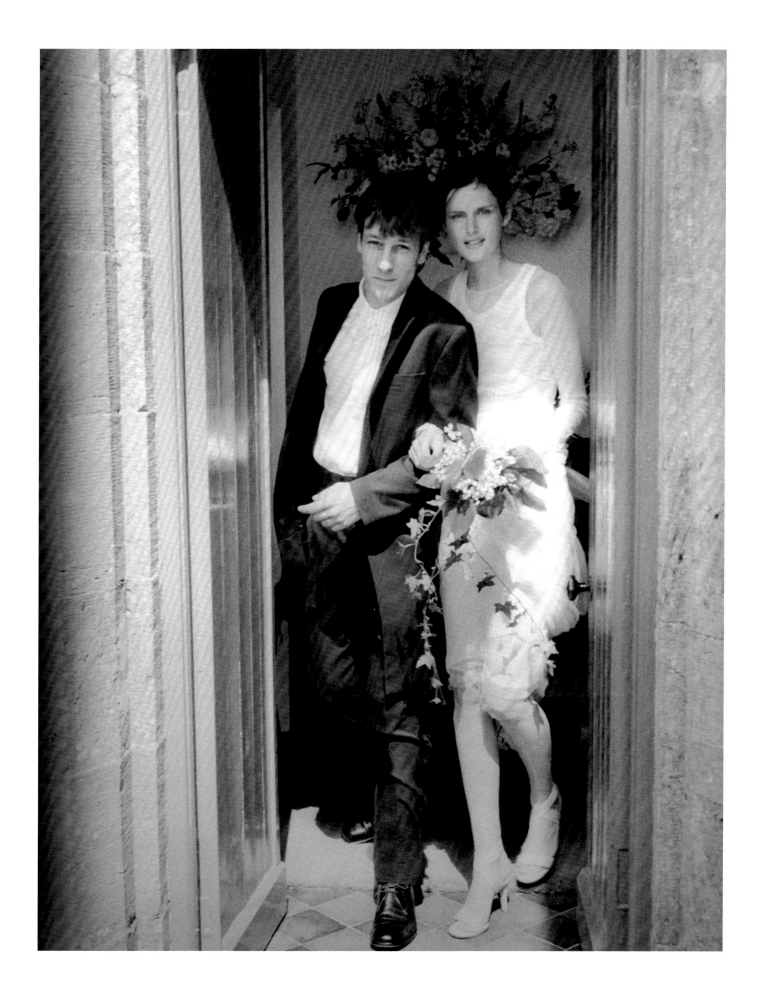

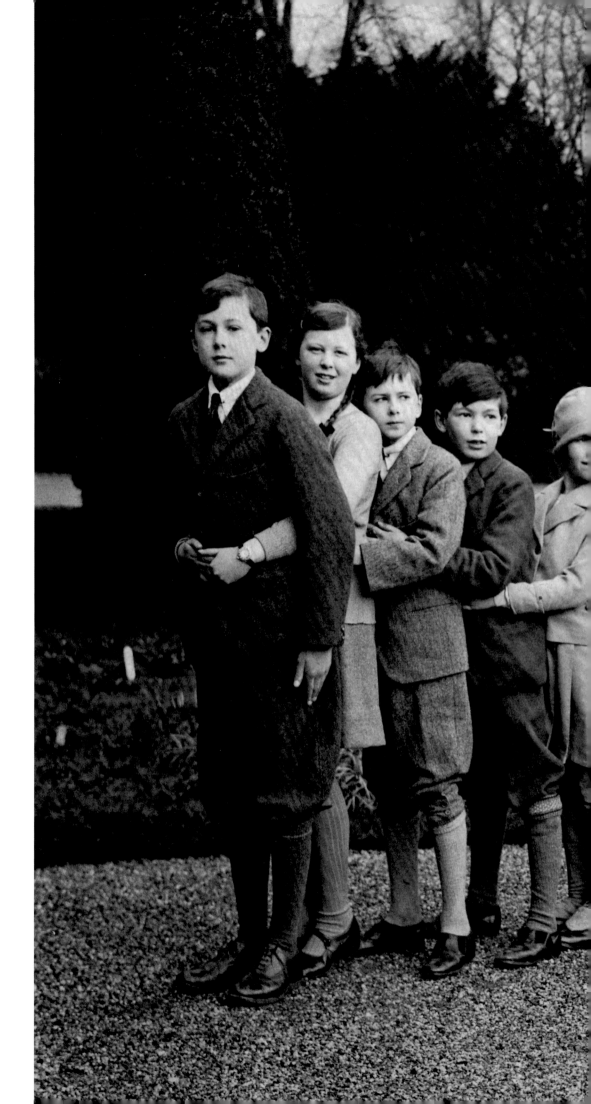

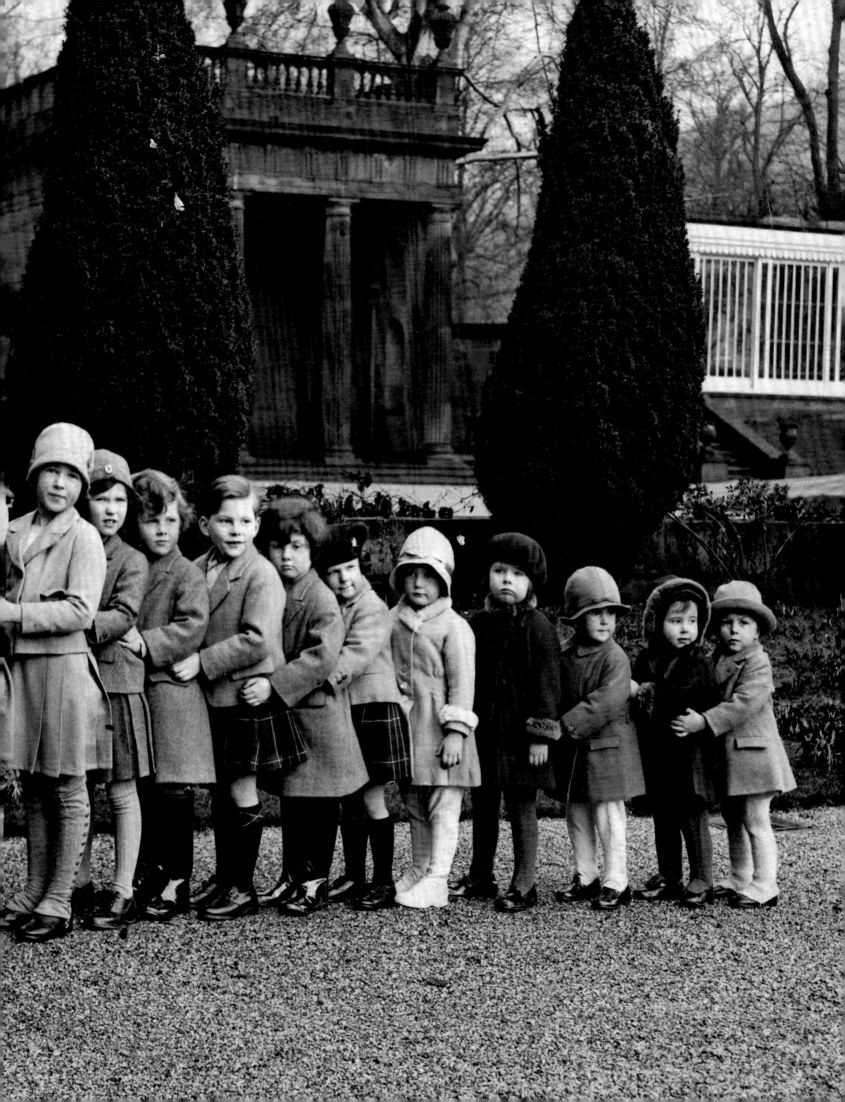

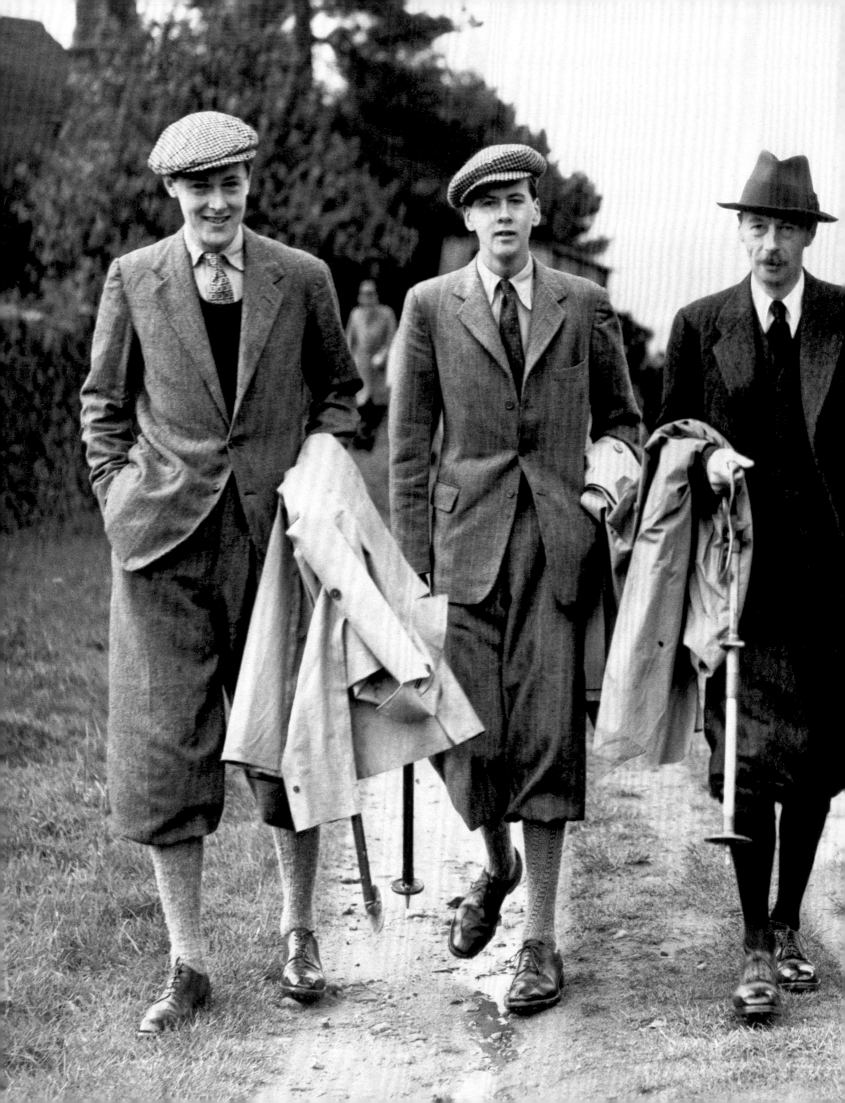

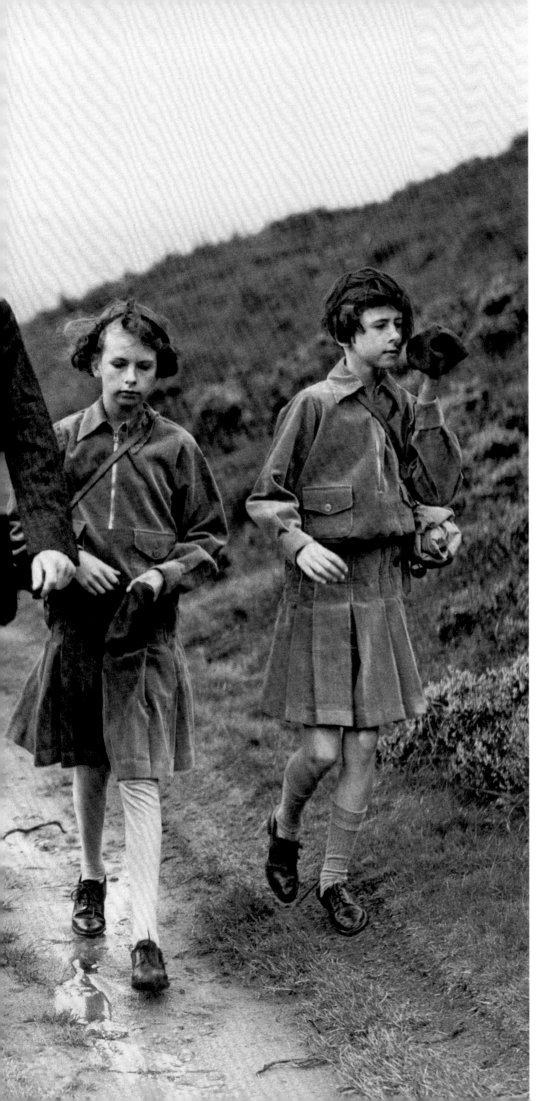

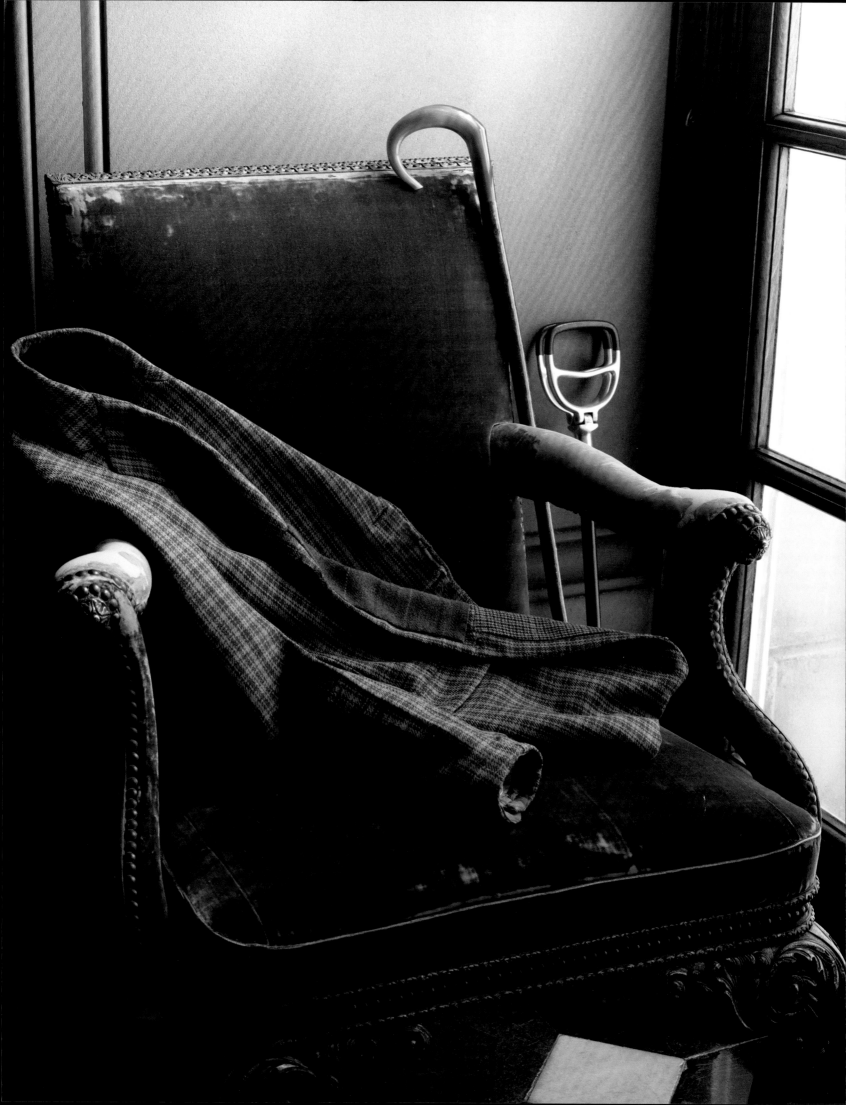

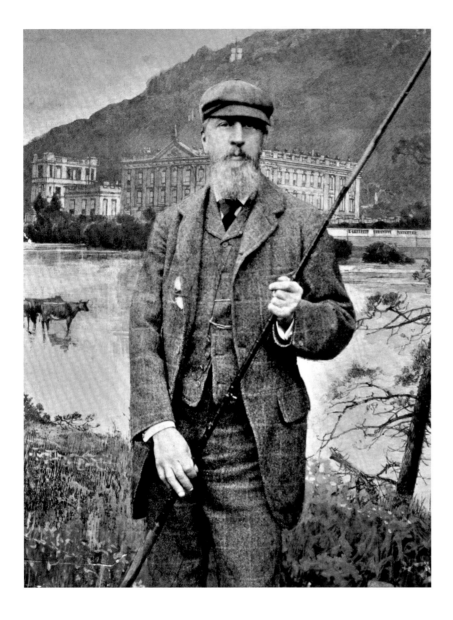

with white tie for a dinner at the Royal Academy, walking from his London home on Chesterfield Street thusly attired. 'I know people are very oddly dressed now', noted Debo, 'but he must have looked a bit of an apparition.'

The accoutrements of traditional country pursuits are well represented in the collection, and again reveal the characters of their wearers. Even the Devonshire tweed – mallard blue window-pane check over an earthy-brown ground – has been subtly customised by the family members (fig. 67). The 10th Duke had a passion for fishing and 'begged plumes from the hats of women friends', to make his own flies. 'Picking one up', wrote Debo, '[he] would sigh with nostalgia and say things like, "Ettie Desborough, Ascot, 1921." Once the flies were ready, he lay in the bath imagining he was a salmon while Edward, the butler, pretending to be a fishing rod, jerked them over his submerged head. The ones the Duke judged most attractive were used on his stretch of the Blackwater in County Cork at the start of the salmon fishing season.'

Andrew inherited his father's passion, dressing for the river with characteristic panache in one of his trademark motto jumpers, a checked flannel shirt, and the flourish of a printed cotton bandana at the neck (fig. 77). Debo, meanwhile, took up shooting at the age of 30 (fig. 65). 'Women guns were rare 60 years ago', she recalled, 'and initially I was regarded with suspicion all round.' 'Better give it up', her sister Nancy Mitford teasingly counselled, 'It'll ruin your looks.' 'I like the battle with the weather', Debo protested, and her long-time ladies' maid Christine Thompson has recalled that for shooting, Debo was heavily layered with a Barbour jacket, shirt, cardigan, silk roll-neck vest and woollen stockings and undergarments worn over cotton ones. A lipstick was always packed in a small purse next to the first aid plasters.

Those recurring death duties necessitated economies, but cherished garments have long been expected to see sterling service. For the important festivities held to celebrate William Burlington's 21st birthday in 1990, Debo ordered a new dress from Hardy Amies for the evening garden party and for the ball itself wore a dress that Balmain had made for her 30 years earlier. The latter was sleeveless, and its strident dye had proved somewhat fugitive over the years, so Debo remedied the situation by having Christine Thompson make her a dramatic evening wrap in two shades of fuchsia-pink taffeta that covered both her arms and the dress's faded back. The stole was attached to the dress,

63 *(opposite)* Favourite tweed jacket of the 11th Duke of Devonshire, heavily repaired, laid on George II walnut and parcel-gilt armchair, circa 1735.

64 *(above)* Studio portrait of the 8th Duke of Devonshire, 1880s.

65 *(following pages)* Deborah Devonshire at Bolton Abbey, 1960s.

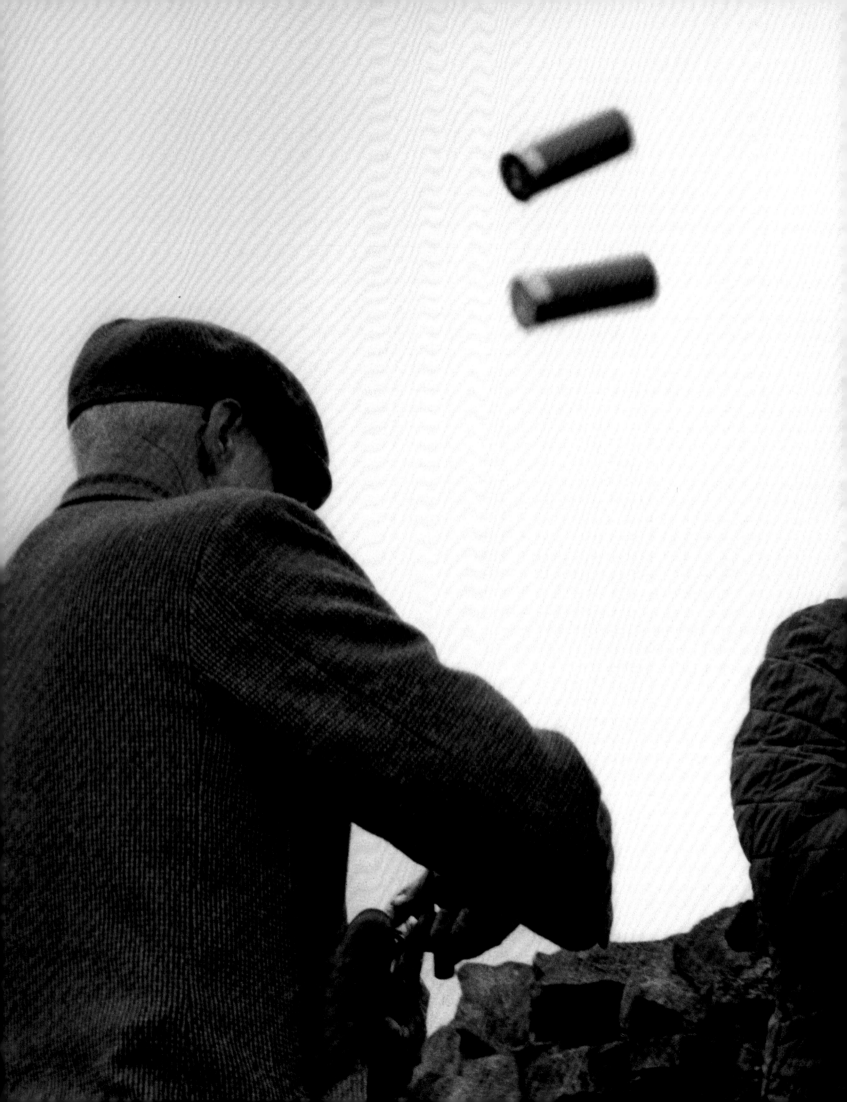

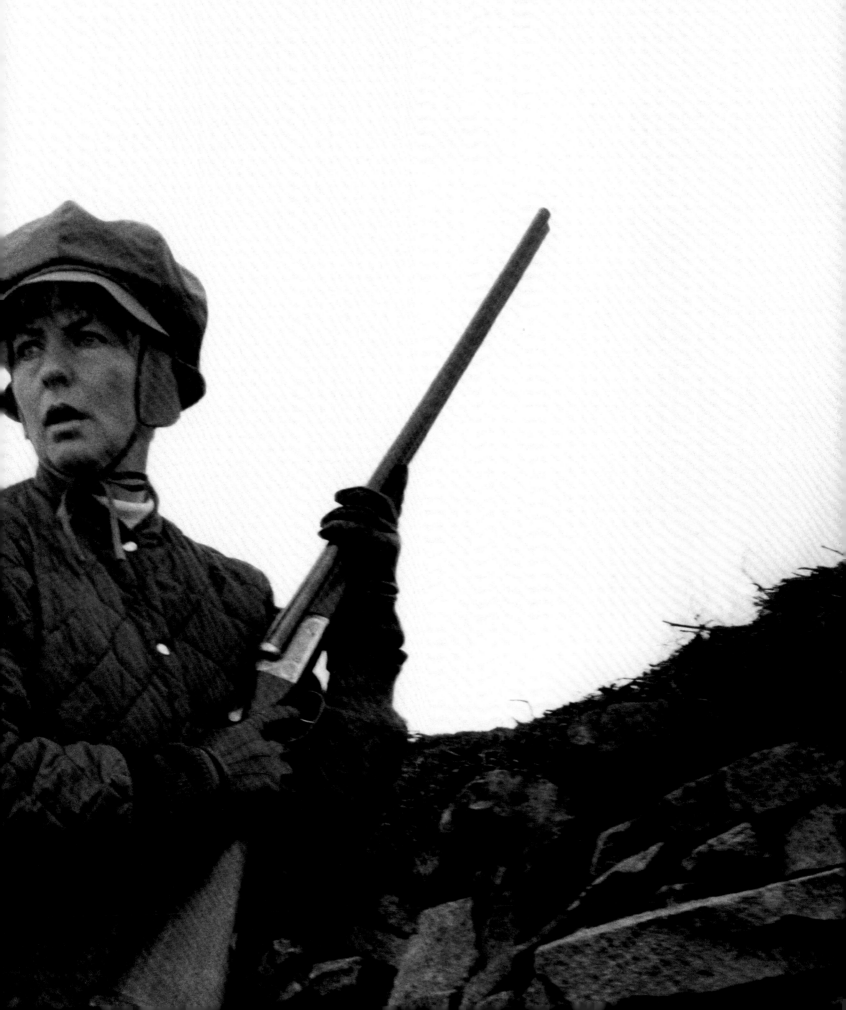

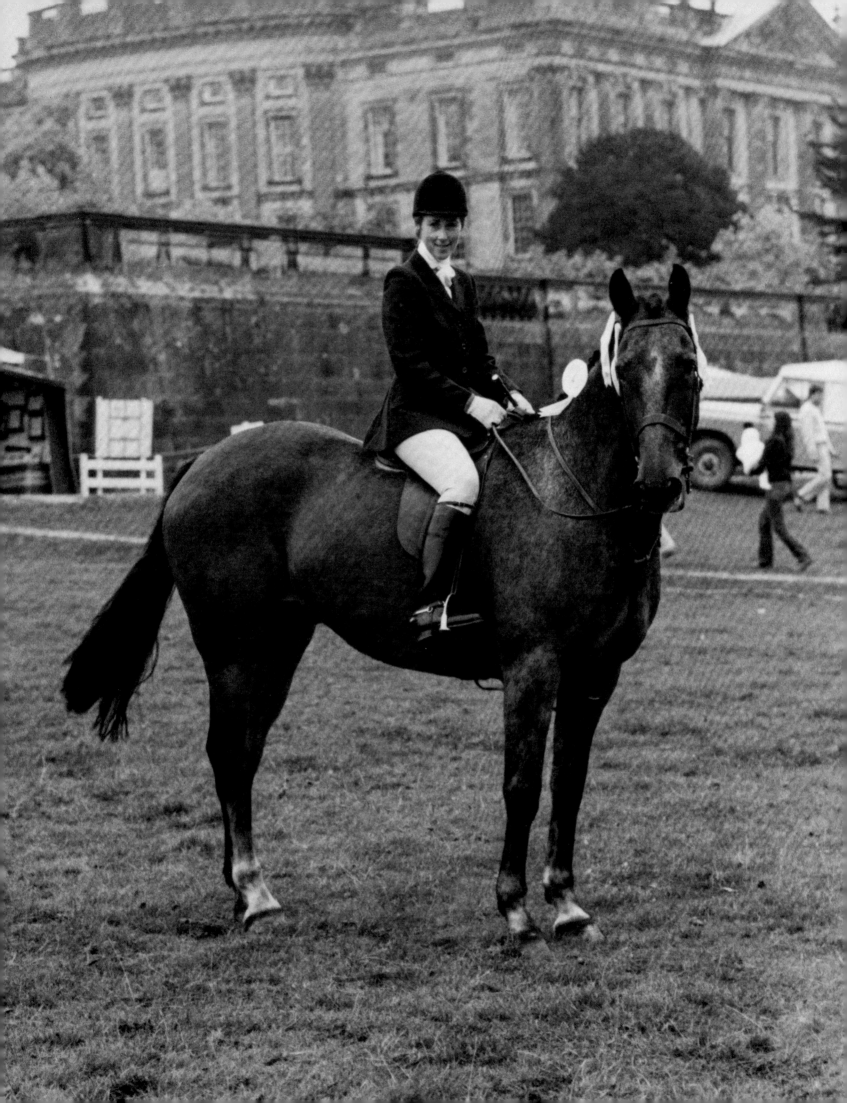

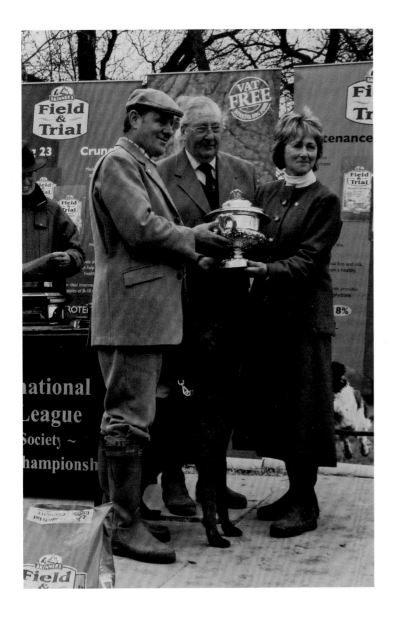

so Debo had to be hooked into it – and out of it again, when she finally retired at 4.40am. Bruce Weber memorably photographed her wearing this ensemble whilst feeding her beloved chickens (fig. 122).

Christine Thompson also made Debo one of her favourite ensembles, based on the 1864 portrait of Lady Frederick Cavendish (currently at Holker Hall), by William Blake Richmond, itself evocative of a Renaissance robe, with organza sleeves caught in puffs. This was worn with a 'cardinal' cape in either black or red, and the bug brooches that Debo amassed, clustered over its bodice or neatly lined along the closing seams of the tabard (fig. 133). The ensemble was originally intended to be worn at a dinner for the American Ambassador. 'She wanted something that nobody else had', Thompson explained, which was 'why you had homemade.' As a debutante, the many clothes required by Debo for the season had to come out of her annual £100 allowance, so evening dresses were run up by Gladys the maid for £1 a pop using fabric from John Lewis. '[A]lthough I envied girls with dresses by Victor Stiebel, mine were always unique', she observed philosophically.

Mary Feeney, a maid at Lismore Castle, was taught dressmaking by Adele Astaire's mother, Ada. Adele was soon enthusing about Miss Feeney's skills to Duchess Mary, not least the prices, which at £2 for a dress, and £4 for a suit in 1945 were as modest as their maker. Miss Feeney later 'became a great friend' of Debo's, who brought her over to Chatsworth for ten weeks a year and 'wore her creations at both the grandest and humblest occasions and always felt happy in them.' Feeney was even commissioned to make the wedding dress for her daughter, the botanical artist Lady Emma, in 1963. Mary Feeney created a gown of no small chic and some great ambition, made from a lace flowered with tulle ribbon and incorporating a 25-foot train.

The 10th Duke, presumably not so strapped for funds as his inheritors, was nevertheless conspicuously poorly dressed. '[H]is tailors bore the suitable name Cutter & Rook', noted his son Andrew wryly, whilst Debo observed that, 'He wore paper collars, did not possess an overcoat and would stand, oblivious of the weather, in the freezing wind on Chesterfield Station in a threadbare London suit.' His ready-rolled Turkish cigarettes, meanwhile 'smouldered away merrily in Eddy's coat pocket and made some decent holes, blackened around the edges; these became part of the suit, which he would never have dreamed of replacing.'

'I imagine I care so much about all things sartorial because my father was the worst dressed man in the world', Andrew noted, and in reaction he certainly became something of a dandy, sporting straw boaters with pale grey suits for Goodwood Races, and

66 *(opposite)* The Duchess of Devonshire on Lancer at the Triathlon Finals at Chatsworth, 1982.

67 *(above)* The Duchess of Devonshire receiving the winner's trophy at the Retriever Championship, 2009.

suits made by Jarvis & Hamilton of what *Country Life's* James Knox described as 'pinstripes of gangster strength.'

The Duke's famed motto jumpers (fig. 76), made by Lords of Burlington Arcade, included such playful aphorisms as NEVER MARRY A MITFORD and NEVER ARGUE WITH A CADOGAN, whilst FAR BETTER NOT was the phrase of usual recourse for the 8th Duke 'when people – colleagues, civil servants – came up with schemes, proposals or plans', as Andrew noted.

Other jumpers bore the names of the Duke's favourite places: CAREYSVILLE, for instance, the fishing lodge near Lismore, as well as the sites of his legendary treks. LYKE WAKE WALK recalls a 39-mile hike across the North Yorkshire moors in 1978. Sir Patrick Leigh Fermor wrote to the Duke following a walking expedition in Peru in 1981: 'It's suddenly come to me in a flash what ought to be written on the Peru jersey: SIERRA DE HUANTAY! Correct, romantic, euphonious, mystifying; in fact, perfect.' (On this trip, Leigh Fermor wrote home to describe the Duke's dandy flair flourishing even in these far-flung climes. 'Andrew wears a dashing betting jacket of bold-green plaid, extremely smart crocodile shoes and a white silk tie with a blue pattern bought in Cuzco.')

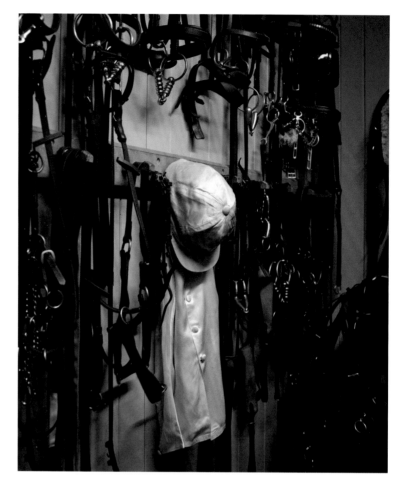

The 11th Duke's most celebrated racehorses were memorialized on straw-coloured jumpers, including PARK TOP – '[A]n owner's dream', as he himself wrote – who won La Coupe at Longchamp, the Cumberland Lodge Stakes and, memorably the King George VI and Queen Elizabeth Stakes, both at Ascot; GAY GEORGE ('named by an innocent Irish farmer'), who won the Scottish Champion Hurdle in 1982; and TEAPOT ROW. Stoker, meanwhile, recalls these horses' memory in cufflinks that bear their names, gifts from his father.

In 1874 Victor Cavendish wrote to his wife Evelyn noting that, 'All the servants now wear the state livery here at Chatsworth (fig. 2). It looks rather well but must be very uncomfortable.' Entertaining at the house was splendid. On the eve of the First World War, the vicar of Edensor's wife Christine O'Rorke, herself dressed by Worth in crimson velvet, records the magnificence of a Christmas dinner party attended by Queen Mary: '[I]t was more like a scene on the stage than anything else I can think of – the beautiful gowns, the well dressed hair, & above all the magnificent jewellery… many of the ladies hardly seemed to have on low dresses, their necks were so covered with ornaments!'

Until 1924, the footmen were also obliged to powder their hair for such a party, and the state livery was worn until 1938 if there were more than six guests to dinner. At Chatsworth, Andrew would always change for dinner, even if he and Debo were dining alone. The 11th Duke's valet, Henry Coleman Snr, was as invaluable to him as Christine Thompson and Mary Feeney were to Debo. Henry Coleman began working

68 *(above)* Devonshire racing silks in the tack room.

69 *(opposite)* Row of children's jodhpur boots in the Front Hall, standing in front of *Flying Childers* by James Seymour, circa 1722-1725.

70 *(following pages, left to right)* Attributed to Adam Frans van der Meulen, *Equestrian Portrait of the 1st Duke of Devonshire*, circa 1670.

71 Glen Luchford, still from Gucci's Cruise 2016 campaign shot at Chatsworth.

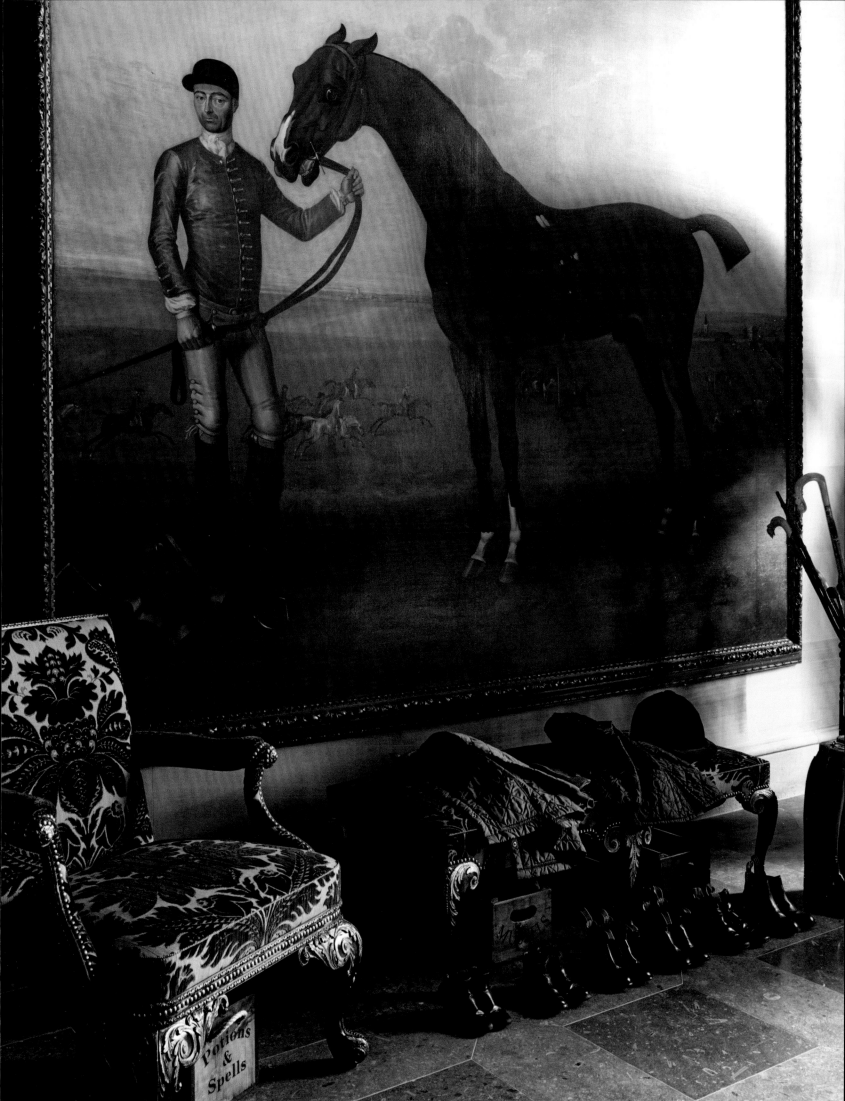

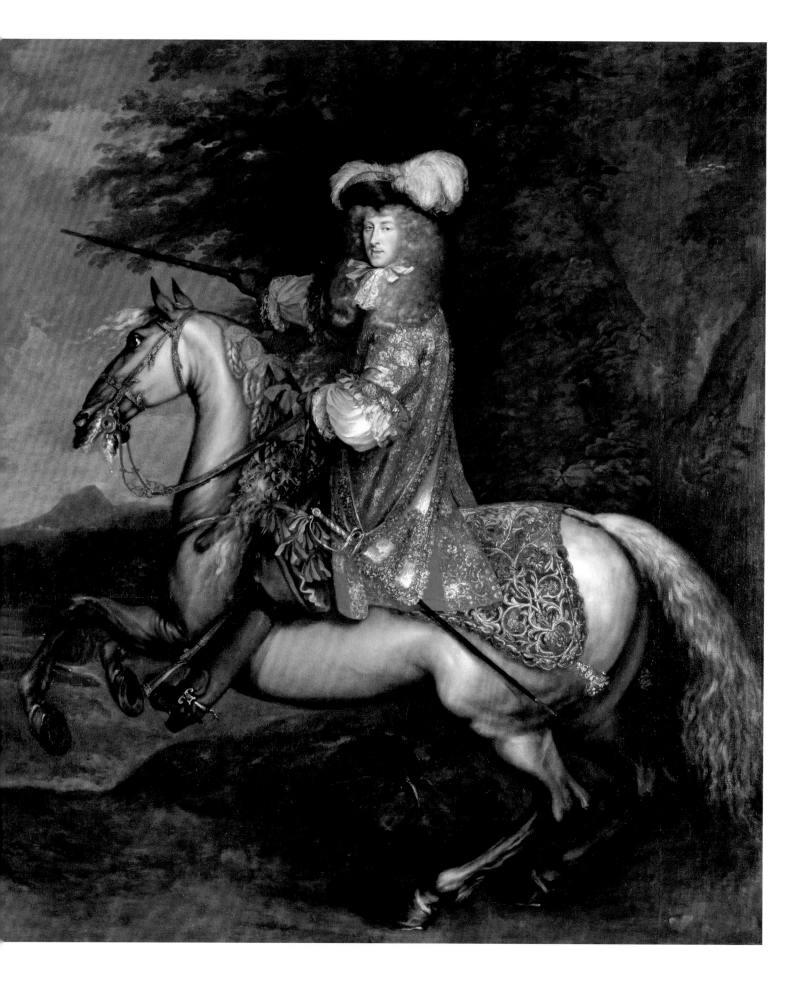

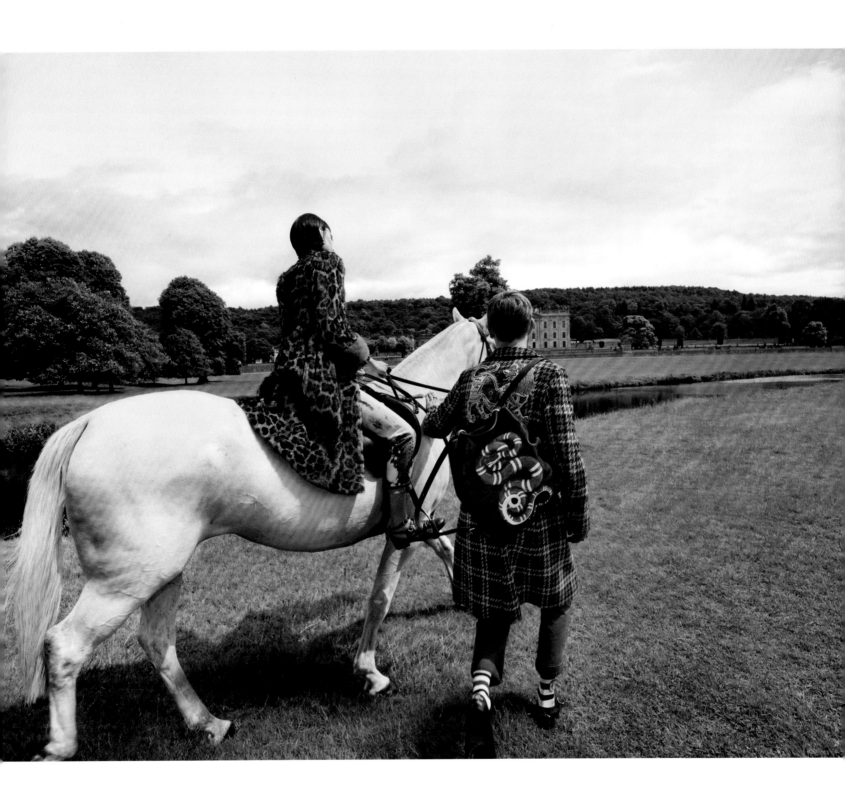

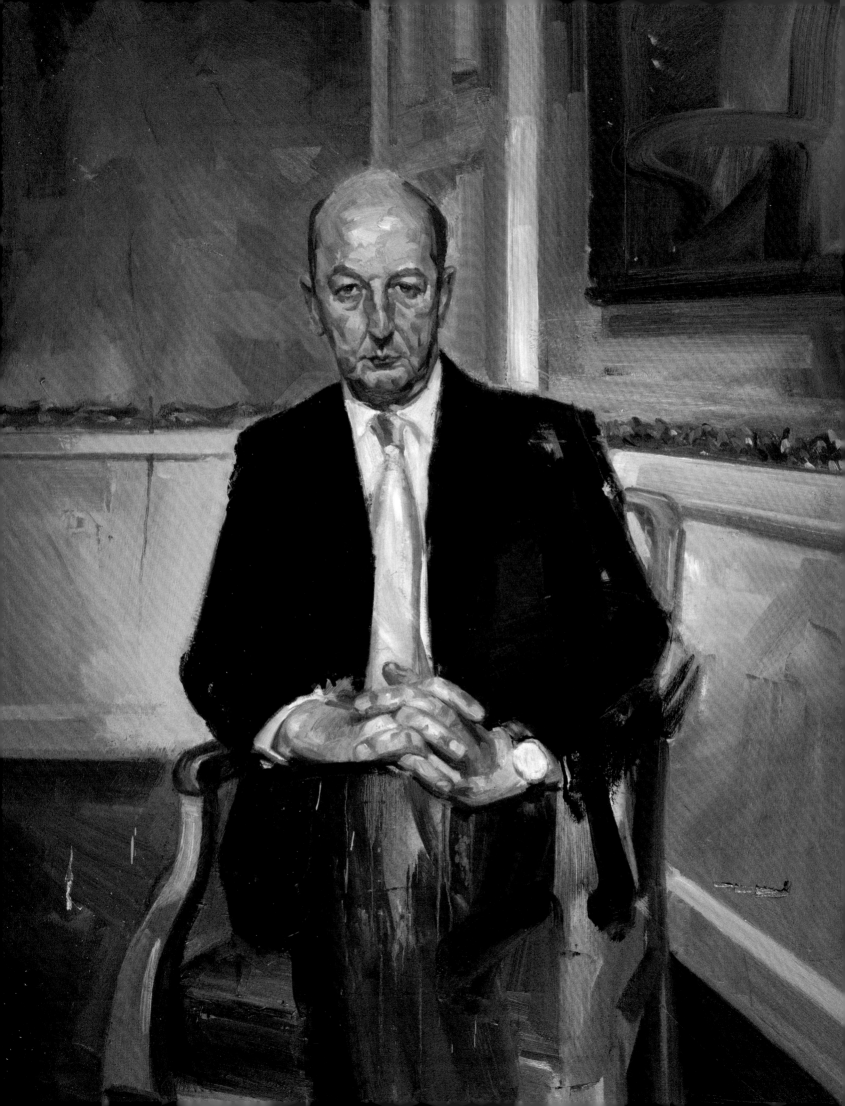

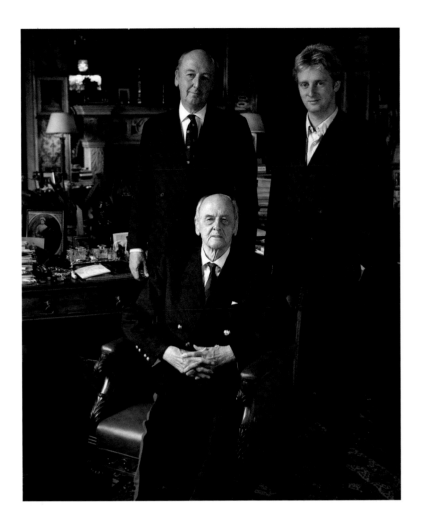

at Lismore Castle in 1963 at the age of 16, and was the butler at Chatsworth by the time he was 21 years old.

It was Coleman who initiated the considerate and stylish laying out of the Duke's clothes. The coat (Andrew abhorred the word 'jacket') would be draped over the chair's back, the trousers laid on its seat with the shirt on top (starched collar attached to the collarless shirt with its brass stud, and cufflinks already threaded through so the Duke had only to put his hands through the cuffs), and the socks next to the shirt, with the shoes laid beneath the chair.

He thoughtfully laid out gifts, such as handkerchiefs, if he knew the giver was coming to visit, and scrupulously maintained the clothes, scrubbing the Duke's muddied shoelaces with Fairy Liquid and a wire brush, for instance. Some of the Duke's clothing, however, defied rational repair. Andrew loved one of his tweed coats so much that as its elbows and edges frayed with age and use, it was patched with random scraps of mismatched tweed until it resembled nothing so much as a piece of traditional Japanese '*boro*' (fig. 63). When the scales on his crocodile Lobb shoes began to peel off with age, they were carefully sewn on with tiny blanket stitches, whilst his embroidered slippers from the same establishment were so beloved that they were worn until threadbare and patched up with scraps of leather like ancient holy relics (fig. 18). (Debo, meanwhile, wore slippers emblazoned with the likeness of Elvis Presley (fig. 81), who had been the unlikely object of her veneration since she came across a television documentary about him in the late 1970s.)

In other respects, however, the 11th Duke could indulge in sartorial extravagance. The Devonshire racing colours – 'straw' – are the oldest registered on the Turf (fig. 68), and can be seen worn by the groom in the circa 1723 James Seymour painting of the horse 'Flying Childers' (fig. 69). Andrew paid homage to these colours by ordering yellow socks by the dozen from Turnbull & Asser, the establishment that also furnished his cream silk pyjamas, embroidered with a ducal coronet hovering over the Devonshire 'D' on the breast pocket and also ordered *en masse* (fig. 18). When the pyjama bottoms wore out, however, they were consigned to a drawer in the Sewing Room to be used for mending. 'I had a terrible day two years ago when the Duke of Marlborough's grapes beat mine in the fruit show', Andrew playfully told the *Observer Magazine*'s Lynn Barber in 2002, 'and I got back to the club to read in the *Evening Standard* that the Duke of Beaufort was the best-dressed duke. That *was* a bad day!'

Stoker also experimented with the dandy fashions of his 1960s youth, acquiring shirts at Mr Fish, and a moss-green evening suit and a swaggering, ankle-length tweed coat from Blades, the store that Rupert Lycett Green established in a handsome bow-fronted

72 *(opposite)* Tai-Shan Schierenberg, *The Duke of Devonshire*, 1997.

73 *(above)* The Duke of Devonshire, 11th Duke of Devonshire, Earl of Burlington (left to right), 2001.

74 *(page 96)* Sir Godfrey Kneller, *The 1st Duke of Devonshire*, circa 1680-1685.

75 *(page 97)* Tim Walker, Stella Tennant in an evening dress by Riccardo Tisci for Givenchy, Autumn/Winter 2007. Originally published in Italian *Vogue*, August 2007.

76 *(page 98)* Wool jumpers by Lords, commissioned by the 11th Duke of Devonshire, 1980s.

77 *(page 99)* The 11th Duke of Devonshire, fishing on the Blackwater, circa 1986.

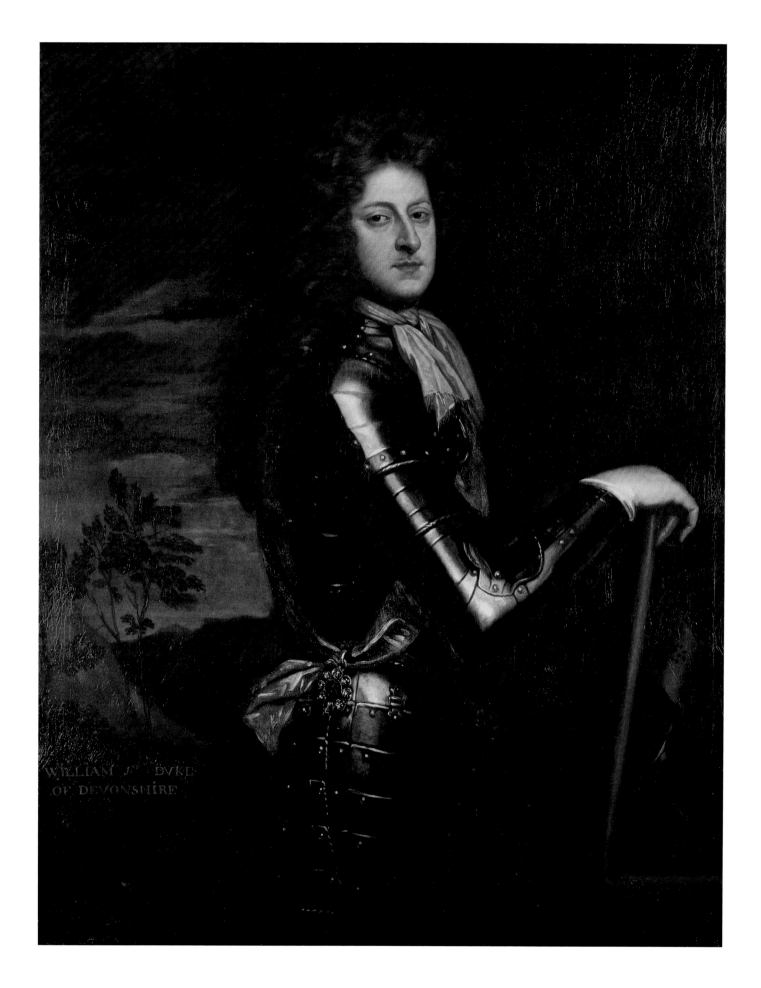

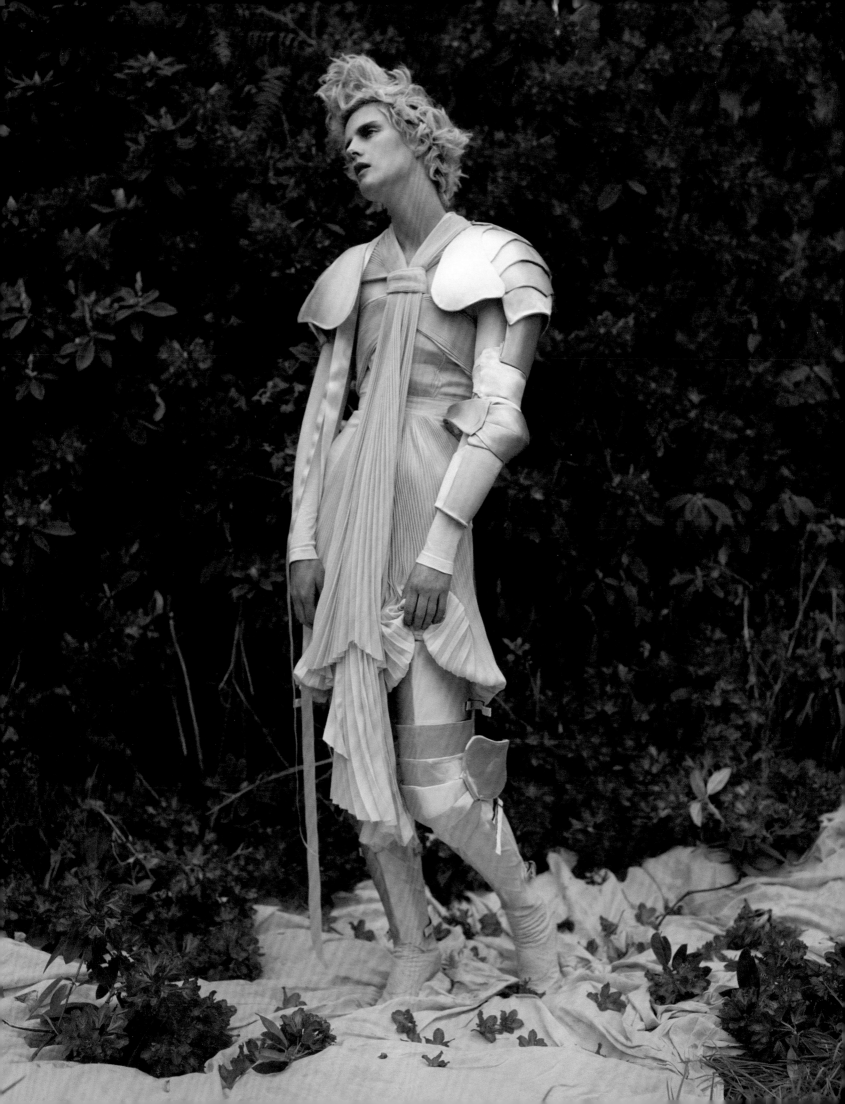

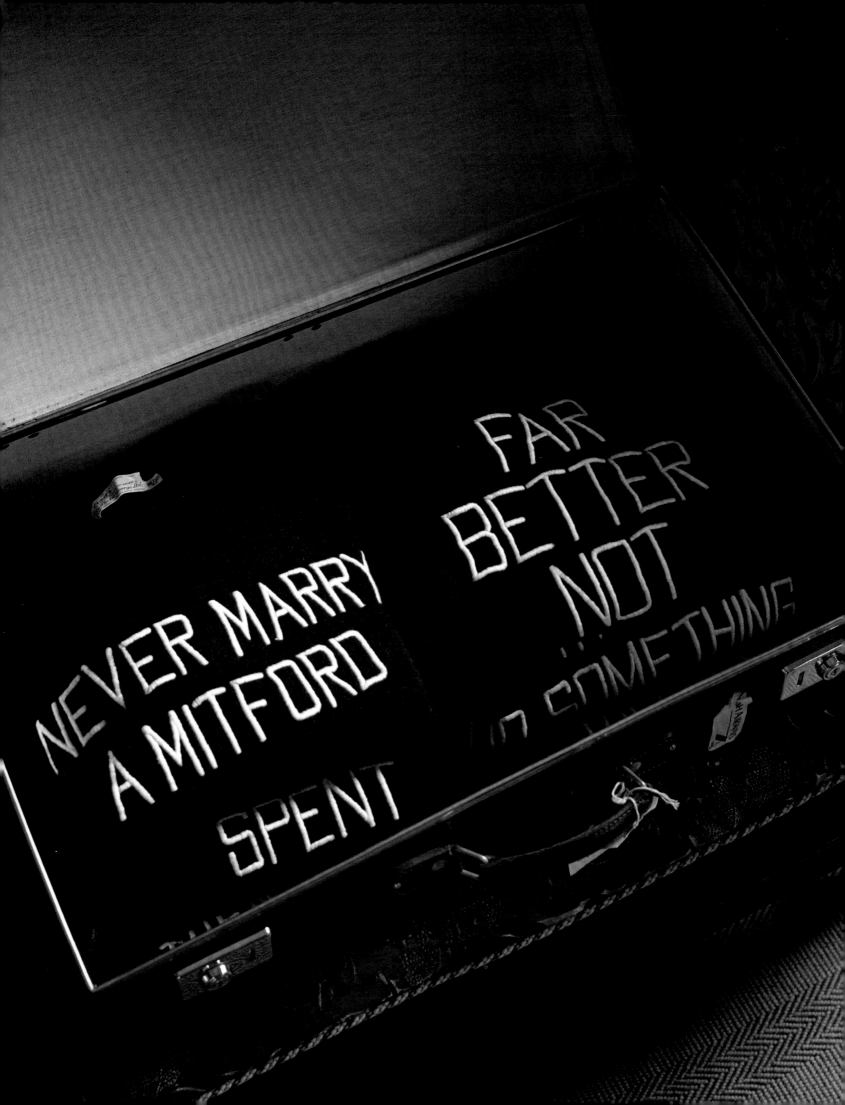

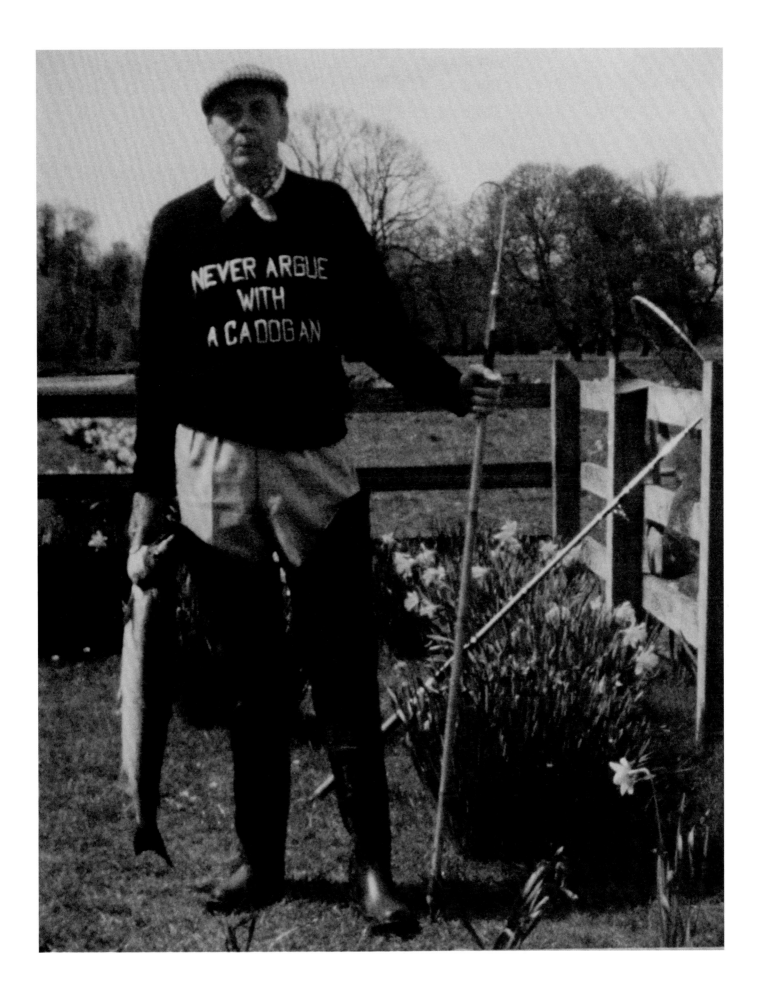

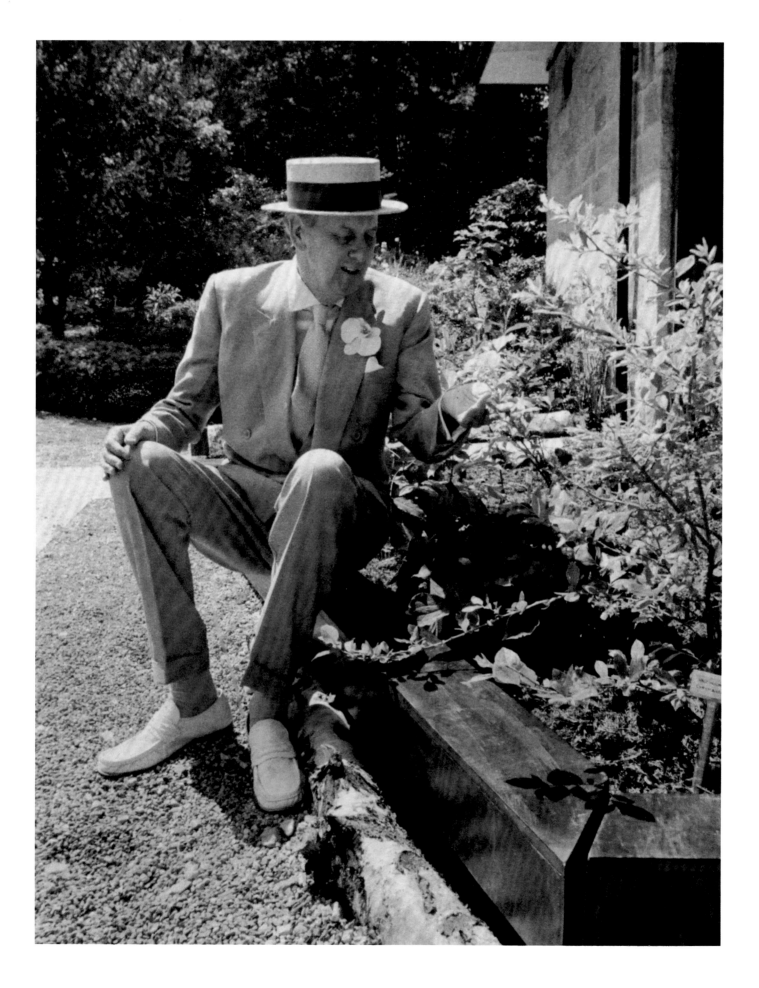

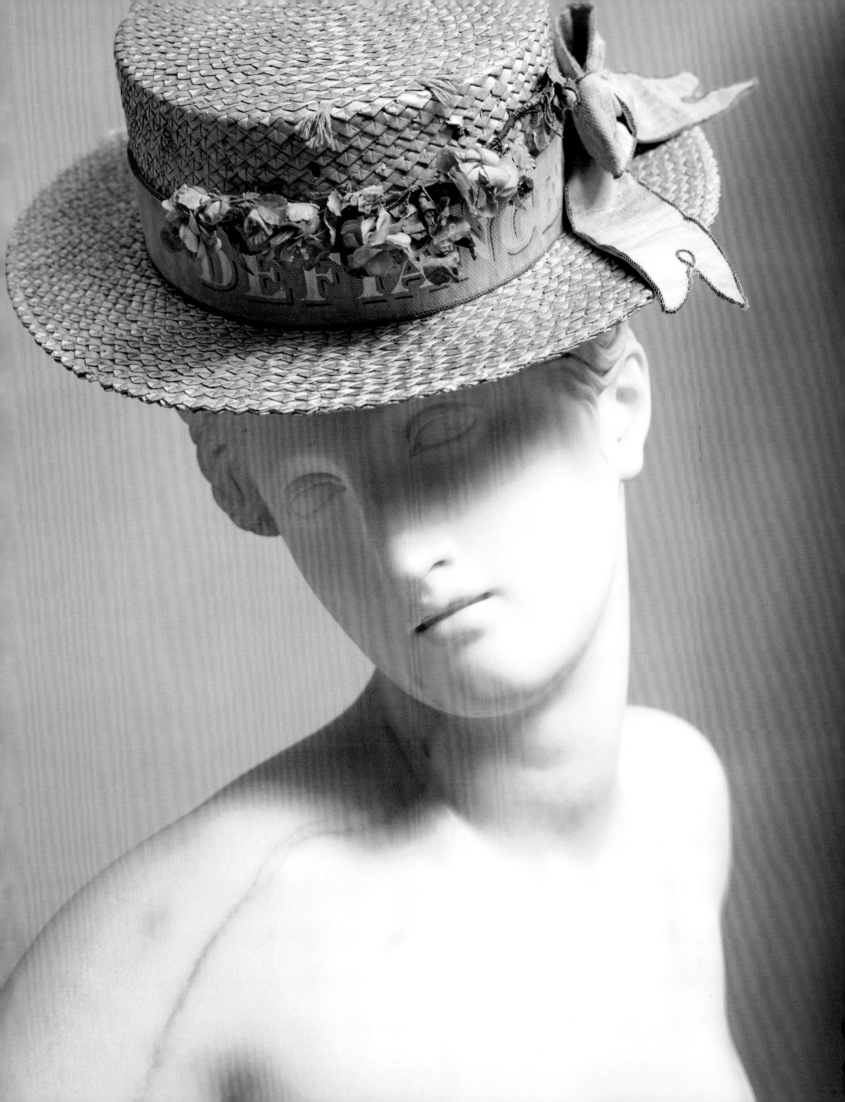

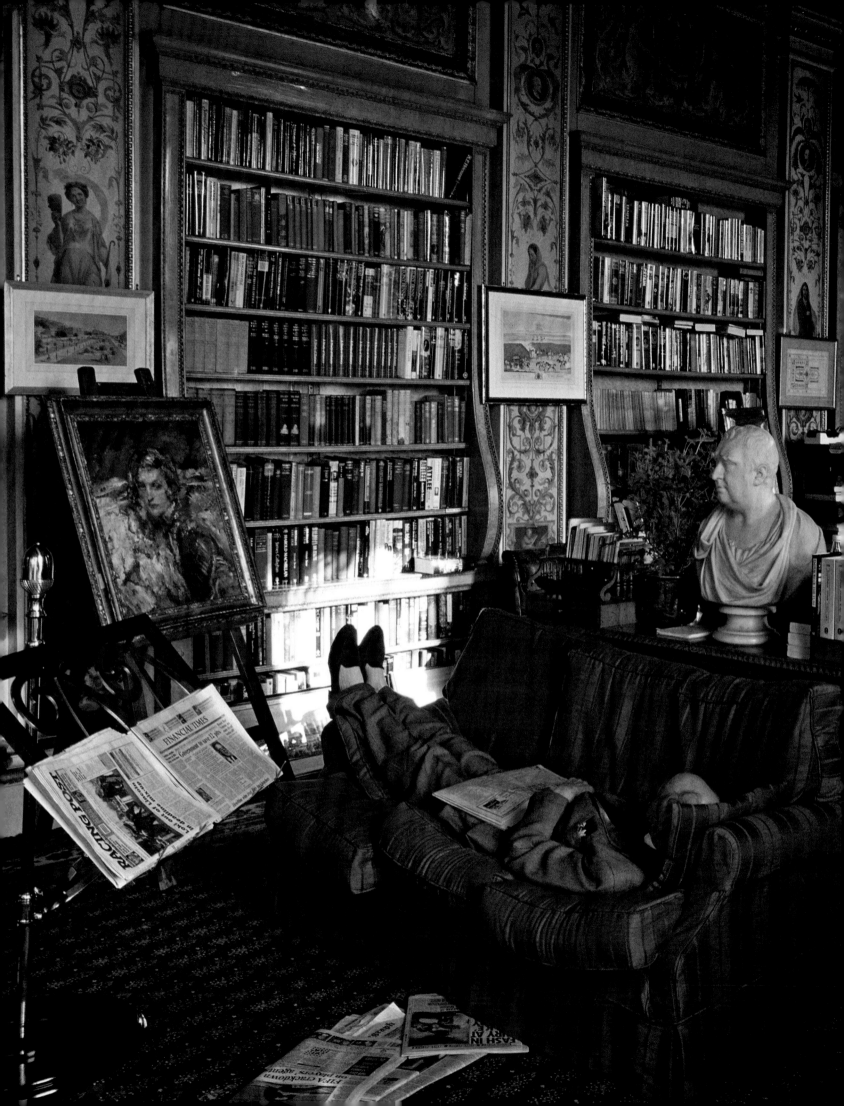

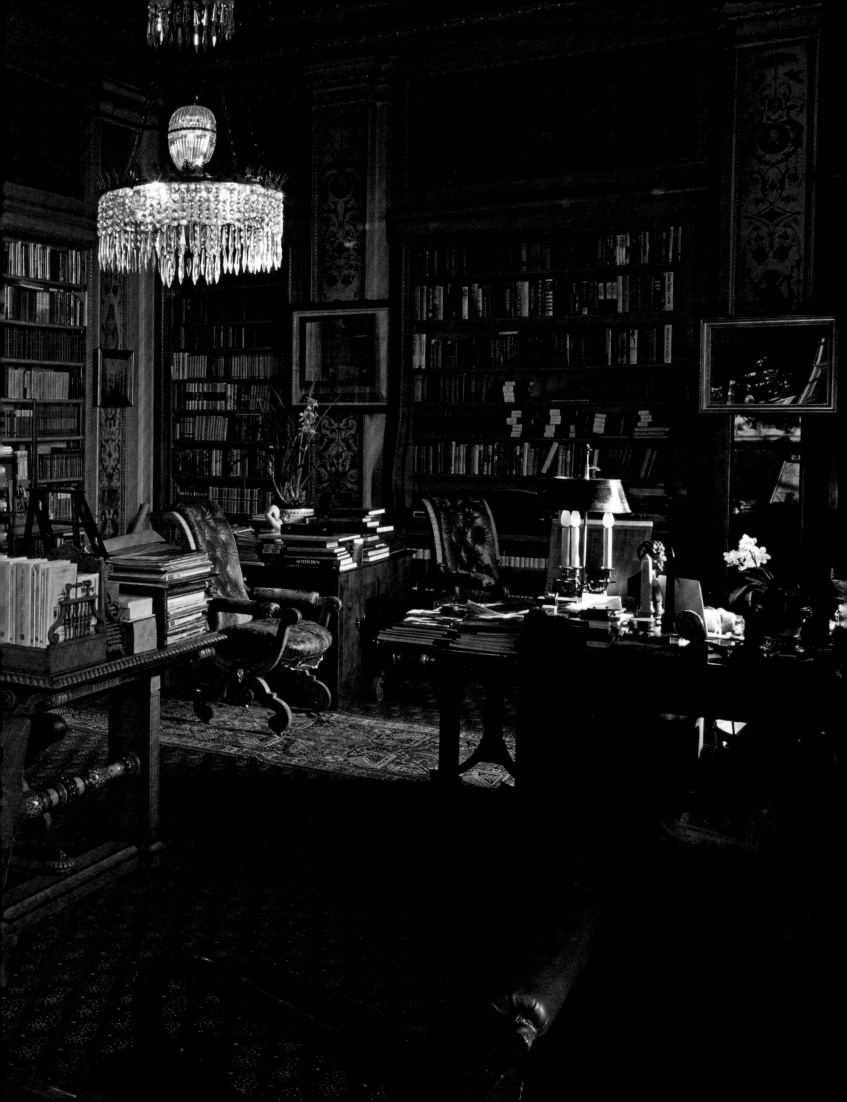

eighteenth-century townhouse on Burlington Gardens and whose motto was, 'For today rather than the memory of yesterday.' In turn, William Burlington shopped at Voyage, the 90s hippie-chic store so exclusive that at one point customers needed membership cards to shop there.

'The contrast between modern forms and materials, and this space steeped in history is one we enjoy', Stoker has written, referring of course to the stimulating interventions inside and out by contemporary artists and sculptors that he and Amanda have initiated, but he might equally have been referring to the exciting dynamics between the clothes the Cavendish family have chosen to wear in this storied setting.

The truth seems to be that from all that dandy swagger, to an embarrassment of muddied tweed, from the cradle's lace and eyelet to the graveside's mourning black, Chatsworth, ever mutating itself, seems to offer a welcome to all. It is a place that relishes the stories that clothes tell.

78 *(page 100)* The 11th Duke of Devonshire at Compton Place, Eastbourne, 1995.

79 *(page 101)* Eton 'Defiance' straw hat, E C Devereux, 1930s.

80 *(pages 102-103)* Christopher Simon Sykes, the 11th Duke of Devonshire in his sitting room (Lower Library), 1995.

81 *(opposite)* Velour slippers with Elvis portrait by Stubbs & Wootton, much loved by Deborah Devonshire.

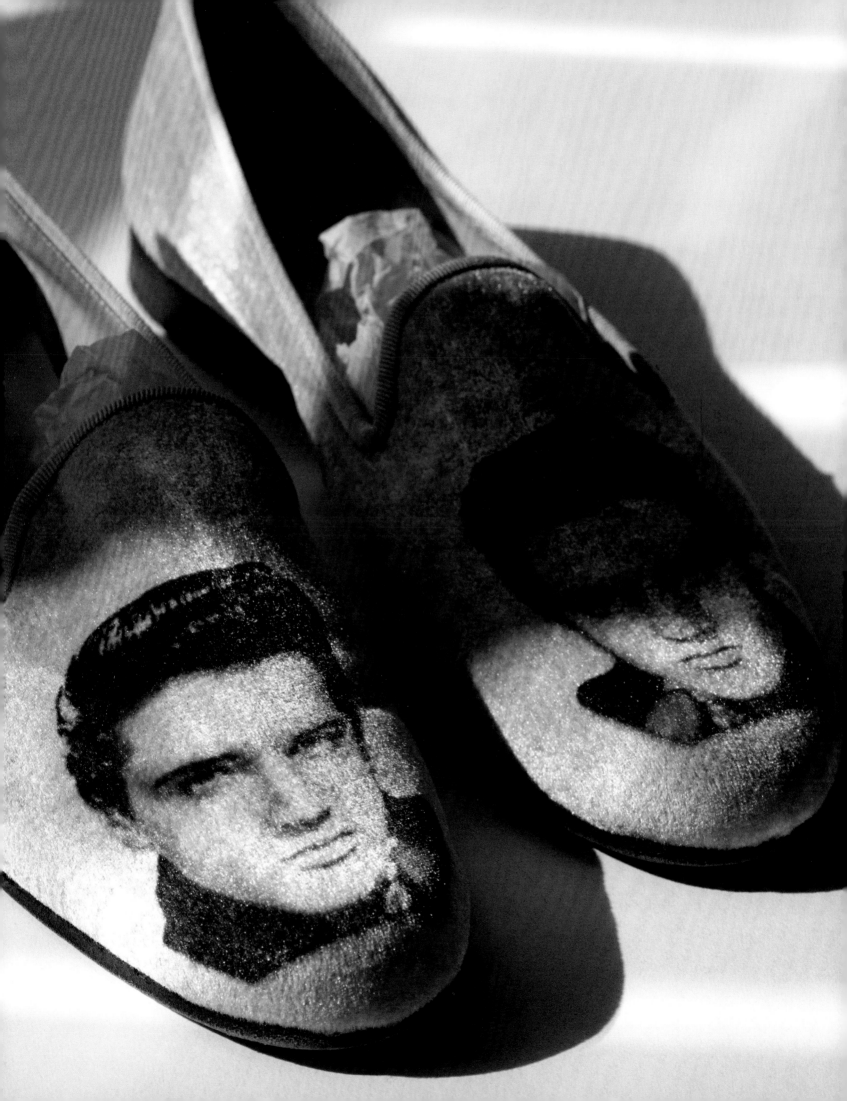

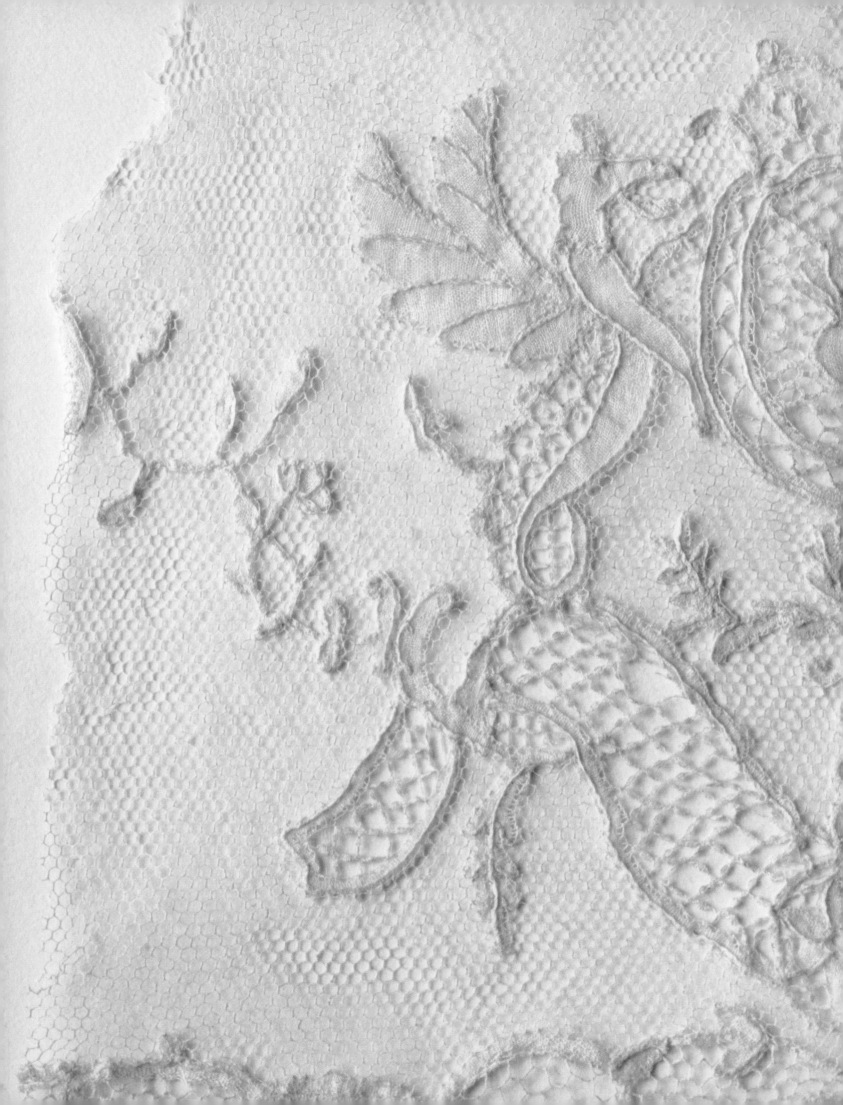

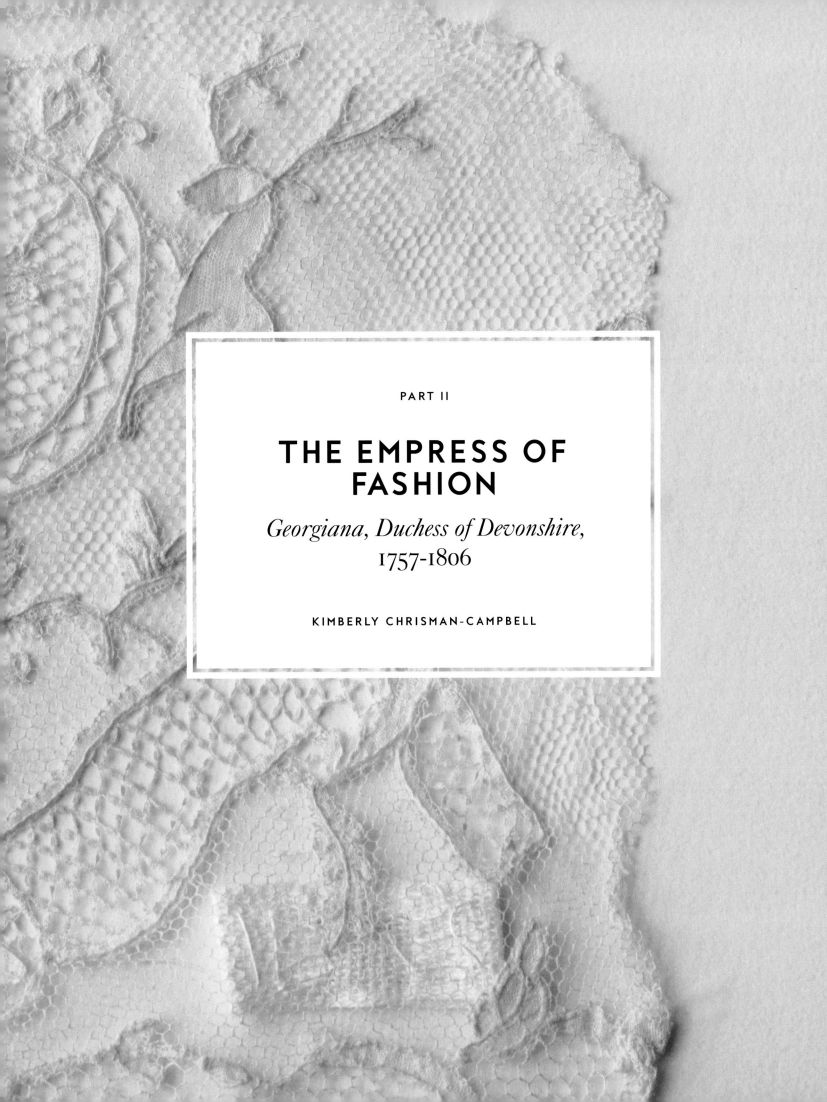

PART II

THE EMPRESS OF FASHION

Georgiana, Duchess of Devonshire, 1757-1806

KIMBERLY CHRISMAN-CAMPBELL

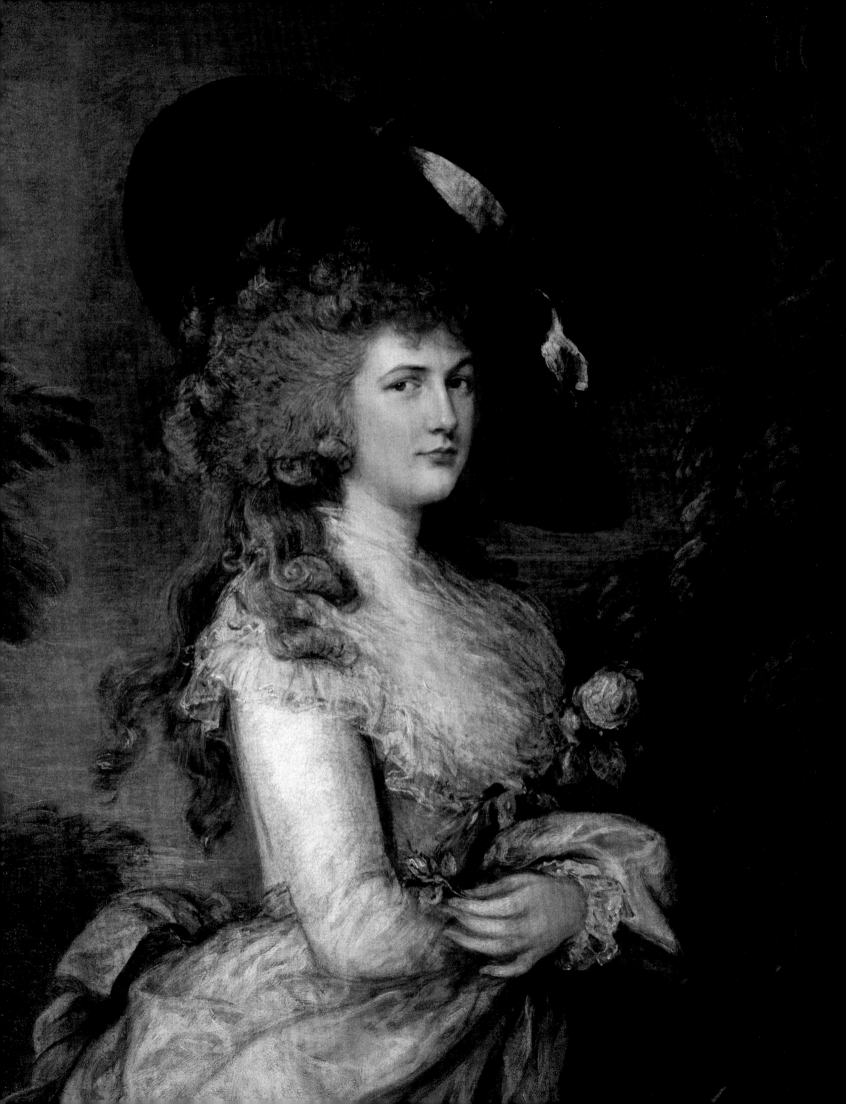

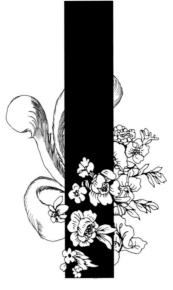

f the court of Versailles was the centre of taste and fashion in the eighteenth century, the court of St James was the 'residence of dullness', in the damning phrase of a visiting Prussian dignitary[1]. Rather than the conservative court, English fashion was led by an elite group of aristocratic women in the circle of the Prince of Wales, who presided over a rival 'court' of powerful, pleasure-loving Whigs opposed to the ruling Tory party. Among these titled luminaries, one name was (and still is) paramount: Georgiana, Duchess of Devonshire, dubbed 'the empress of fashion' by Horace Walpole[2].

From an early age, Georgiana was tutored in the art of dress by a mother whose renowned intellect and piety did nothing to dampen her own love of fashion. Almost as soon as her daughter's illustrious marriage to the 5th Duke of Devonshire was arranged, Countess Spencer turned her energies to the important business of assembling a magnificent trousseau, spending £1,486 on gowns, riding habits, shoes, fans, hats, mantles, undergarments and other accessories in the two months preceding the ceremony on 5 June 1774[3]. Kid gloves, silk stockings, caps and handkerchiefs arrived by the dozen. The soon-to-be-Duchess ordered stays from Hector Flamand of Golden Square, hoop petticoats from Hornby and Harris of Soho, lace from John Misbury of St James's Street and muslins from Hatchett and Payne of Covent Garden.

Many of these fashion dealers were French, or at least pretended to be; Paris was the epicentre of style, then as now. A Pierre Langlois provided 65 pairs of shoes and slippers, many with lavish gold or silvery embroidery and stylish contrasting heels. Flamand printed 'from Paris' at the head of his invoices and advertised his stays as '*alamode de Frances*' [sic]; other bills were written entirely in French[4]. But Georgiana patriotically patronized long-time suppliers to the English establishment, as well. Van Sommer, Paul and Niccolls of Pall Mall – 'Silk Weavers to their Majesties' – provided her with hundreds of yards of 'Lustring', a reflective silk. And she purchased lace, artificial flowers and other trimmings from Elizabeth Beauvais, the French-born milliner to Queen Charlotte[5].

The wedding itself was a quiet, clandestine affair, attended only by a few family members. The gossips got their first glimpse of the bride three weeks later when she attended her first Drawing Room at St James's Palace as a married woman. As was customary, she wore her gold and white wedding dress, along with 'very magnificent' diamonds, a gift from her husband[6]. The new Duchess of Devonshire was vivacious, self-assured, inventive, effortlessly elegant and wildly rich – qualities which made her a natural fashion leader (and more than compensated for her lack of conventional beauty). As a celebrity with connections in the highest social and political circles, Georgiana was well placed to influence other women, both of her own class and of the middle and lower ranks. But her exalted position gave her license to take fashion risks that would have left women of lesser status exposed to ridicule.

For example, she popularised the much-maligned 'high heads' of the 1770s. These elaborate hairstyles are the most conspicuous features of late-eighteenth-century portraits and fashion plates. Contrary to popular belief, women did not wear wigs. Instead, they augmented their natural hair with false hair and padding as well as *poufs*: confections

82 *(opposite)* Thomas Gainsborough, *Duchess Georgiana*, 1785-1787.

83 *(following pages, left to right)* J Lockington, *Lady All-Top*, May 15, 1776.

84 Sir Joshua Reynolds, *Georgiana Cavendish, Duchess of Devonshire*, circa 1775-1776.

85 *(Pages 112-113)* Mario Testino, Stella Tennant in an evening dress by John Galliano for Christian Dior Haute Couture, Spring/Summer 1998, set design by Patrick Kinmonth. Originally published in American *Vogue*, May 2006.

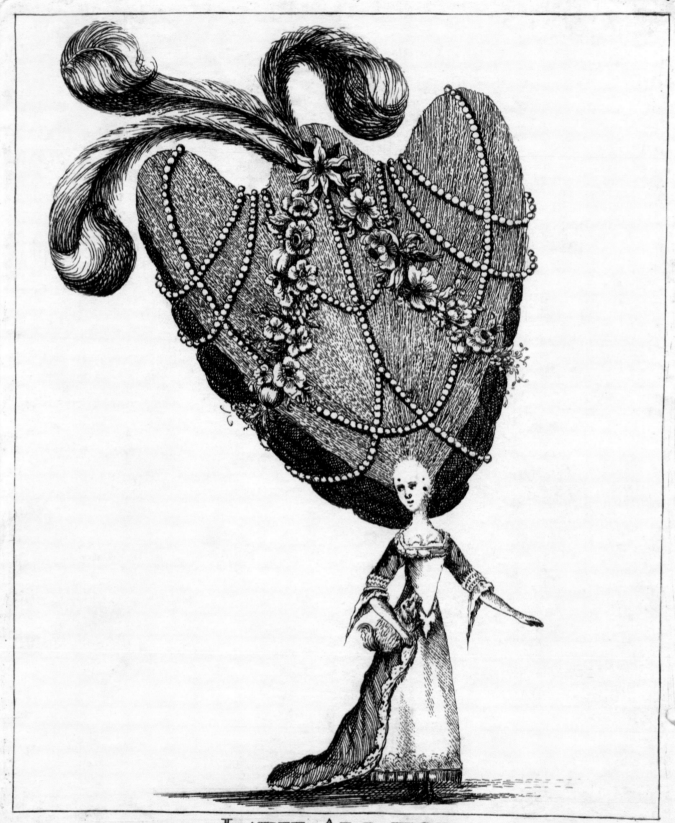

LADY ALL-TOP.

Pub.d according to Act of Parl.t May 15 1776 by J. Lockington Snug Lane Golding quare

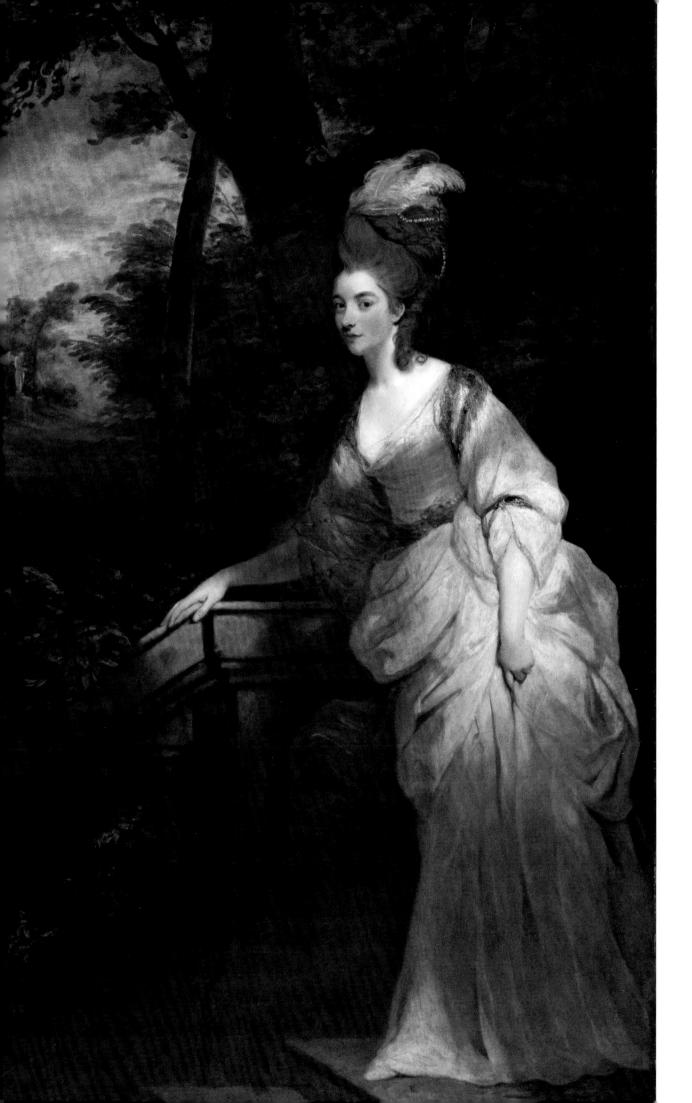

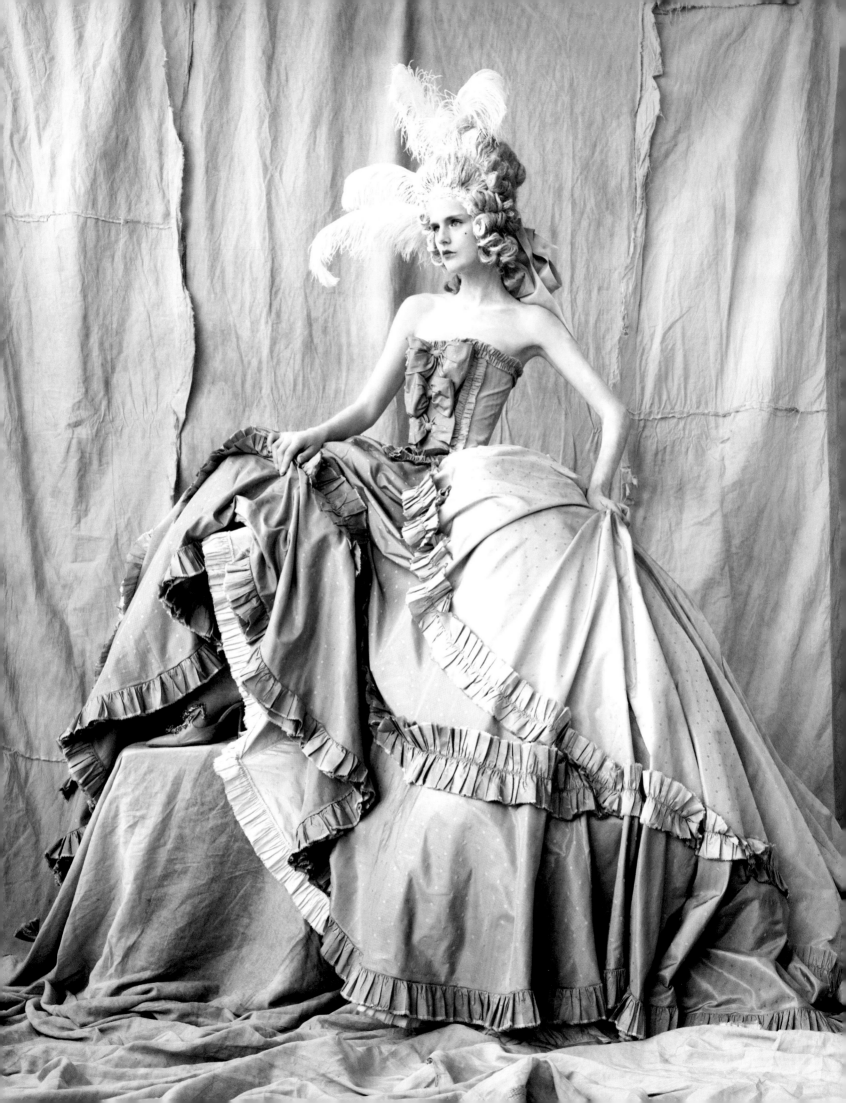

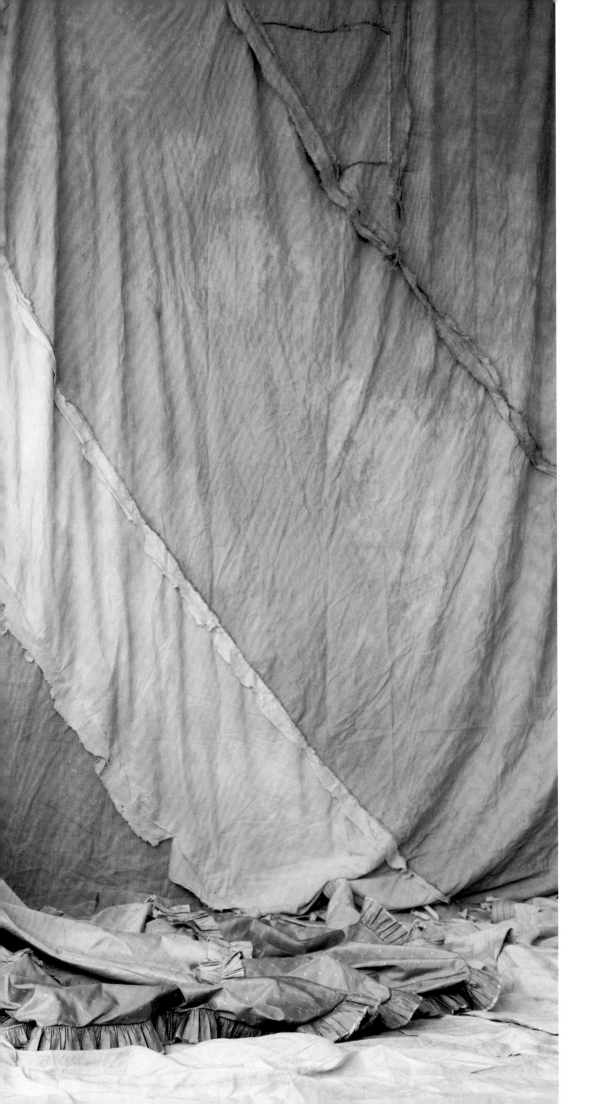

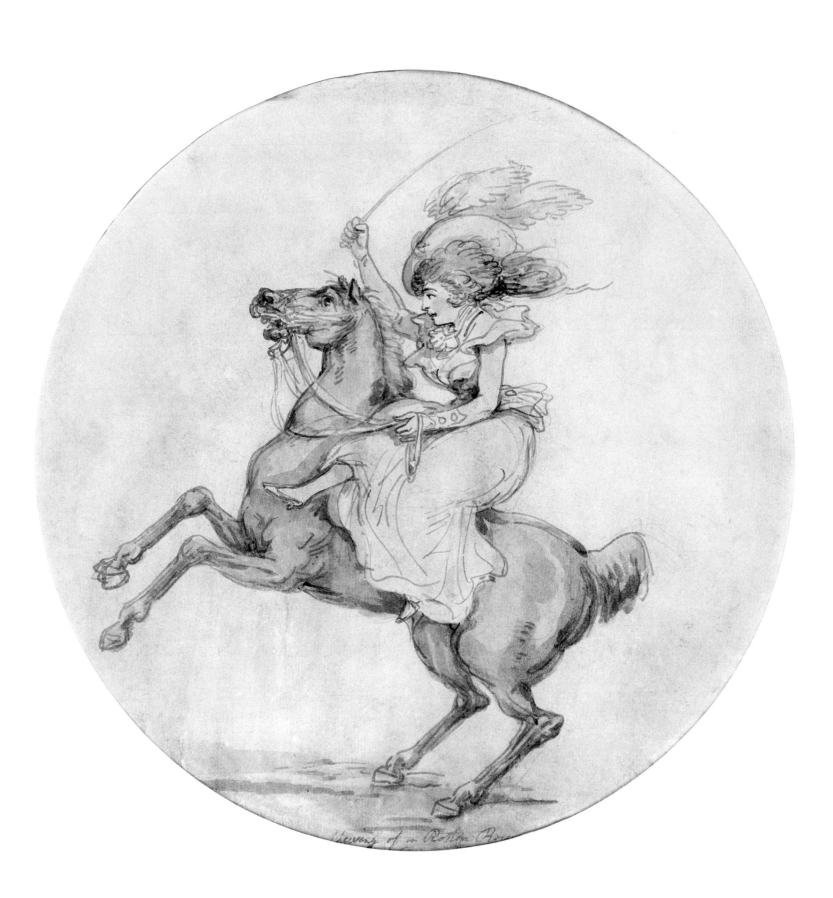

of feathers, flowers, ribbons and other ornaments nestled in sculptures of scented powder and pomade.

The trend began in Paris, where Georgiana had several well-placed informants[7]. In November 1774, her friend Lady Clermont wrote to her from Paris with news of a surprising fashion trend started by Madame de Boufflers: 'There is no describing her head dress & of all young people. They sit at the bottom of their coaches as they have not room if they sit on the seat[8].' As she was unable to describe the new headdress, Lady Clermont drew a picture of it in the text of her letter. It was not long before Georgiana began wearing similar high, feathered coiffures. Previously associated with actresses, the style gained respectability and aristocratic cachet thanks to the duchess. In her portrait by Joshua Reynolds (circa 1775-1776), exuberant white and pink ostrich plumes crown Georgiana's intricate coiffure (fig. 84). Though her gown is a fanciful blend of Turkish and classical references typical of the costumes worn at masquerades, her coiffure would not be out of place in an English drawing room – or a French one, for that matter.

As the fashion for feathers spread, Georgiana took pains to ensure that hers were larger than anyone else's. In March 1775, Mrs Delany wrote to a friend in the country: 'Nothing is talked of now so much as the ladies' *enormous* [headdresses], more suited to the *stage* or a *masquerade* than for either *civil* or sober societies. The three *most* elevated plumes of feathers are the Duchess of Devonshire, Lady Mary Somerset and Lady Harriet Stanhope, but some say Mrs Hobart's exceeds them all[9].' Georgiana had recently appeared at Hampton Court wearing 'two plumes 16 inches long, besides three small ones', an amused observer reported, adding: 'This has so far outdone all other plumes, that Mrs Damer, Lady Harriet Stanhope, &c., looked nothing[10].' Incensed, Lady Stanhope, Lady Ailesbury and Mrs Damer travelled to France, the original source of the fashion:

> They have returned in fine feathers, but the Duchess of Devonshire has still the highest. One lady tried all places to get one longer than those of the Duchess, but without success, till she luckily thought of sending to an undertaker; he sent word back his hearses were all out, but they were expected home in a few days, and then he hoped to accommodate her ladyship[11].

This seemingly frivolous sartorial rivalry may have had a more serious political dimension; feathered hairstyles were particular to the Whig party. As Mary Moser noted, 'The Queen and her ladies never wear feathers. They say here that the minority ladies are distinguished from the courtiers by their plumes[12].' Lady Louisa Stuart remembered that the Queen:

> thought it her duty to declare how highly she disapproved of them; and consequently for two or three years no one ventured to wear them at Court, excepting some daring spirits either too supreme in fashion to respect any other kind of pre-eminence, or else connected with the Opposition, and glad to set her Majesty at defiance. So an *Ostrich* Feather… had the glory of becoming treasonable[13].

Georgiana – being both 'supreme in fashion' and a loyal Whig – refused to be daunted by the Queen, nor by the satirists and moralists who condemned the style. As the *Morning*

86 *(opposite)* Thomas Rowlandson, *Showing Off in Rotten Row: 18th Century*, circa 1780-1795.

115

Post reported: 'Many other females of distinction have been made to moult, and rather than be laughed at any longer, left themselves featherless; while her Grace, with all the dignity of a young Duchess is determined to keep the field, for her feathers increase in enormity in proportion to the public intimations she receives of the absurdity[14].' So firmly associated was Georgiana with 'high heads' that the 1776 satire *Lady All-Top* (fig. 83) is likely a pun on Althorp, the Spencer estate.

Clearly, Georgiana had a flair for headgear. In the summer of 1779, she visited the Continental resort town of Spa, returning to England by way of Versailles, where the 'chapeau à la Devonshire' – also known as the 'chapeau à la Spa' – instantly became all the rage. According to the French fashion magazine *Galerie des Modes*, *'cette mode fût apporté de cette ville à la Cour de France, et y avait été portée par Mme Devonshire*[15] (fig. 27).' The plumed hat combined the exuberant trimmings of the pouf with the novelty of the hat, an accessory previously worn primarily by men in France and considered to be quintessentially English. On 3 November 1779, the Marquis de Boisgelin bought his niece a 'chapeau à la Devonshire' from Rose Bertin, *marchande de modes* to Marie Antoinette and other ladies of the court, as well as Georgiana herself[16]. The hat of 'English' white straw had a large pink satin ribbon tied in a bow around the turned-up crown and a 'panache' of ten black feathers, four white feathers and a little bunch of *aigrettes*[17].

This chic chapeau was not Georgiana's only sartorial namesake. On 21 October 1782, the *Morning Herald and Daily Advertiser* reported: 'The Duchess of Devonshire, it is said, means to introduce a head piece which is to be neither hat, cap, nor bonnet, and yet all three, a sort of trinity in unity, under the appellation the "Devonshire Whim"[18].' And, in circa 1785, Thomas Gainsborough painted Georgiana's portrait in another wide-brimmed, feather-trimmed hat, allegedly of her own design (fig. 82). When the portrait was exhibited, women immediately began to demand copies of the 'Duchess of Devonshire's picture hat[19].' Within weeks, the style had crossed the Channel. In 1786, the *Galerie des Modes* introduced an entirely new 'chapeau à la Devonshire.' Though it bore only a slight resemblance to the hat in Gainsborough's portrait, it was similarly broad-brimmed and be-plumed, and pointedly paired with a *robe à l'anglaise*, a gown with a fitted bodice inspired by English fashions[20]. By this time, 'à la Devonshire' had become synonymous with 'à l'anglaise' in France, and 'anglomanie' – the craze for English dress, politics and pastimes – was sweeping the country.

Georgiana would not return to Paris until 1789; however, she kept abreast of French fashion. In 1783, she became one of the first Englishwomen to wear the *robe à la Turque*,

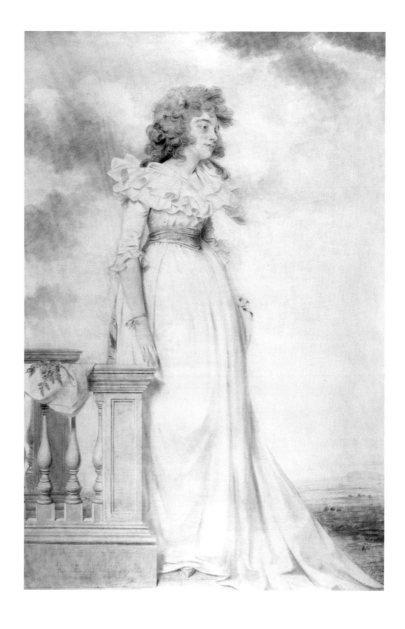

87 *(above)* John Downman *Duchess Georgiana*, 1787.

88 *(opposite)* Mme Yevonde, Deborah Devonshire in a costume she wore to the Beistegui Ball in Venice, inspired by a John Downman watercolour of Duchess Georgiana, 1951.

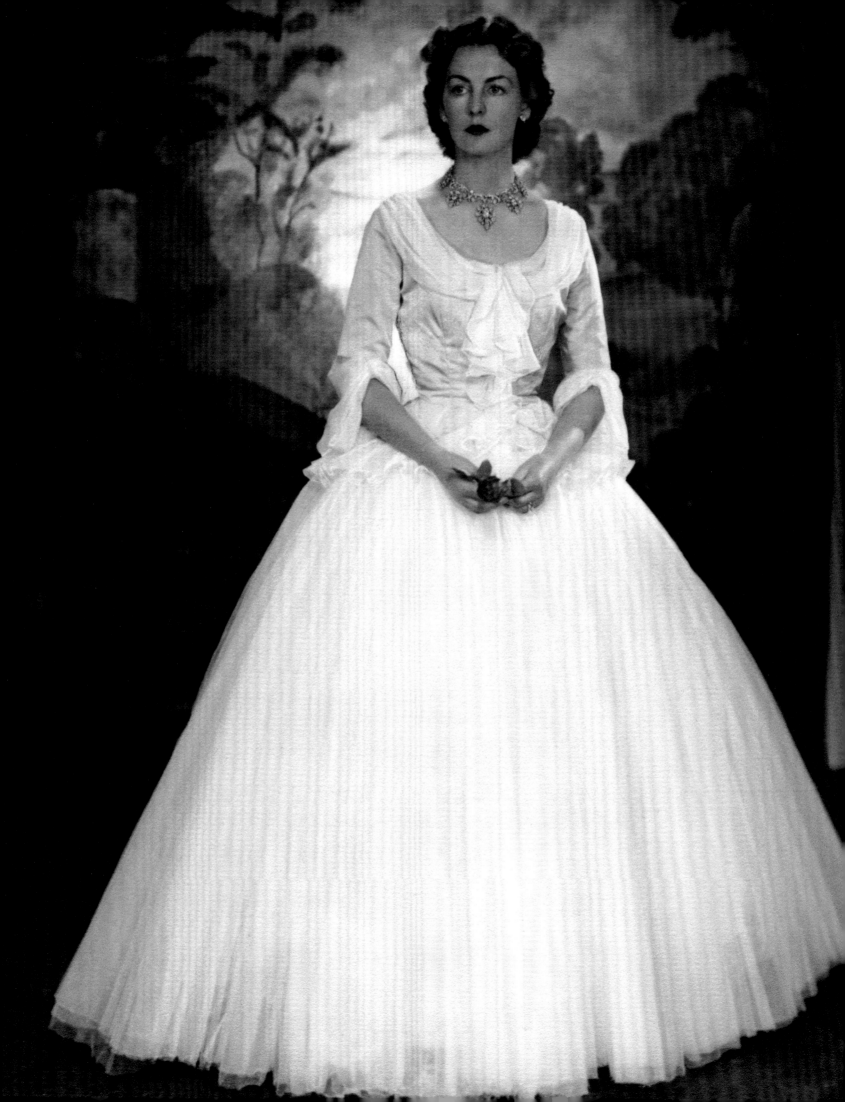

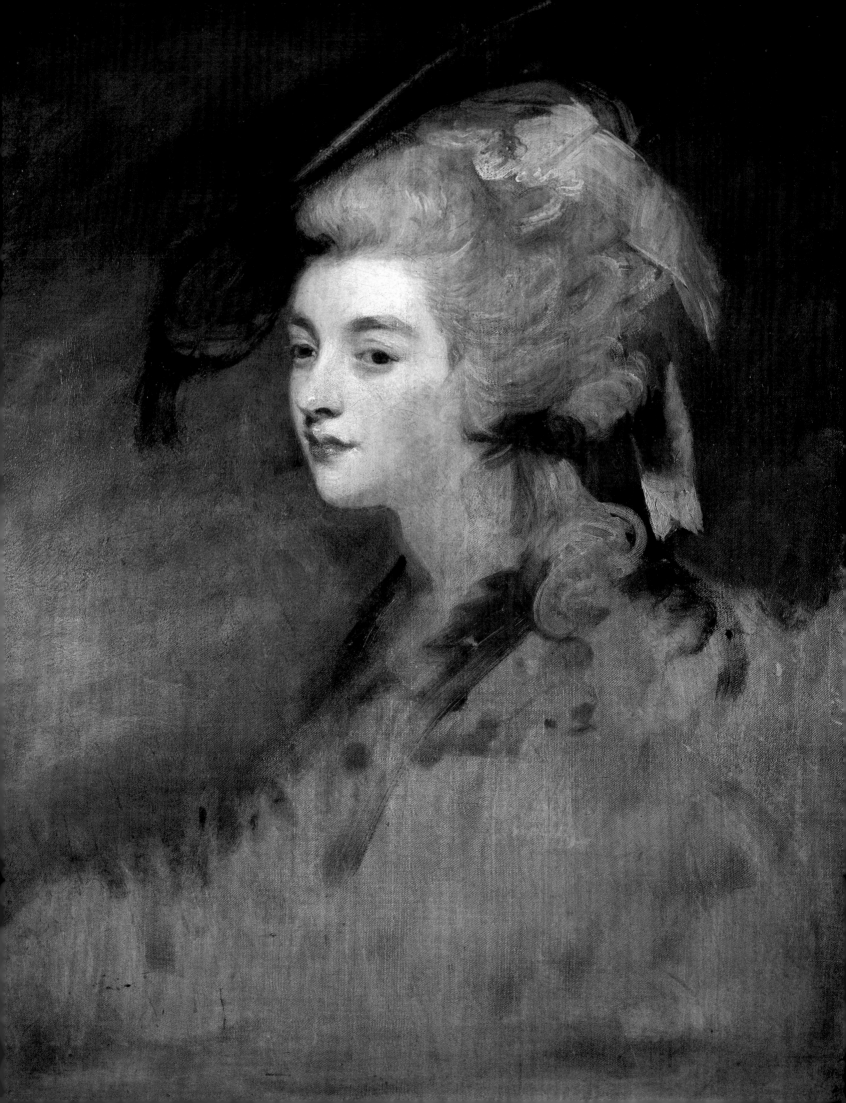

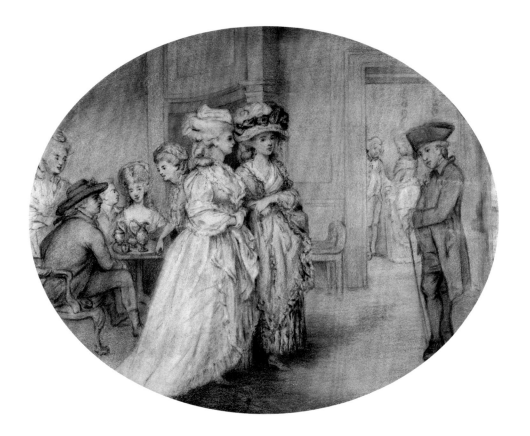

first seen in Paris in 1779; the gown's short over-sleeves and exotic trimmings alluded to Ottoman styles. For her daughter's christening, she donned 'a habit turc, of Lace (all joining lace trimd [sic] with Brussels) apron & cc. to suit & all white[21].' The following year, at Lady Lucan's assembly, Georgiana and her sister Harriet wore '*robes turques*', Lady Louisa Stuart reported, adding, 'I don't think I ever saw new fashions set in with such a vengeance, except in the year when feathers and high heads first began[22].' Once again, Georgiana was in the vanguard of an all-conquering trend; she and Harriet often dressed alike, doubling the impact of their innovative fashions (fig. 90). In February 1785, they attended a party at Carlton House – the London residence of the Prince of Wales – looking 'very smart', as Georgiana informed her mother, in 'night gowns of my invention – the body & sleeves black velvet bound with pink & fastend with silver buttons The pettycoat light pink, & the *Shift* apron & handkerchief crape bound with light pink & large chip hats with feathers & pinks[23].'

Marie Antoinette remained a friend and correspondent. In 1783, the queen scandalised French society by posing for a portrait in a plain, informal white muslin gown, the so-called '*chemise à la reine*[24].' The style's simplicity and informality evoked the pastoral ideal so prevalent in eighteenth-century art and literature, notably the writings of philosopher Jean-Jacques Rousseau, as well as the relaxed elegance of English fashions. She sent Georgiana some 'muslin Chemises with fine lace', which Georgiana wore to a concert on a warm August evening in 1784[25]. Soon, the once-shocking chemise gown became the fashionable female uniform in both countries. As Britain's *Lady's Magazine* reported in 1787: 'All the Sex now, from 15 to 50 upwards… appear in their white muslin frocks with broad sashes[26].' Georgiana may wear one of the queen's gifts in Downman's 1787 watercolour (fig. 87).

If the chemise gown was the quintessential French garment, its English equivalent was the riding habit. With its cut, textiles, trimmings and accessories inspired by menswear, it was originally adopted by women for riding, hunting, travelling and other active pursuits. By the 1780s, however, it was considered appropriate for a variety of

89 *(opposite)* Sir Joshua Reynolds, *Duchess Georgiana*, 1780 and later.

90 *(above)* After John Raphael Smith, *The Promenade at Carlisle House*, late eighteenth century.

increasingly formal occasions. Though worn throughout Europe, it was synonymous with English style, and was even regarded as a sartorial expression of English democratic values.

But the riding habit was no less criticised than the chemise gown. The playwright and critic John Gay argued in 1713 that it should be called 'the *Hermaphroditical*, by reason of its Masculine and Feminine Composition[27].' And novelist Samuel Richardson admonished young women that 'one cannot easily distinguish your Sex by it. For you neither look like a modest Girl in it, nor an agreeable Boy… A cock'd Hat, a lac'd Jacket, a Fop's Peruke, what strange Metamorphoses do they make![28].'

It was true that riding habits tended to blur gender distinctions; when the Duchess of Queensbury wore one during her Continental travels in 1734, she was 'called Sir upon the road above 20 times[29].' But they also carried controversial political associations. When Georgiana actively campaigned for Charles James Fox in the 1784 Westminster election, political caricatures invariably depicted her wearing a uniform-like riding habit, often in buff and blue, the colours adopted by male and female Whigs as well as by George Washington's Continental Army, which the Whigs supported against the British crown. Georgiana is known to have worn riding habits on horseback, as she does in Rowlandson's presumed drawing of her titled *Showing off in Rotten Row*, a reference to the popular bridle path in Hyde Park (fig. 86). But she had a history of deploying them for patriotic purposes, too; in the summer of 1778, when British militias gathered at Coxheath in anticipation of a French invasion, she had led a daily cavalcade of 'beauteous Amazons' wearing riding habits '*en militaire*, in the regimentals that distinguish the several regiments in which their Lords, etc. serve[30].' Similarly, the *Morning Herald* reported that 'Ladies of Fashion, in the interest of Mr Fox's election, are distinguished by wearing a feather in exact imitation of a fox's brush[31].' Whether or not Georgiana ever wore such an ornament, they appear in many caricatures of her, often paired with riding habits.

Georgiana's flair for fashion advanced her social and political ambitions, but it would also be her undoing. Her mounting debts and failing health increasingly kept her out of society. While most of her money troubles were caused by gambling, shopping also played a role, as indicated by the financial advice her mother gave her in 1790: 'Try only for the next 6 Months not to buy… a hat a Cap a gown & cc or to suffer any tradesman Milliner or Mantua maker or hairdresser to come near you – I am sure if you are in Earnest you have things enough of every kind to last you for years[32].'

Though Georgiana continued to take a lively interest in fashion, she was no longer the socially prominent trendsetter she had once been. In 1796, a serious illness left her frail and scarred, with a blind and drooping right eye. She immediately changed her hairstyle, but it would take more than a strategically placed bunch of curls to hide the damage[33]. Though she lived another ten years, she never regained her influential position before dying on 30 March 1806, at the age of 48. Nonetheless, the *Morning Chronicle* eulogised her as an English style icon: 'For no less than 33 years have we seen [the Duchess of Devonshire] regarded as the glass and model of fashion[34].'

91 *(opposite)* Maria Cosway, Duchess Georgiana as Diana, circa 1781-1782.

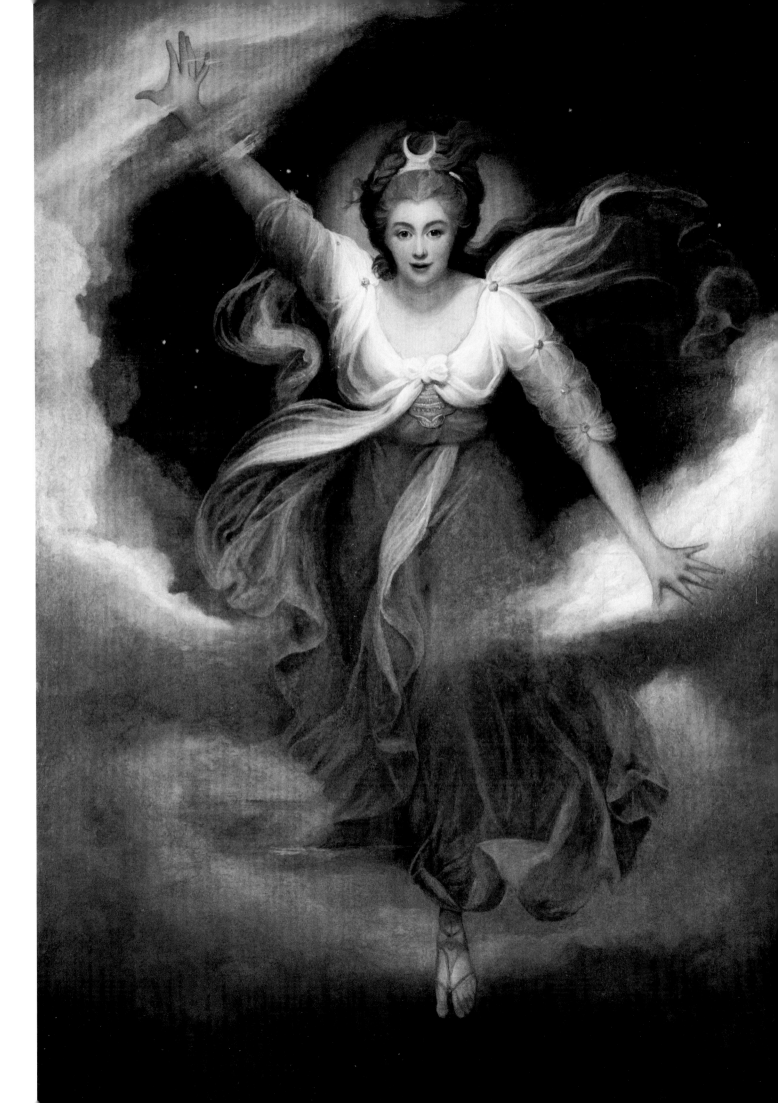

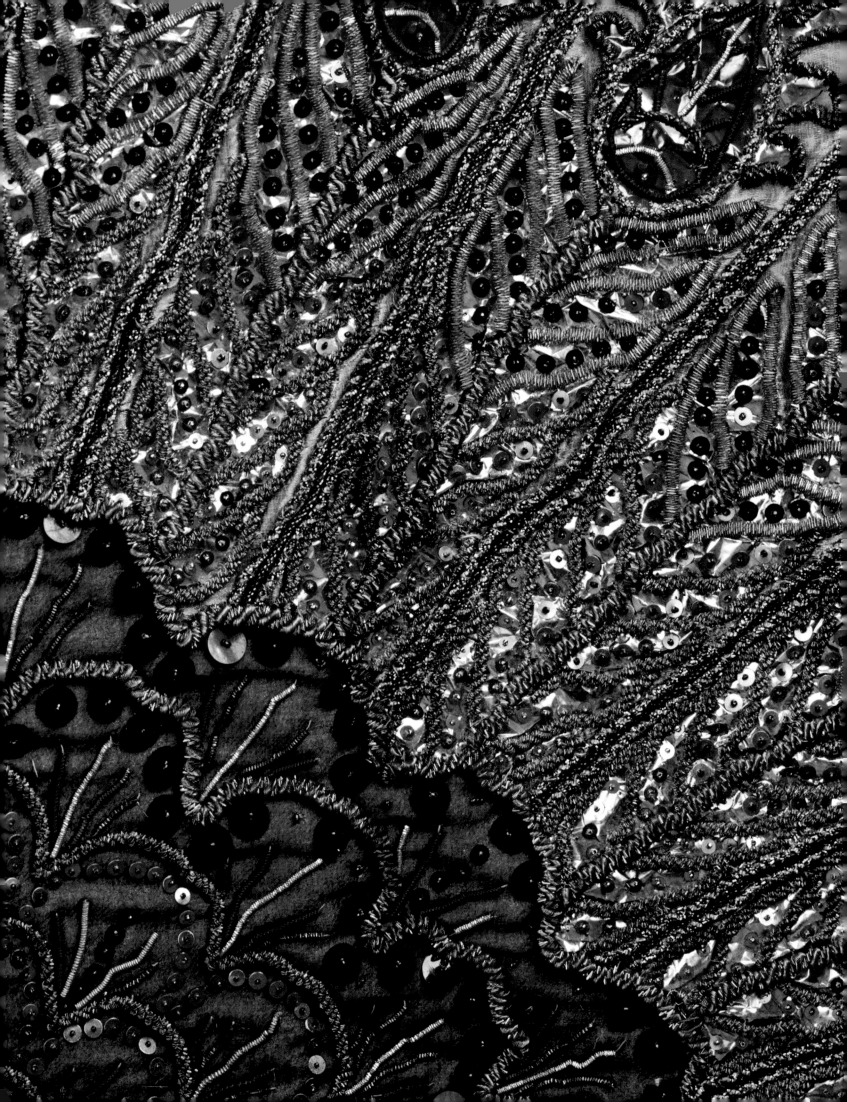

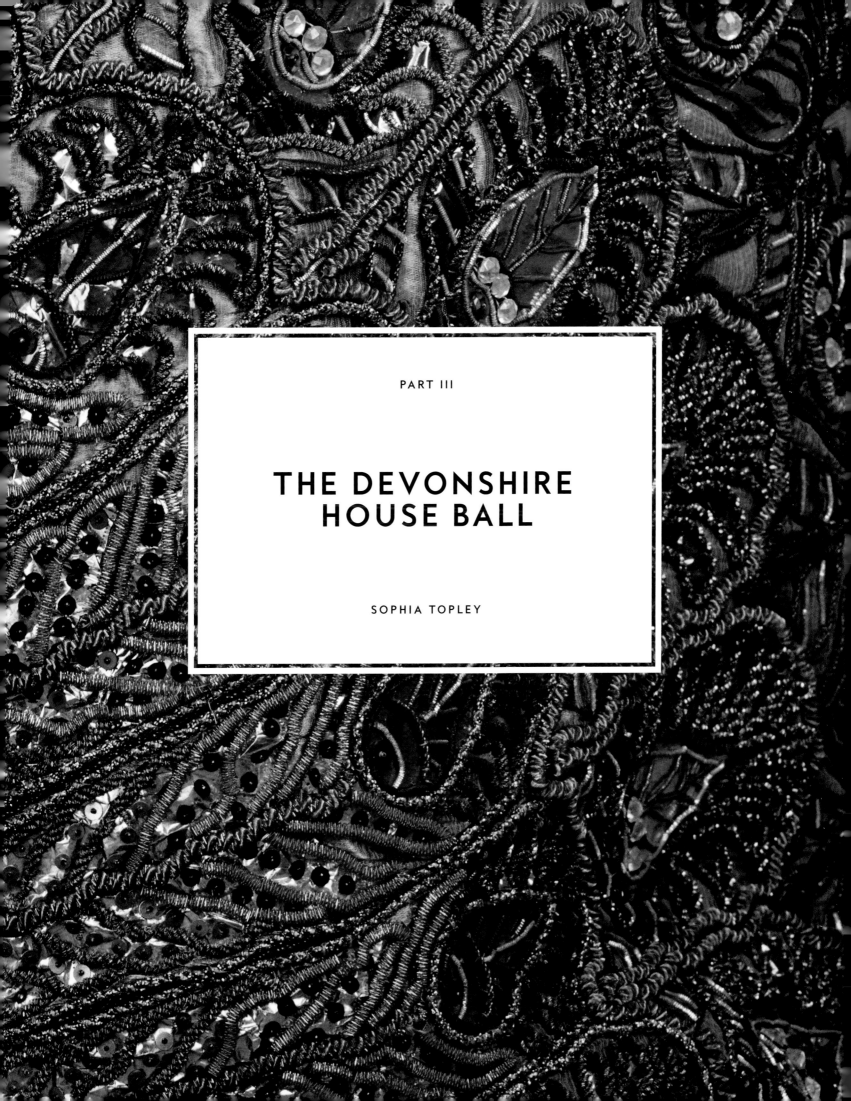

PART III

THE DEVONSHIRE
HOUSE BALL

SOPHIA TOPLEY

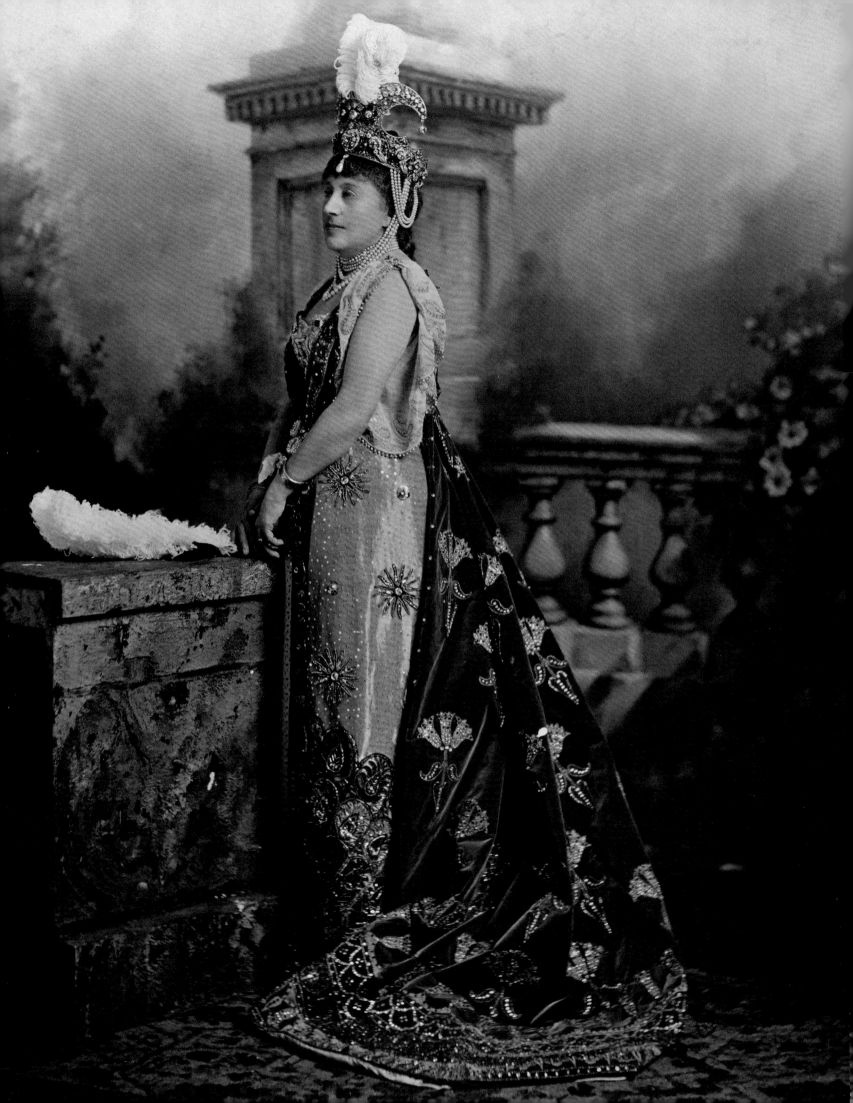

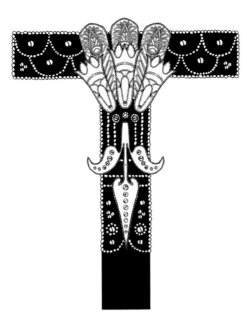

he history of fancy dress goes back many centuries. Costumed masked balls were a feature of sixteenth-century Italy, and were especially popular in Venice, with the custom spreading across Europe.

Legend has it that a Swiss count, John James Heidegger, introduced public subscription masked balls from Venice to London in the early years of the eighteenth century. The masked balls were held in theatres and assembly rooms, and later in public gardens, such as Ranelagh and Vauxhall. Costumes varied from masks and dominoes (an all-enveloping hooded cloak) to characters from commedia dell'arte and Medieval court dress, French huntsmen and various national dress.

The fashion for fancy dress parties was further endorsed by Queen Victoria and Prince Albert. In 1842 they gave a Plantagenet ball, followed in 1845 by one requiring costumes in the style of early Georgian dress, and then a Restoration ball in 1851.

So popular were such parties that in 1887 a book appeared called *Fancy Dresses Described, or What to Wear at Fancy Balls*. It contains, 'Several hundred characters, which a long and varied experience has proved to be the favourite and most effective, are here described, with every incidental novelty introduced of late years.' Following are suggestions for every imaginable costume with detailed instructions of how to achieve the best effect, starting with Amy Robsart, Anne Boleyn and the Queen of the Amazons right through the alphabet to Yseult of Ireland, Yachts, Zenobia and Zurich.

Devonshire House in Piccadilly (figs. 97, 101,102) was designed by William Kent for the 3rd Duke of Devonshire, and built between 1734-1740 replacing the house on the site which had been destroyed by fire in 1733. It became famous as a political centre during the tenure of the 5th Duke of Devonshire, who was remembered chiefly as the husband of the fascinating and much loved Georgiana.

Their son, the 6th Duke, or the Bachelor Duke, as he became known, made a number of structural changes and redecorated the property extensively, leaving only his mother's blue and white boudoir untouched in her memory. It was an ideal place for entertaining, with a large courtyard with room for carriages to turn, thus avoiding the traffic jams which occurred around houses which were entered directly from the street. It also had a large garden, and the building itself was on a scale big enough to comfortably contain a large crowd.

Every season the 8th Duke of Devonshire and his Duchess Louise gave a number of parties and entertainments, including an annual dance the night after the Derby, but Queen Victoria's Diamond Jubilee in 1897 was the perfect opportunity to give the ball of the century. Since fancy dress was all the rage, Louise decided to give her guests plenty of scope for imagination, and stipulated on the invitation that dress should be 'allegorical or historical costume before 1815.'

Some guests preferred to keep their outfits a surprise. Others got together and organised their costumes to join a court or procession. Lady Tweedmouth led the English Court of Elizabeth I; Lady Londonderry the Court of Maria Theresa; Lady Ormonde

92 *(opposite)* Lafayette (Lafayette Ltd), Duchess Louise as Zenobia, Queen of Palmyra, wearing a costume by Jean-Philippe Worth for the House of Worth, after a design by Attilio Comelli, 1897.

93 *(following pages, left to right)* Lafayette (Lafayette Ltd), the 8th Duke of Devonshire as Emperor Charles V, wearing a costume by Alias, 1897.

94 Fancy dress costume by Jean-Philippe Worth for the House of Worth, after a design by Attilio Comelli, worn by Duchess Louise as Zenobia, Queen of Palmyra, 1897.

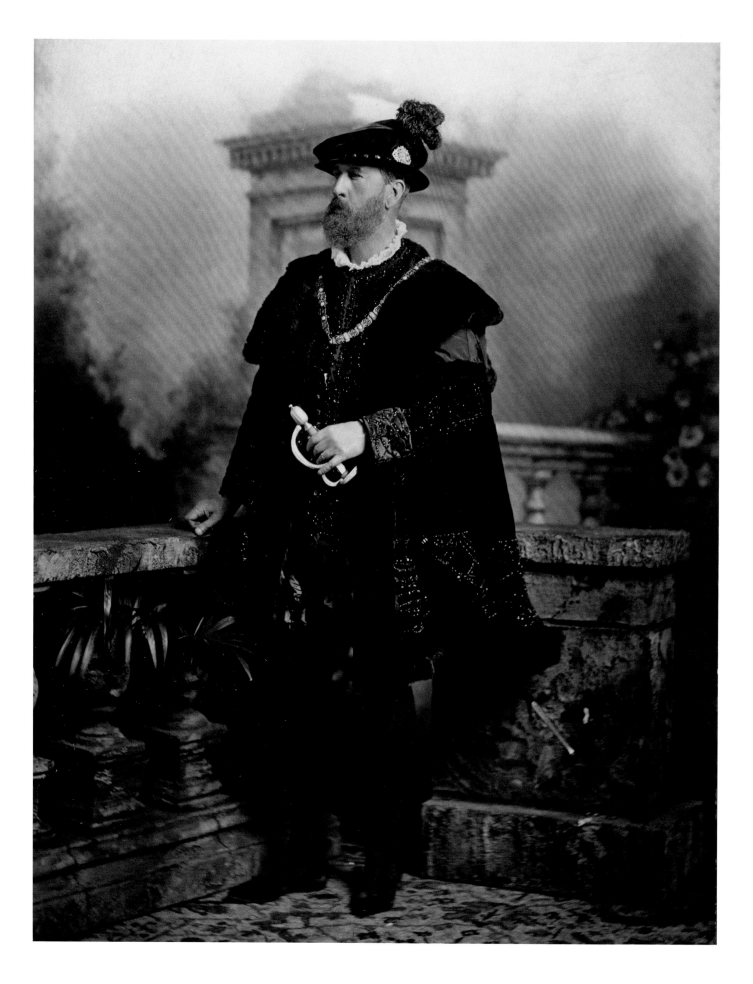

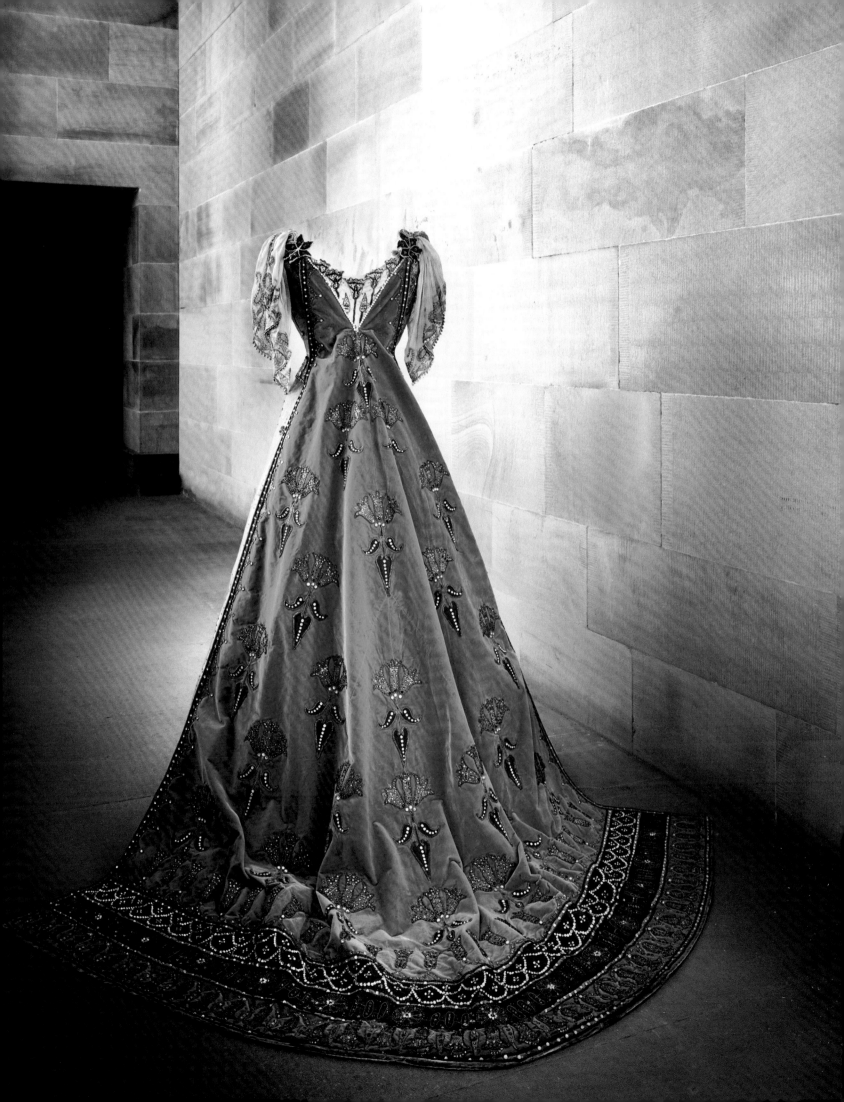

went as Queen Guinevere with the Knights of the Round Table; the Russian Court of Catherine the Great was headed by Lady Raincliffe and the Court of Louis XV and XVI had the Countess of Warwick as Marie Antoinette (there was some irony in this, as Lady Warwick had converted to socialism – well, a version of it – after a blistering attack by Robert Blatchford, editor of the left-wing paper the *Clarion*, on the extravagance of her fancy dress ball at Warwick Castle in 1895. She later offered her estate in Essex, Easton Lodge, to the Labour Party, and when they refused, to the TUC). Costumiers such as Nathans of Coventry and Alias of Soho Square provided 100 costumes each, and many of the ladies were dressed by fashionable couturiers Mrs Mason and Mrs Nettleship (mother-in-law of Augustus John).

For her costume, the hostess chose the Parisian house of Worth, founded by Charles Frederick Worth in 1858, and then under the creative direction of his son, Jean-Philippe Worth (fig. 94). The famous Parisian couturier could be relied on to produce something both original and beautiful. She opted to portray Zenobia, Queen of Palmyra, and the outfit was indeed striking and original (fig. 92). The skirt of gold gauze, appliquéd with tinsel medallions and peacock plumes

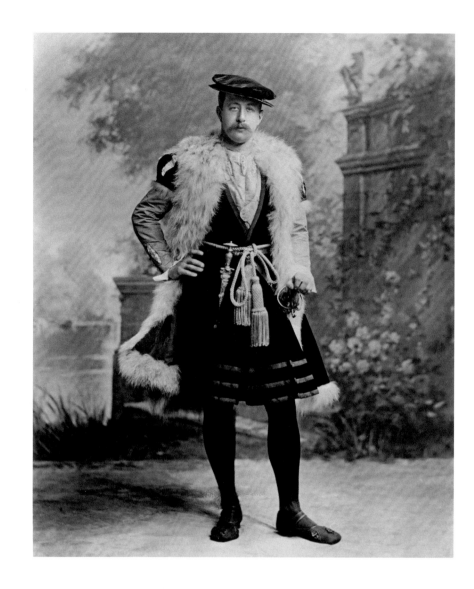

worked in bright foils, wire coils and spangled with sequins, was worn over an ivory satin underskirt wrought over with silver thread and diamonds. Attached to the shoulders was a long graduated train in the most vivid emerald-green velvet, appliquéd with velvet and gold work in an Eastern design and studded with jewels.

Louise was of substantial size, but M Worth's talent ensured that she looked imposing and stately rather than fat. The Duke's outfit was less ostentatious but equally impressive; he went as the Holy Roman Emperor, Charles V (fig. 93), his costume copied from the portrait of that monarch by Titian.

Most of the men took their costumes at least as seriously as the women – the reason, according to Lord Dunraven, being that in everyday life men were restricted in their dress and a fancy dress ball was the only occasion in which they could give full flight to sartorial fantasy, although some men had complained about not being able to go in standard military uniform. The Duke of Marlborough took this theory to extremes and went to Paris where, according to M Worth, he requested 'something new under the sun which shone on the Worth establishment.'

95 *(above)* Lafayette (Lafayette Ltd), the 9th Duke of Devonshire as Ambassador Jean de Dinteville in Holbein's 1533 painting, *The Ambassadors*, 1897.

96 *(opposite)* Lafayette (Lafayette Ltd), Duchess Evelyn as a Lady of the Court of Marie Thérèse, 1897.

97 *(following pages, left to right)* The ballroom at Devonshire House, circa 1910.

98 Regency simulated rosewood and parcel-gilt seat furniture by Morel & Hughes from Devonshire House, now in the Library at Chatsworth.

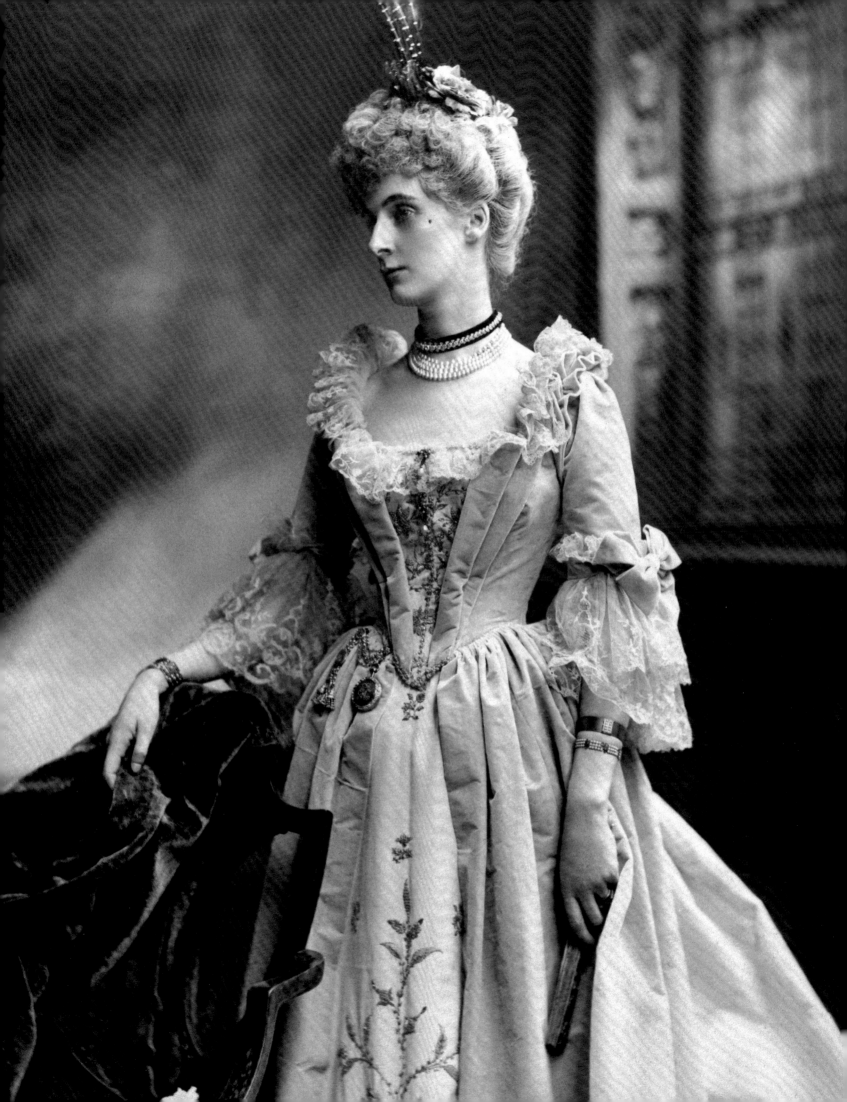

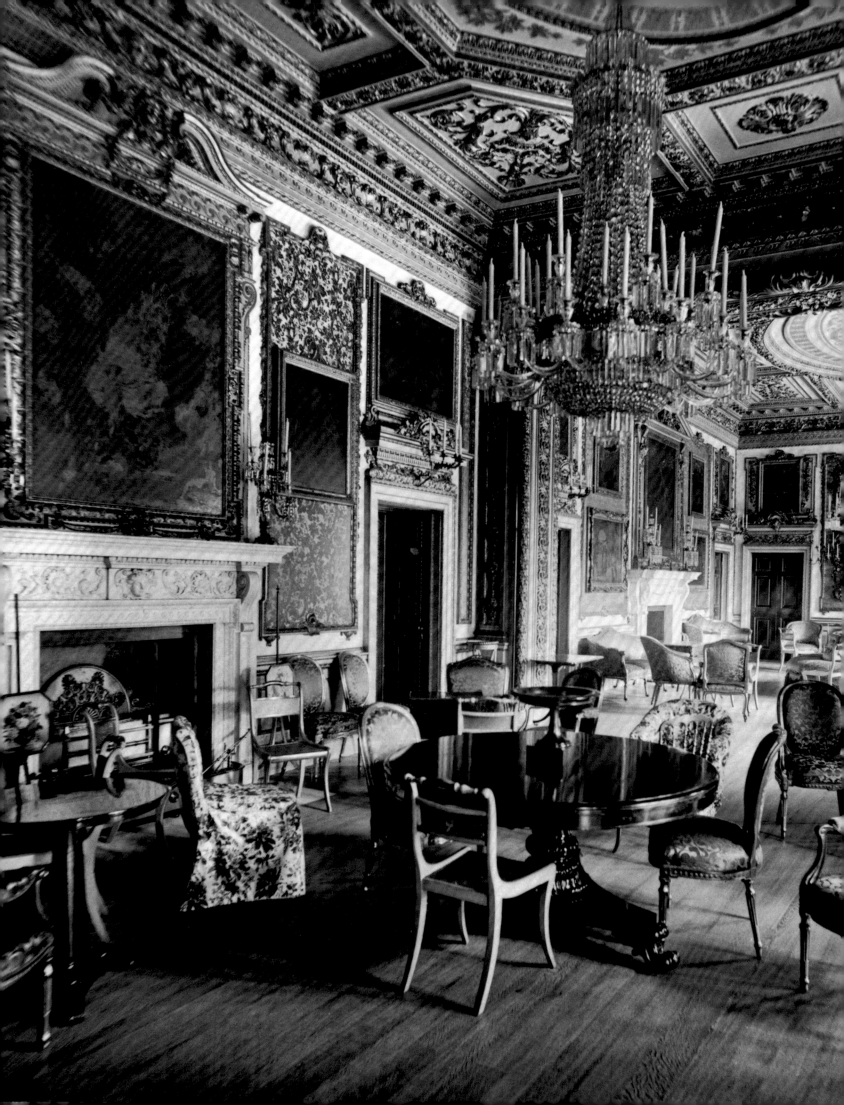

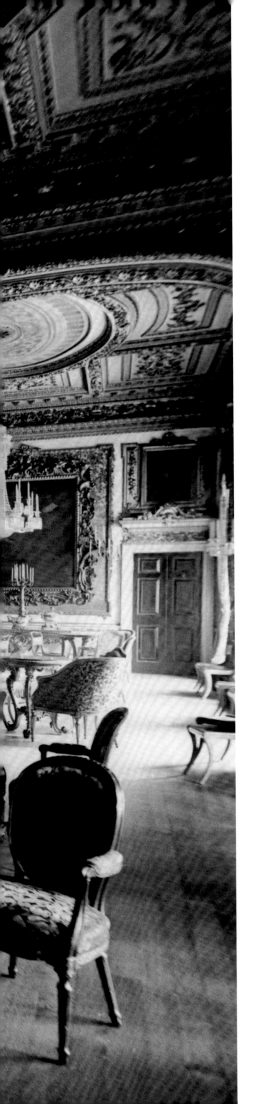

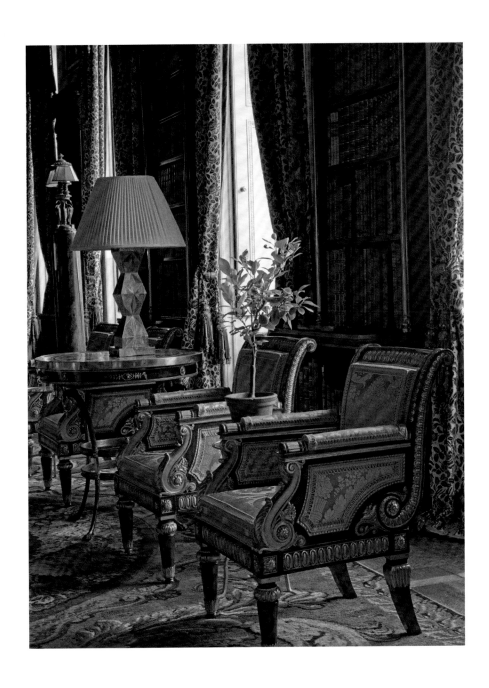

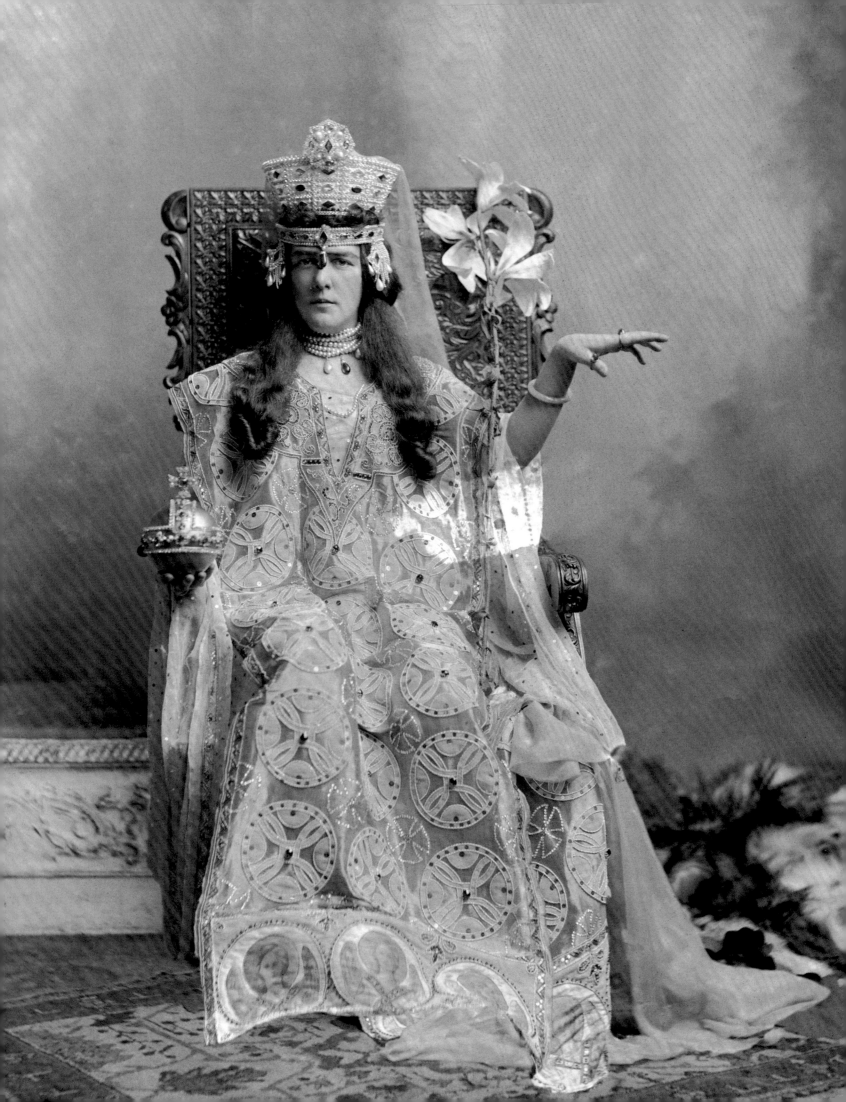

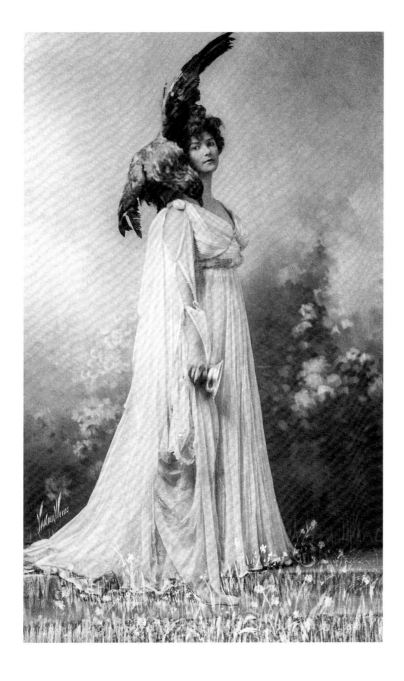

He and his famously beautiful wife Consuelo, then seven months pregnant, went as the French Ambassador and his wife at the Court of Catherine of Russia, and his costume took several employees nearly a month to make, each pearl and diamond being sewn on by hand, resulting in a bill for 5,000 francs – a huge sum for one night's entertainment.

Another American heiress was Mrs Arthur Paget, née Minnie Stevens. She chose Cleopatra and also asked Worth to make her costume (fig. 37). There were two other Cleopatras, including Lady de Grey, but if Minnie Paget was disappointed, then she could take consolation from the *New York World*'s loyal report: 'When she [Minnie Paget] entered, people accustomed to the greatest displays of jewels that world had ever known, gasped with wonder and astonishment. Lady de Grey's dress, although it cost $6,000, was quite eclipsed by Mrs Paget's costume.'

She was not the only guest to find herself duplicated: Lord Dunraven went as Cardinal Mazarin, commenting, 'and was quite pleased with myself until late in the evening Henry Irving arrived as another Cardinal. That was a beastly shame and quite put my nose out of joint, for though I was a good presentment of Mazarin in particular, Irving was certainly a better one of Cardinals in general.'

For some guests, the ingenuity of their outfits turned out most impractical once in the crush of the party. Sybil, Countess of Westmorland represented Hebe with a large stuffed eagle on her shoulder, which proved a major encumbrance (fig. 100). Mrs Reginald Talbot, dressed as Valkyrie, suffered a bad headache from her metal-winged helmet but did not dare remove it lest she could not redo her hair. The Duchess of Portland, splendid as she looked as the Duchess of Savoy, also suffered from the weight of her wig, and her husband as Duke of Savoy avoided a nasty incident when his yellow cotton wool moustache caught fire as he lit a cigarette.

Mrs Ronalds, a famous singer and close friend and mentor of Sir Arthur Sullivan, managed ingenuity without inconvenience. She attended the ball as Euterpe, 'the Spirit of Music', in a yellow satin dress embroidered with bars from Verdi's *Ballo in Maschera* with a cloak of green and white satin embroidered with musical instruments. On her head she wore a crown of diamonds in the shape of a lyre surrounded by sparkling crotchets and quavers, lit by electricity by means of a tiny battery hidden in her hair.

The Queen herself was too frail to come to the ball, but many of her family enthusiastically entered into the spirit of it all. The Prince of Wales was stout but dignified as a Grand Prior of the Order of St John and his wife represented Marguerite de Valois accompanied

99 *(opposite)* Lafayette (Lafayette Ltd), Lady Randolph Churchill as Empress Theodora, wearing a costume by Jean-Joseph Benjamin-Constant and House of Worth, 1897.

100 *(above)* Henry Van der Weyde, photogravure by Walker & Boutall, the Countess of Westmorland as Hebe, photogravure 1897, published 1899.

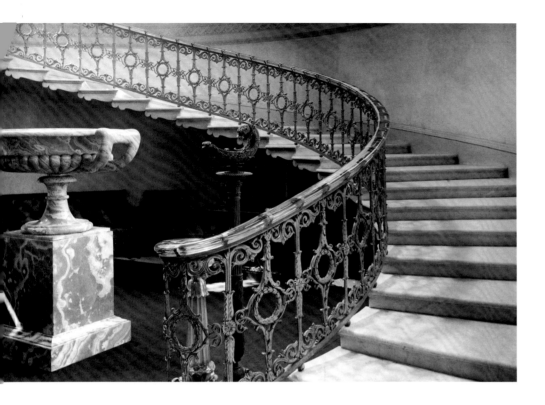

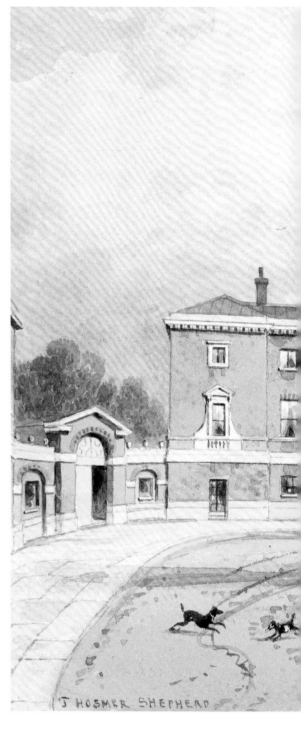

101 *(left)* The Crystal Staircase at
Devonshire House, circa 1910.

102 *(above)* Thomas Hosmer
Shepherd, *Devonshire House*,
1844.

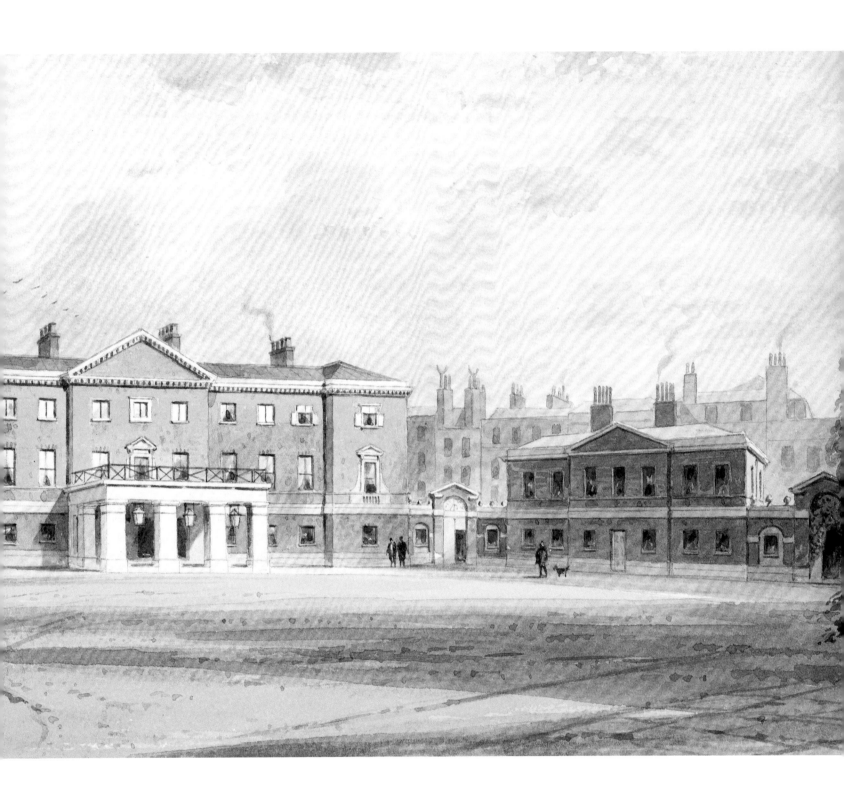

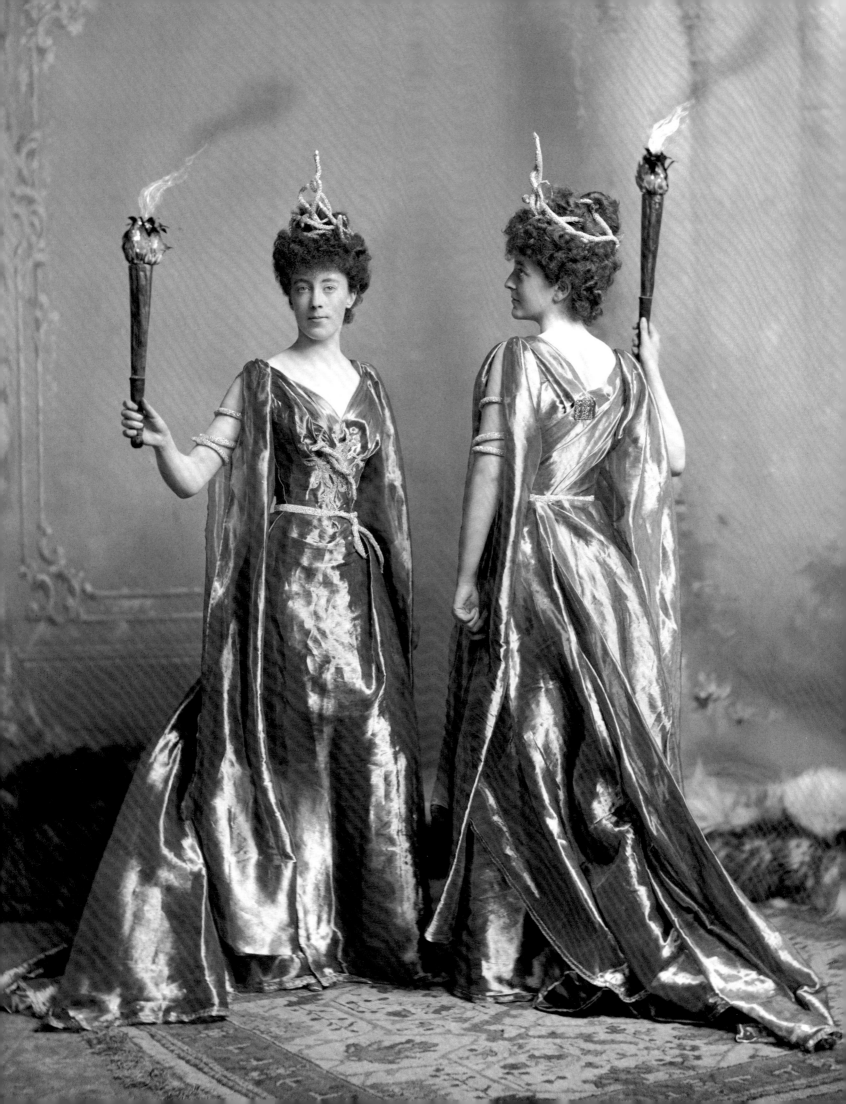

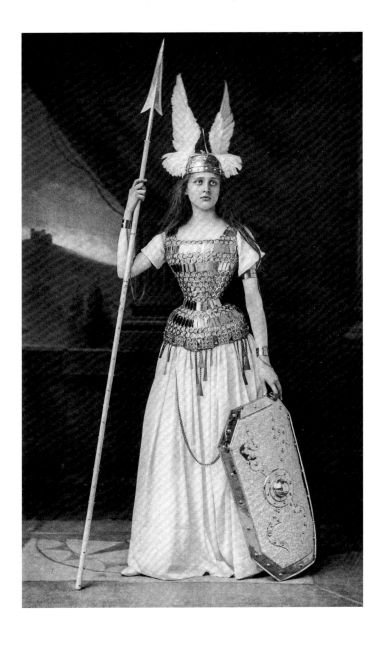

by two of her daughters, Princess Maud and Princess Victoria, as ladies of Marguerite's court.

Such an event required extensive planning and attention to detail. The housekeeper aided by two secretaries was in charge of organisation inside the house with precise instructions from the Duchess on menus and all arrangements. It is unlikely the Duke took much part in the planning, as he was well known for his slothfulness. On one occasion he was woken by a footman with the news that the house was on fire to which he replied, 'then it is your job, not mine, to put it out' and went back to sleep.

Then there was the mammoth task of organising costumes for the staff, as the Duchess had decided that they should all be in fancy dress. Those hired from outside were to wear Elizabethan and Egyptian costumes from a theatrical outfitter and, for the Devonshire House staff, the men were to be dressed in the blue and buff Devonshire livery of the eighteenth century and the maids in Elizabethan sprigged frocks.

Most of the furniture was removed from the reception rooms and chairs were placed around the edge of the ballroom with the parquet floor polished until it gleamed. The huge chandeliers were taken down and each piece of crystal was washed and polished and new candles fitted.

Flowers arrived early on the day of the party, and by the afternoon each room was a mass of orchids and exotic plants from Paxton's great conservatory at Chatsworth. The large marble *tazza* in the hall was filled with water lilies, and there was even a Night Flowering cactus, a tropical plant whose flowers bloom at night and last a few hours before dying by morning. There was dancing to mazurkas, waltzes and Hungarian *csárdas* by composers such as Brahms, Strauss and Sousa after which, at around midnight, supper took place in a large marquee in the garden.

On each table were palm fronds after the fashion set by the Savoy Hotel the previous year, and hidden in these fronds and the flower arrangements around the marquee were tiny electric lights which gave a glittering, fairy-like appearance to the room. This was a novelty in 1897, and the Duchess was taking a risk, as in these early days of electricity, hostesses who chose this form of lighting were apt to find their parties plunged into darkness without warning. Fortunately, at this event all was well.

Round the tables was a bizarre mixture of characters from every century and country, historical and fictional. Dante's Beatrice (Countess of Mar and Kellie) sat next to d'Artagnan (William James) and Archbishop Cranmer (Lord Rowton), while a Roundhead Soldier (Herbert Asquith) made conversation with Marie Antoinette (Countess of Warwick) and Esther, Queen of Israel (Countess of Dudley). Nearby, Will Somers (Henry Holden) chatted to Merlin (Mr Hall Walker) and Medusa (Mrs Hope Vere) whilst being

103 *(opposite)* Lafayette (Lafayette Ltd), Lady Lurgan and Lady Sophie Scott as Furies, wearing costumes by Mrs Mason, 1897.

104 *(above)* Alfred Ellis, photogravure by Walker & Boutall, Mademoiselle Henriette de Courcel as Valkyrie, photogravure 1897, published 1899.

served by an Egyptian slave. It is fortunate that cultural appropriation did not exist in 1897.

Not until the early hours did the party break up, and the sun was rising when the guests finally got their coats and called for their carriages. For Lady Randolph Churchill (fig. 99) and her sister there was still one last excitement: on their way to their house near Marble Arch they met a travelling circus from which a camel put its head into their brougham and, according to Mrs Leslie, was amazed by the strangely dressed occupants.

For those who had attended, the rest of the season's entertainments must have seemed flat. The ball was a hot topic of conversation, both in the lead up and afterwards – much to the chagrin, no doubt, of those who had not been invited.

The beautiful costumes met various fates; some, as in the case of Chatsworth, still exist, including that of Duchess Louise which is in wonderful condition. Others were cut, the embroideries and lace being used on other frocks; some no doubt found their way into family dressing-up boxes. All Minnie Paget's clothes were sold at auction after she died in 1911 and her acclaimed Cleopatra costume fetched £9.

The Duke died in 1908 followed by the Duchess, who in 1911 suffered a fatal stroke at Sandown races. Devonshire House was a sad victim of social change. The 9th Duke sold it to developers in 1919, knowing full well what its fate would be, and in 1924 it was totally demolished. On the site of the house and garden are now flats and offices.

Fancy dress, on the other hand, lives on. At many 18th and 21st birthday celebrations today, young people must use their imagination for costumes for 'Country Code', 'Alice in Wonderland', 'Carnival', 'Great Gatsby' and so on with the same enthusiasm and ingenuity as the guests at the Devonshire House Ball.

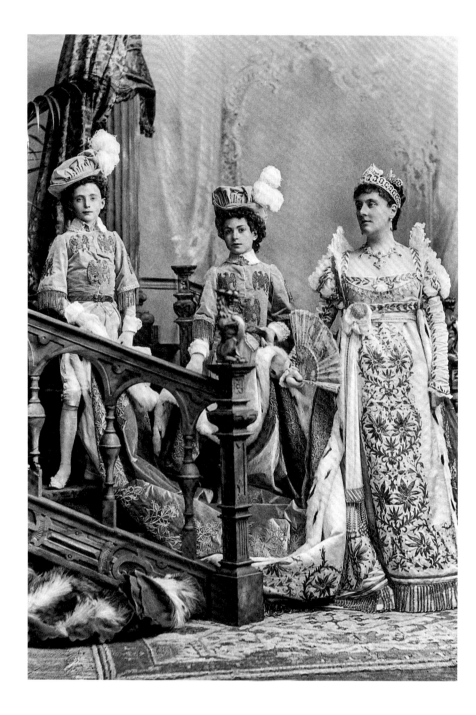

105 *(above)* Lafayette (Lafayette Ltd), photogravure by Walker & Boutall, Marchioness of Tweeddale as Empress Josephine with Lord Arthur Vincent Hay and William George Montagu Hay, 11th Marquess of Tweeddale as pages, photogravure 1897, published 1899.

106 *(opposite)* Lafayette (Lafayette Ltd), Lady Wolverton as Britannia, 1897.

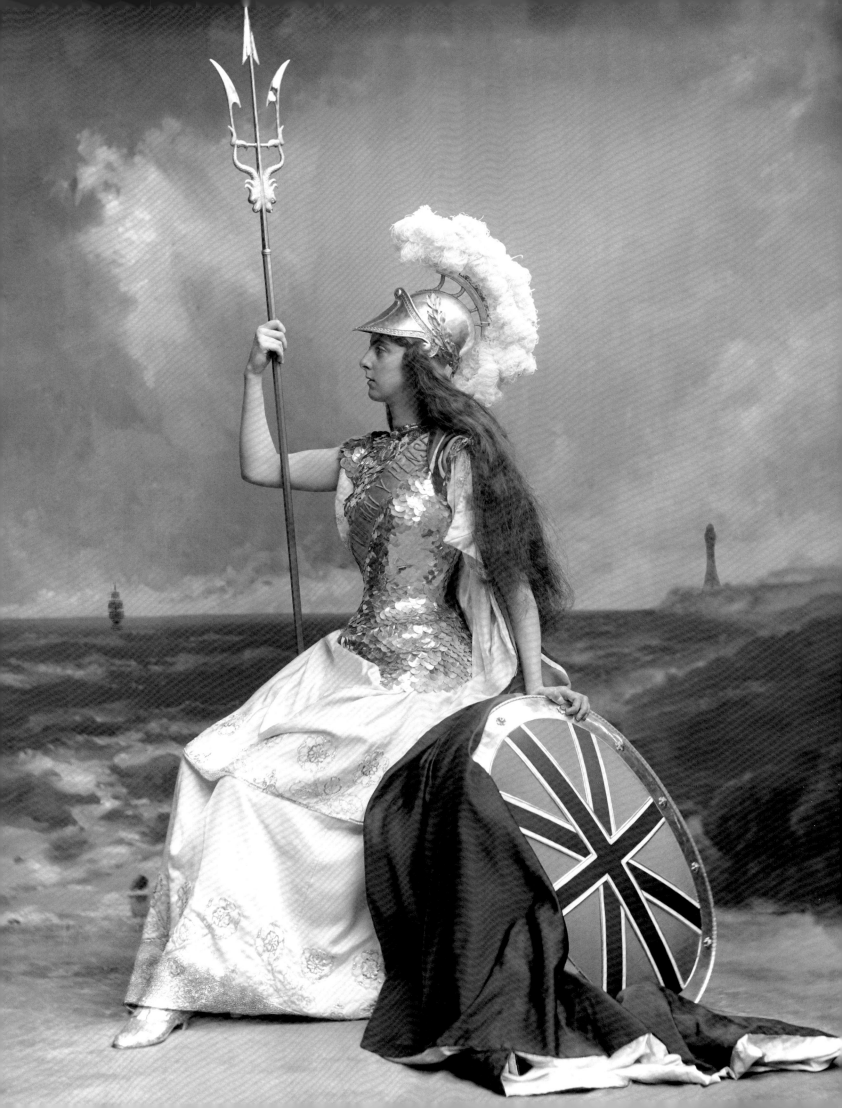

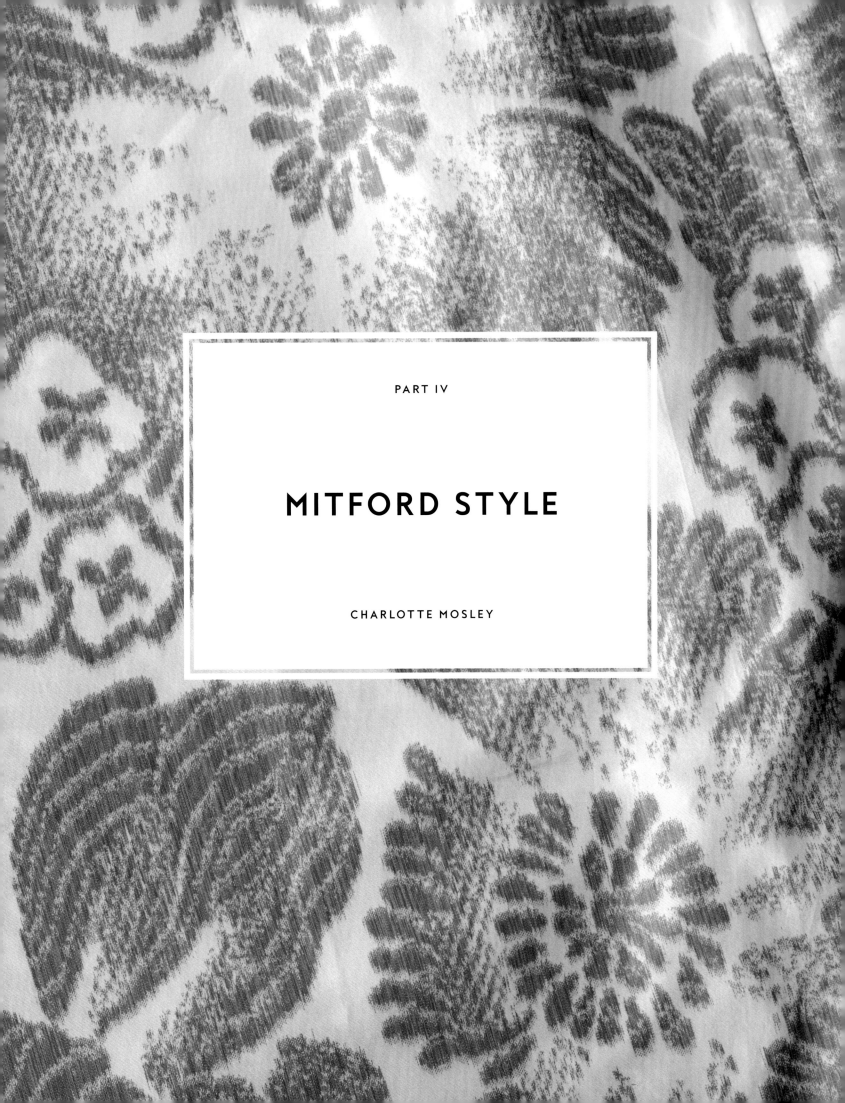

PART IV

MITFORD STYLE

CHARLOTTE MOSLEY

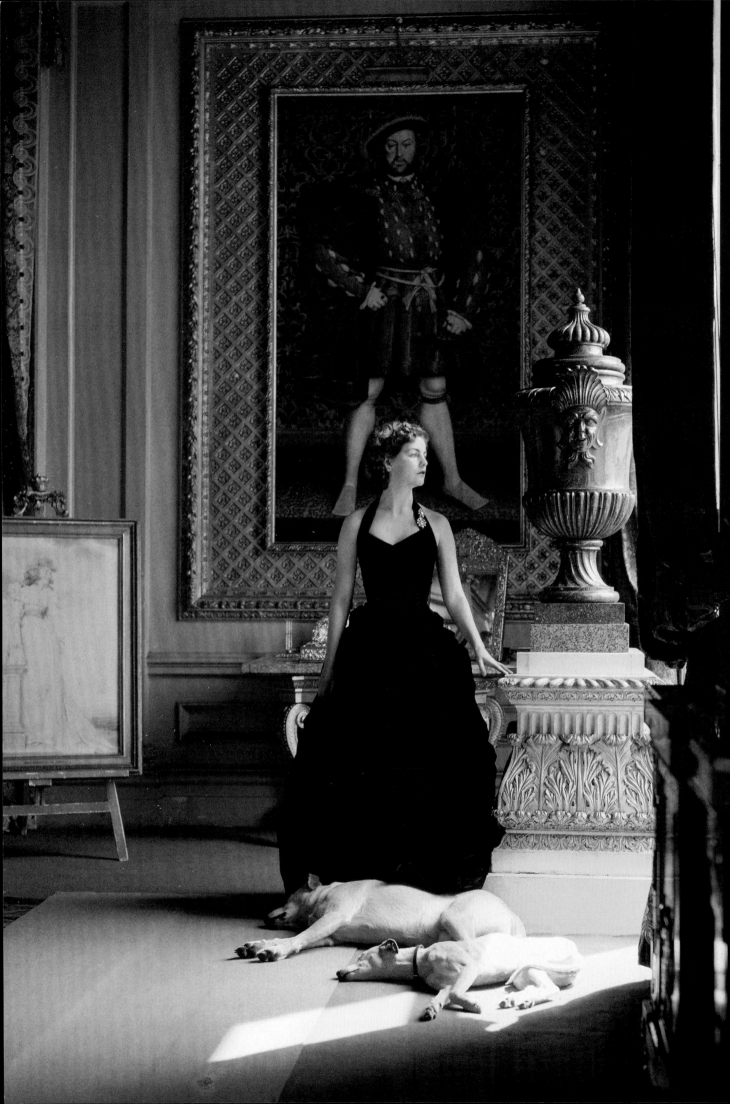

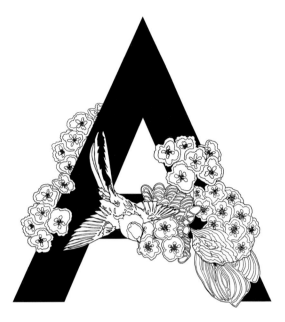

photograph of five of the six Mitford sisters taken in the mid-1930s fixed the 'Mitford style' in the public imagination: tweed suit, Fair Isle jumper, a string of pearls and flat, no-nonsense shoes (fig. 108). How ironic that such a conventional style should be associated with such highly unconventional women. Their lives were anything but ordinary; at the time the photograph was taken, they were defying family expectations and scandalising society with their political views.

But however little the 'Mitford style' might reveal about the women who wore it, certain of its features nevertheless remained constant in their wardrobes. They favoured clothes that were comfortable, practical, long-lasting and, when they could afford it, expensively but discreetly elegant. 'No one is going to look at you', their nanny drummed into them from a young age, even into Diana, the most beautiful of the sisters, on her wedding day. Beyond these shared traits, the sisters were divided – as over many things – into two camps. Nancy (fig. 110), Diana (fig. 111) and Deborah (fig. 107) took a keen interest in fashion; clothes mattered and added greatly to their enjoyment of life. For Pamela, Unity and Jessica, fashion came low on their list of preoccupations.

Pamela, a countrywoman all her life, was the one sister who could be said to have conformed to the 'Mitford style' and, unless dressed up for an occasion, remained faithful to a cotton skirt and cardigan in the summer, and a woollen skirt and quilted jacket in the winter. She was an expert cook, and whereas Nancy remembered occasions by what she had worn, Pamela remembered them by what she had eaten. Unity, the fourth sister, dressed to draw attention to herself, hiring showy costume jewellery for debutante dances and sporting the fascist Blackshirt uniform at a Labour Party rally. Clothes took on importance for Jessica after her elopement, when she found herself short of money and was able to sell her ball gowns for a few pounds. When she first moved to America she worked in an expensive dress shop, but what interested her there were her wages and not the wares, which she could not have afforded anyway. 'Clothes were merely coverings to keep her warm, colours and shapes were thrown together hugger-mugger and made you wonder at her choice', wrote the youngest sister, Deborah. 'Her mind and energies were engaged elsewhere, mainly with people and politics.'

Diana was the first of the sisters to be able to shop for expensive clothes. At the age of nineteen she married Bryan Guinness, heir to the brewing fortune. Her trousseau was homemade, but on their way back from honeymooning in Sicily the young couple stopped off in Paris, where Diana bought a glamorous white faille dress, tied at the back with a huge blue bow, from the dressmaker Louiseboulanger. During her short-lived first marriage, Diana could have all the clothes she wanted. Thereafter she managed on far fewer and, in true Mitford style, made sure they were versatile and would last. She wore a black ottoman coat, the runway model from a late 1940s Schiaparelli collection, for shopping, gardening, funerals and evenings out. She could even have worn it,

107 *(opposite)* Norman Parkinson, Deborah Vivien Cavendish, Duchess of Devonshire, 1952.

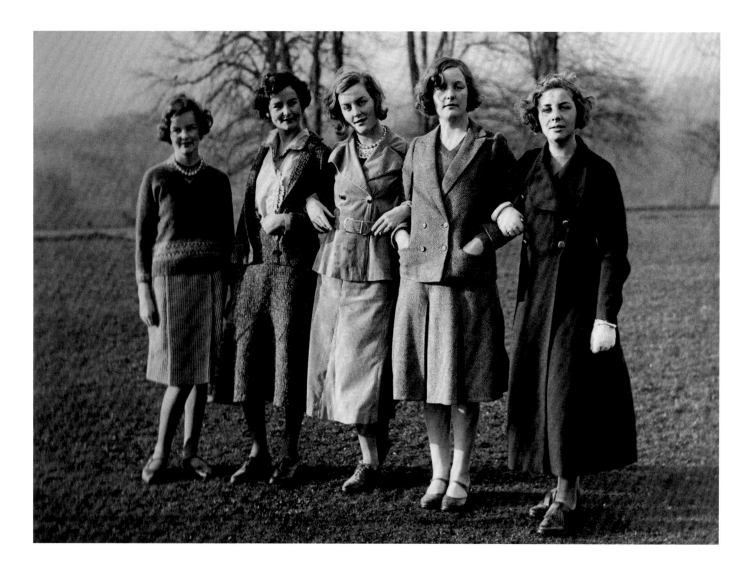

she maintained, to play football. In the last years of her life, she lived in a flat in Paris near the place du Palais-Bourbon, where French *Vogue* has its offices, and as she crossed the square the *Vogue* stylists would gather at the windows to watch her go by. Diana, like the eldest sister, Nancy, looked elegant in whatever she wore. When miniskirts became fashionable in the 1960s, the two sisters decided they had a choice between looking dowdy or ridiculous and they both opted for ridiculous. Their skirts may have inched a fraction above the knee, but neither of them ever looked ridiculous.

Clothes were one of the few things in life that Nancy took seriously. She regarded the great dressmakers as artists whose garments had a signature, and prided herself on being able to recognize and appreciate their creations. 'It's terrible to love clothes as much as I do', she confided to her friend Evelyn Waugh, 'and perfectly inexplicable because I'm not at all vain.' Her passion is not so mysterious if one looks at the sisters' mother, Sydney Redesdale, who also loved clothes and was without vanity, and whose style in dress and decoration was a strong influence on her daughters. Sydney's own mother died when she was seven years old and her father, who loved the sea, dressed his daughter in a thick serge sailor suit, whatever the occasion or season, until she was 18. When Sydney

108 *(above)* Jessica, Nancy, Diana, Unity and Pamela Mitford (left to right).

109 *(opposite)* The Duke of Devonshire's wedding party: Cecil Beaton, Nancy Mitford, Deborah Devonshire, Pamela Jackson, Diana Mosley, 11th Duke of Devonshire (left to right), 28 June 1967.

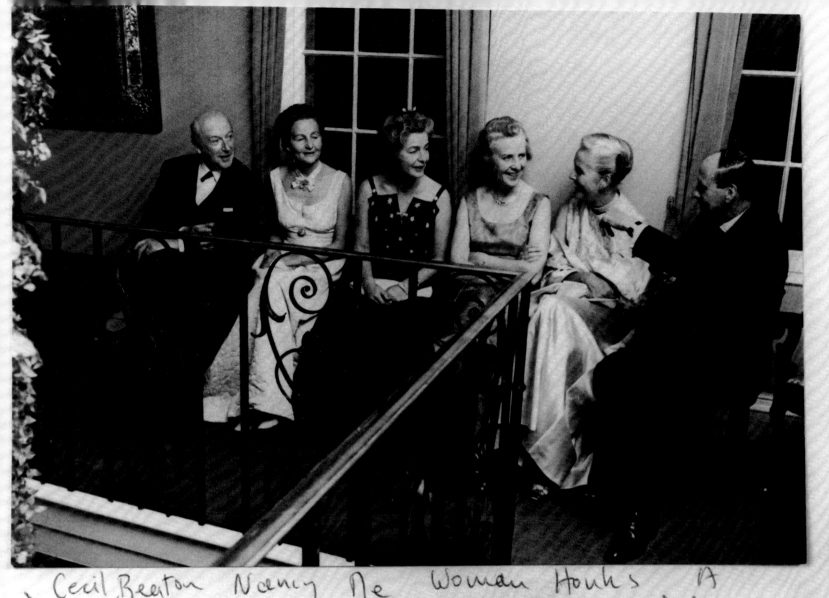

Cecil Beaton   Nancy   Me   Woman   Honks   A
DANCE   after   The   WEDDING

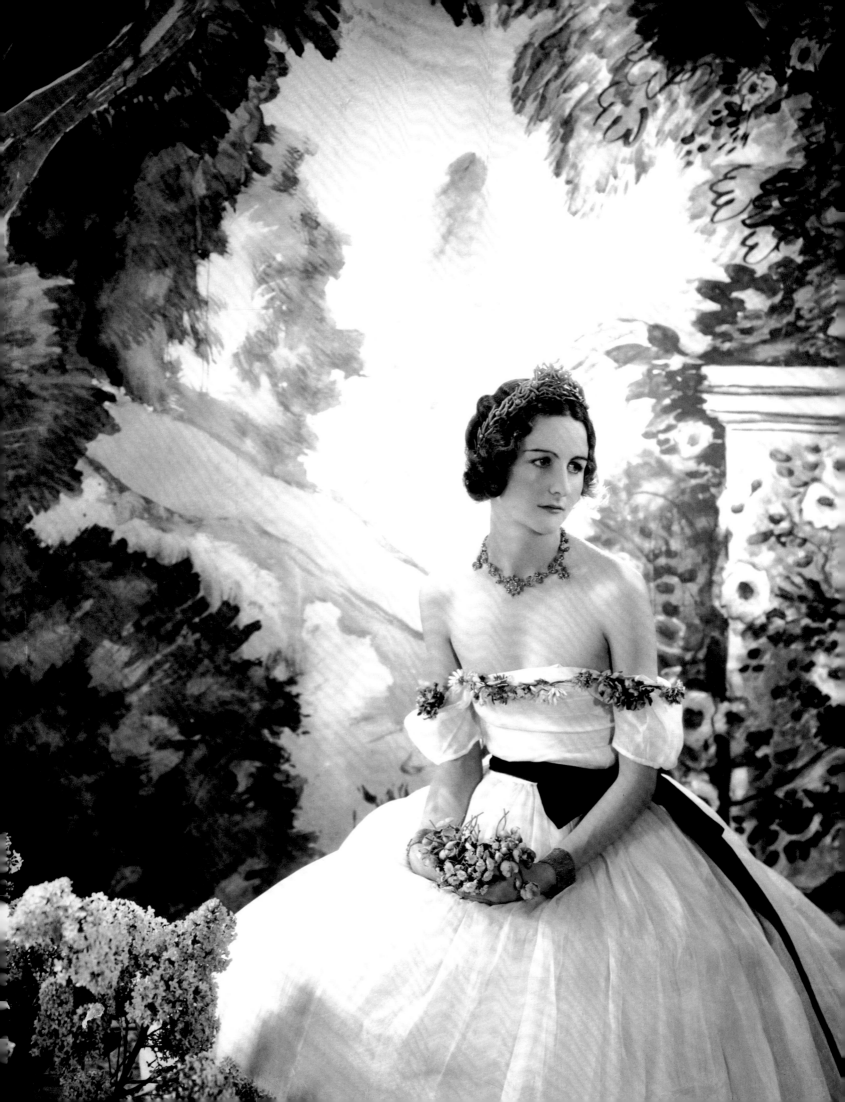

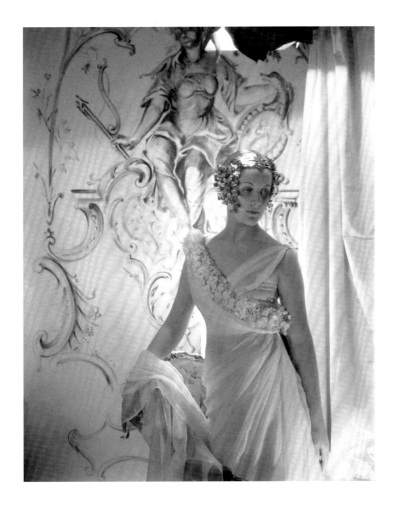

married and was raising a family of seven children on never quite enough money, she could not afford many clothes, but those she had were original and exactly right for her. The pretty uniform she designed for her housekeeper and parlour maid was also original: a blue and white Toile-de-Jouy dress in a traditional bird pattern, a white linen apron and an organdy cap threaded with black velvet ribbon. She had a talent for making herself and her surroundings harmonious, and she too made her clothes last. When Jessica was over from America in 1959, she helped her mother pack up her winter clothes and came across a black silk brocade evening dress. 'This looks awfully familiar', she said. 'Yes, I should think it does', Sydney replied, 'I got it in 1926 for Pam's coming-out dance.'

As a debutante, Nancy went to parties in frocks run up by her mother's retired maid for £1, but she longed for creations from the London dressmakers. Sadly, her husband, Peter Rodd, was feckless and a gambler. But Nancy had natural elegance and looked chic even in homemade or inexpensive outfits.

Her move to Paris in 1946 coincided with the revival of the French fashion industry after the war. Thanks to the roaring success of her novel, *The Pursuit of Love*, she was at last able not only to satisfy her craving for clothes, but could afford to dress in haute couture. No sooner had she arrived in the city than she went on a shopping spree. After combing through several collections, she settled on the *couturière* Madame Grès and splashed out on three day dresses, a printed suit, a coat, two evening dresses and four hats, including 'an utter dream' of a white satin boater embellished with an aigrette. 'I've even ordered a ball dress', she wrote to her mother. 'You never saw such a dress.' Made of black velvet and tied at the waist with a black chiffon sash, the huge skirt contained, wrote Nancy with customary exaggeration, 'fifty metres of stuff.'

When Christian Dior opened his couture house in 1947, Nancy was one of his earliest foreign clients. The tiny waists and full skirts of the New Look suited her tall, slim figure and she treated herself to a design called 'Daisy' from Dior's first collection. 'The skirt has sort of stays at which one tugs until giddiness intervenes', she reported to Diana, 'the *basque* of the coat stuck out with whalebone.' Three months later and after several fittings, the suit was delivered and was 'a dream.' Later that year, Mogens Tvede, a Danish architect married to Dolly Radziwill, Nancy's closest friend in Paris, painted a portrait of Nancy wearing 'Daisy', looking the epitome of Parisian chic (fig. 114).

Over the years, Nancy bought from Piguet, Schiaparelli, Lanvin and Patou, and was often joined on shopping forays by Deborah and sometimes Diana. Deborah's busy life meant that visits to Paris were inevitably short and clothes had to be chosen swiftly. This brought out the disapproving older sister in Nancy, who complained to her mother, 'Of course Paris isn't arranged for that sort of wild two-day shopping – it takes an age

110 *(opposite)* Cecil Beaton, Nancy Mitford in her costume for the Famous Beauties Ball at the Dorchester Hotel, 1931.

111 *(above)* Cecil Beaton, the Hon Mrs Bryan Guinness (later Lady Oswald Mosley), 1932.

to buy properly here.' In 1964, Nancy even persuaded Jessica, who was feeling flush from the proceeds of her exposé of the American funeral industry, *The American Way of Death*, to visit the Dior boutique. Giving in to Nancy's blandishments, Jessica came away with a black cloqué coat and skirt, describing it as, 'the most expensive day's shopping not only of my life, but my wildest dreams.' Just occasionally Nancy felt a pang of guilt. Was it not wicked to spend so much on outfits that were often 'eating their head off in the cupboard'? But she justified the expense by calculating their annual cost over the years she would wear them. And, above all, clothes lifted her spirits.

Although Nancy never bought from Balenciaga, the king of dressmakers, she did have the opportunity to wear his creations. During the 1950s, Bunny Mellon, one of Balenciaga's best clients, sent boxes of cast-off couture to Deborah's mother-in-law, Mary, Duchess of Devonshire (fig. 130), to distribute to poverty-stricken women in the East End of London. The Duchess allowed the sisters to swap the sumptuous ball gowns and cocktail dresses that arrived from America for decent, unworn clothes of their own. They became known in the family as the 'mercy parcels', and Deborah remembered Nancy and Diana sharing a white satin evening dress to wear on the grandest occasions.

As the youngest of six sisters, Deborah wore mostly hand-me-downs when she was growing up, but her style from an early age was wholly individual. Her attitude towards fashion was relaxed and playful. She had a flair for mixing classical with contemporary, refinement with frippery, while remaining always stylish.

Hats were in fashion when Deborah was a debutante, and she and her friends were never without one. The vogue for witty, wacky headgear – Schiaparelli's collaboration with Salvador Dalí had produced the surreal shoe hat the previous season – tallied with Deborah's taste. For Royal Ascot in 1938, she persuaded Madame Rita, a milliner in Berkley Square, to make her a deerstalker in spotted muslin, instead of the traditional tweed, with earflaps that tied in a white satin bow on top of her head. 'It was ridiculous', she wrote, 'but lots of Ascot hats are ridiculous.' She prized a hat from Rose Valois in Paris, given to her by Evelyn Waugh and that he had chosen and tried on himself (fig. 117). Fashioned in white felt and blue straw, with two white-feathered doves perched on either side, 'It would', Deborah wrote in her thank-you note, 'be a giver of confidence when opening fetes.'

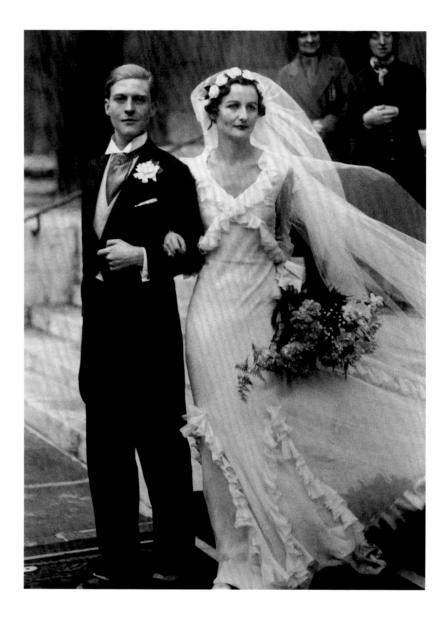

112 *(above)* Wedding of Nancy Mitford and Peter Rodd, 1933.

113 *(opposite)* Mme Yevonde, studio portrait of Deborah Devonshire in her wedding dress by Victor Stiebel, 1941.

114 *(following pages, left to right)* Mogens Tvede, Nancy Mitford, 1948.

115 Mogens Tvede, Deborah Devonshire, 1949.

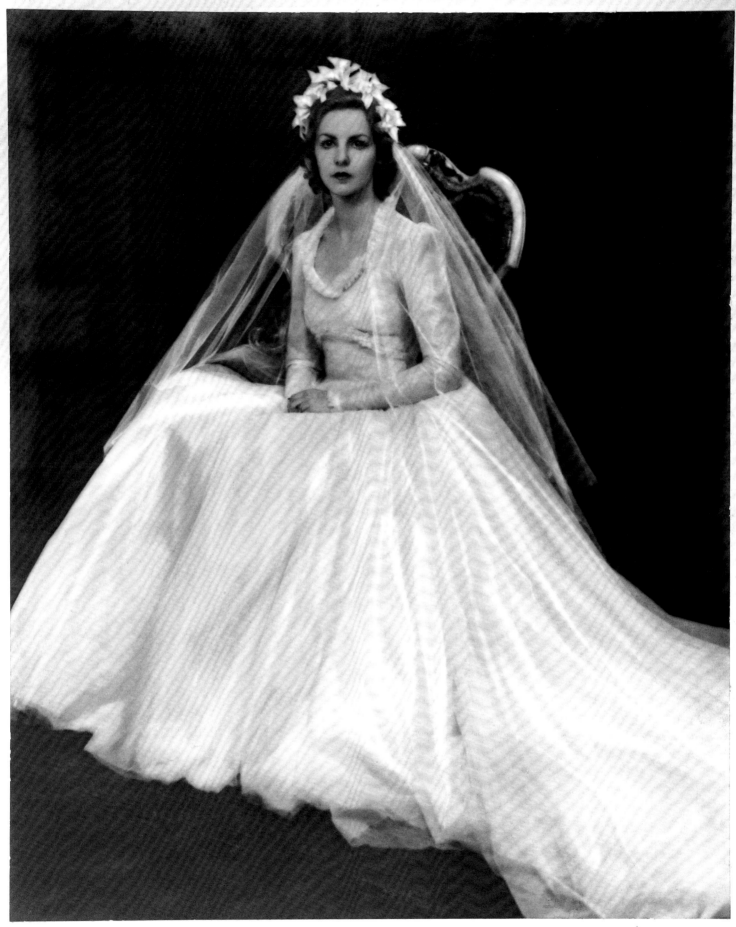

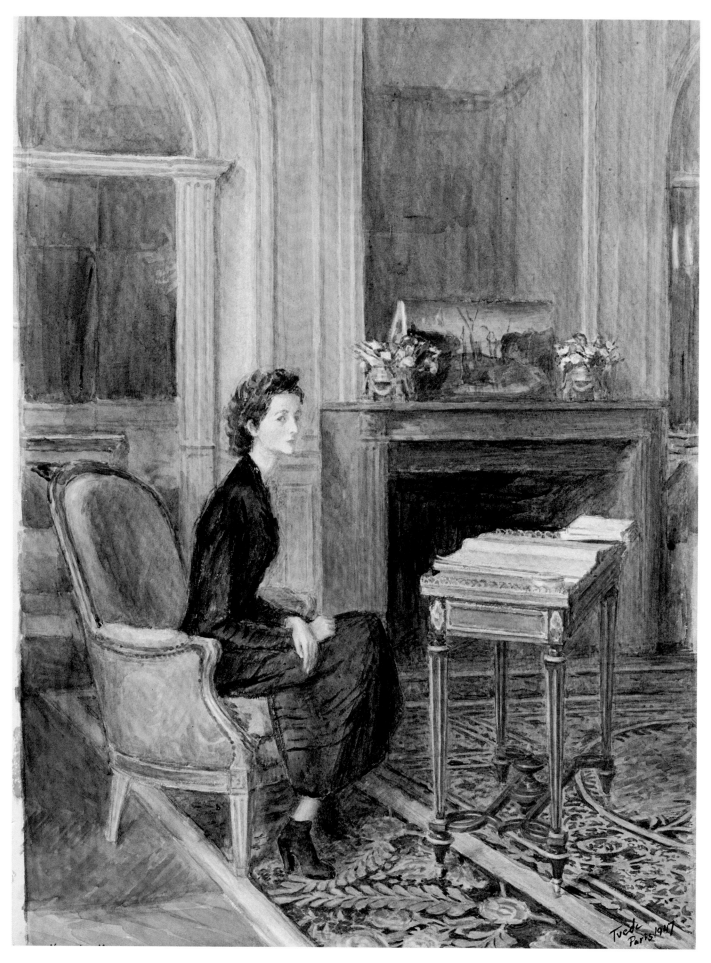

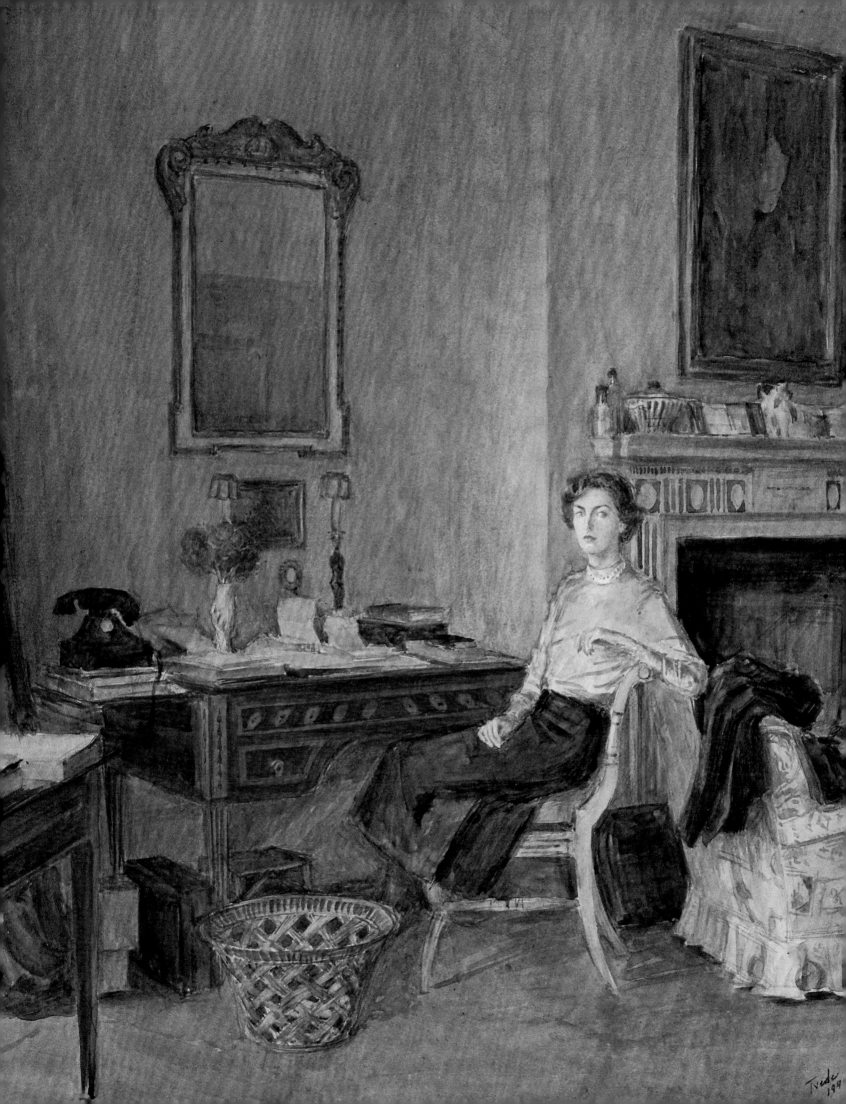

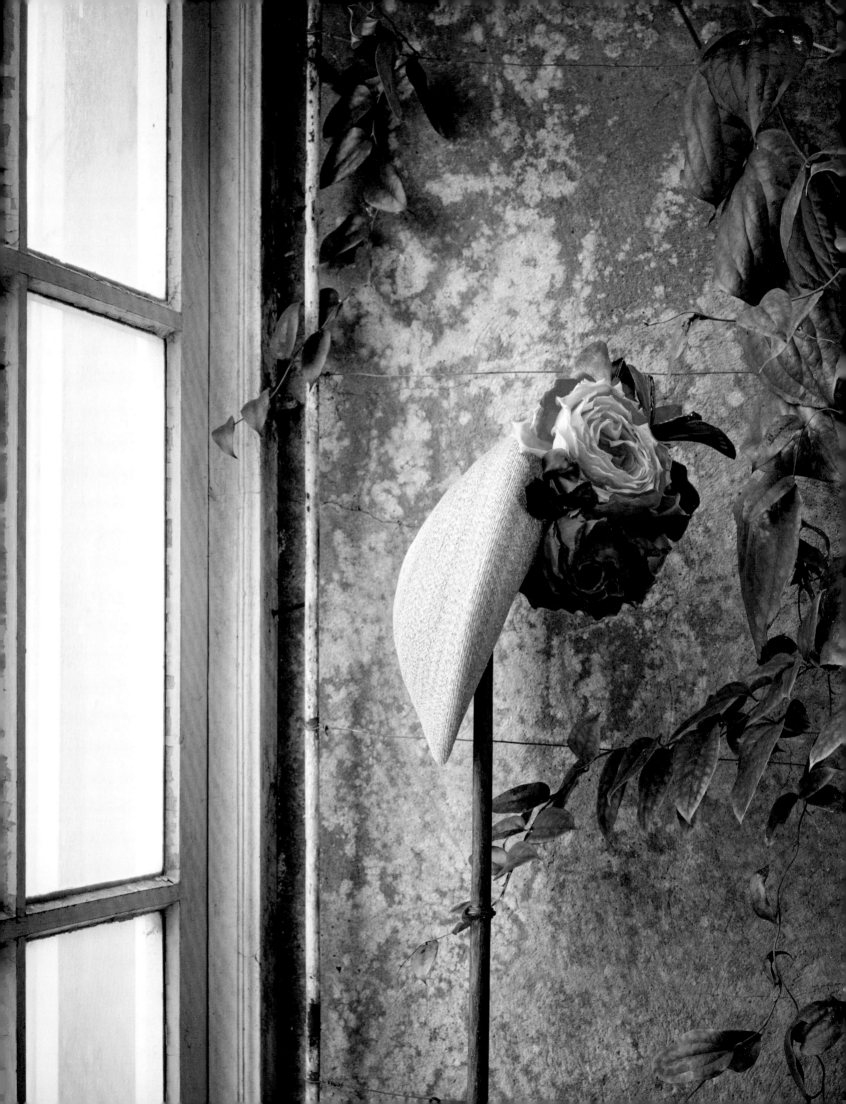

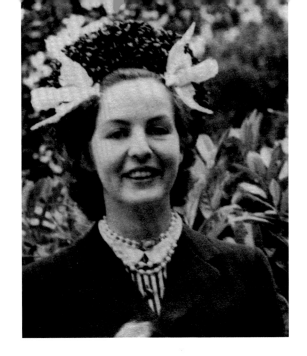

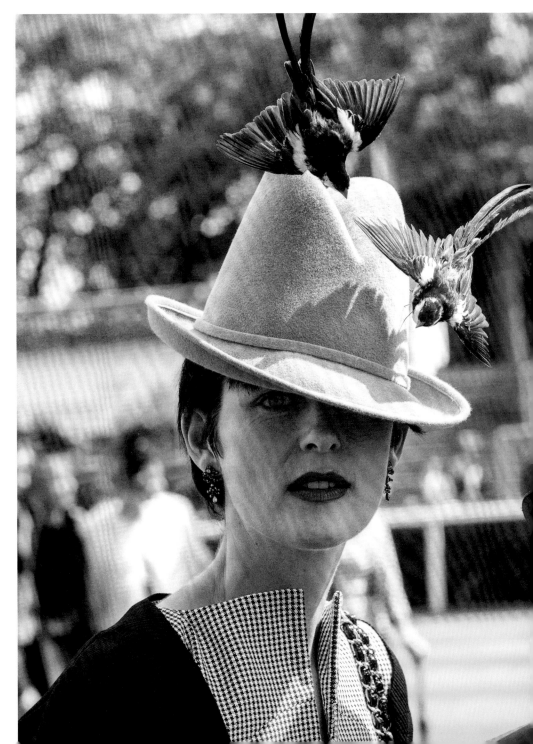

116 *(opposite)* Philip Treacy hat in the 1st Duke's greenhouse at Chatsworth, worn by Deborah Devonshire for the wedding of Prince William and Catherine Middleton, 2011.

117 *(this page, from top)* Deborah Devonshire wearing a Rose Valois hat given to her by Evelyn Waugh, 1945.

118 Stella Tennant wearing a hat by Stephen Jones at the Royal Ascot, 2011.

119 *(following pages)* Mario Testino, Deborah Devonshire and Stella Tennant, Chatsworth House, 2006. Originally published in American *Vogue*, November 2010.

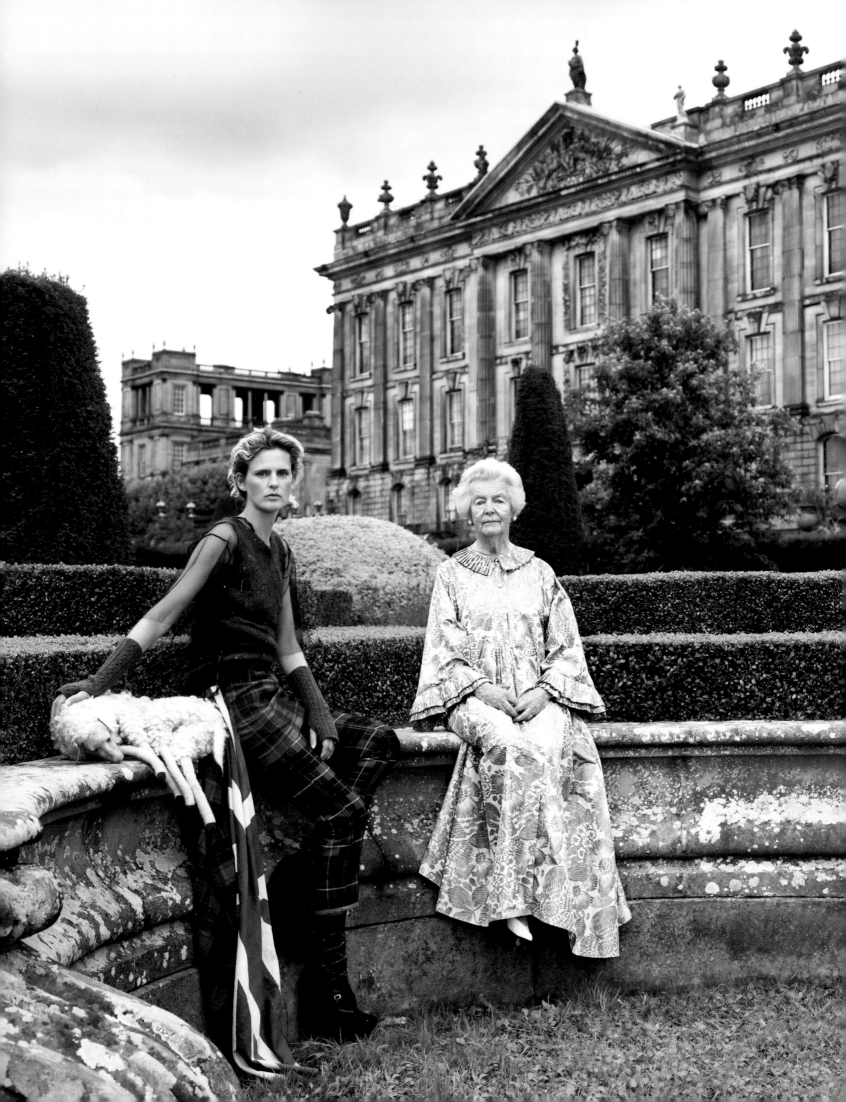

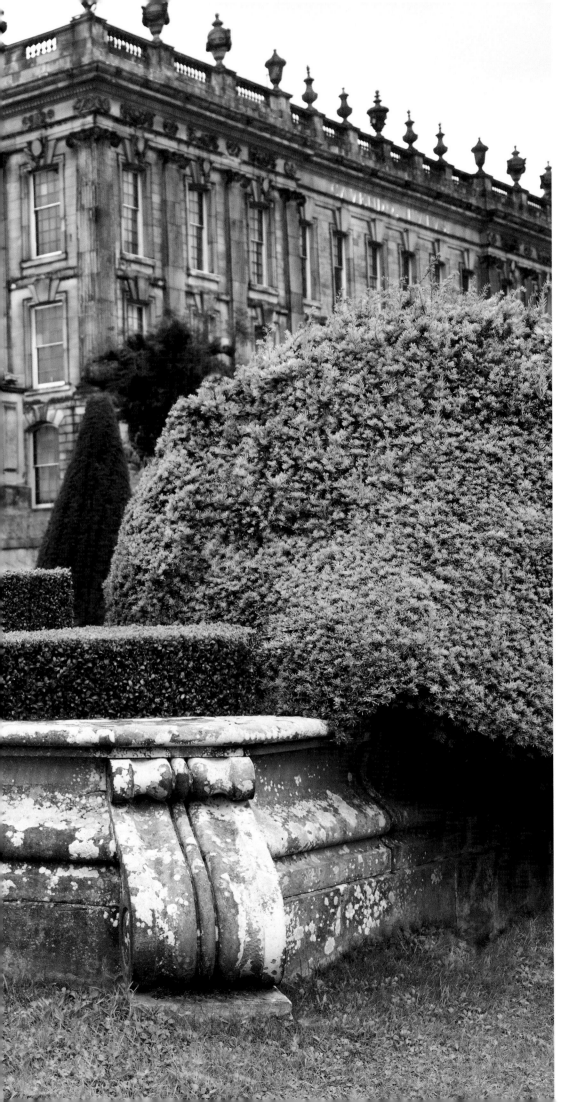

Deborah's first opportunity to dress at a couture house was for her wedding to Andrew Cavendish in 1941, and she knew exactly what she wanted: 'masses & masses & masses of white tulle, tight bodice & sleeves, a skirt such as has never been seen before for size.' The dress came from Victor Stiebel, one of London's top designers, and was finished just in time (fig. 113). Six weeks later, clothes rationing came in and the dress would have required several years' worth of coupons. A close-fitting top and full skirt was the style that Deborah chose to wear for many years: 'I don't mind if that is the fashion or not, it's what suits me.'

'I buy most of my clothes at agricultural shows', Deborah once wrote. 'After agricultural shows, Marks & Spencer is the place to go shopping, and then Paris.' These three shopping meccas supplied many of the outfits required for the hectic and varied life she led after her marriage. As chatelaine of Chatsworth, responsible for the private and public side of the house, she oversaw the kitchens, restaurants, gardens, shops, sewing room, farmyard and, of course, the chicken coops, as well as entertaining friends and undertaking countless public engagements at home and abroad. She also had the good fortune of having two excellent seamstresses at hand to copy, alter or create clothes for her: Christine Thompson at Chatsworth and Mary Feeney at Lismore, the Devonshires' Irish home.

Deborah's trademark everyday uniform was a variation on the 'Mitford style': a plain-colour kilt and wool cardigan, worn over a Turnbull & Asser men's-style shirt in various colours with white cuffs and collar (fig. 123), and Derri boots and a Barbour jacket for the outdoors. Not everyone was impressed by her staple attire. The artist Pietro Annigoni, who painted Deborah's portrait in 1954 (fig. 132), studied her for a long time and in the end decided to portray her in a high white collar and red velvet coat. 'You see', he said, 'your clothes aren't à la mode so it doesn't matter.'

For the grandest clothes, Deborah often went to Paris. In her memoirs she describes shopping in the early days with Nancy:

> She took me to see the clothes at Dior, Lanvin, Jean Dessès, Madame Grès, Balmain and Schiaparelli. Compared to the shops in England, they were fairyland during those early postwar years. A walk down the Faubourg St-Honoré, which we called Main Street, was made impossibly tempting by the window displays and we longed for everything. Usually we looked and longed but did not buy; it was like going to a gallery to admire the pictures.

In 1953, Deborah ordered a pale pink satin ball gown from Christian Dior (figs. 1, 121). She and Andrew had been invited to stay at Windsor Castle for Royal Ascot that year, which required five grand evening dresses. In the same year she bought a Schiaparelli ball gown made of white organza with velvet appliquéd flowers over a silk under-dress in the famous Schiaparelli shocking pink. In 1971, Cecil Beaton asked to borrow it for an exhibition he was curating at the V&A. 'What he meant but did not say', Deborah

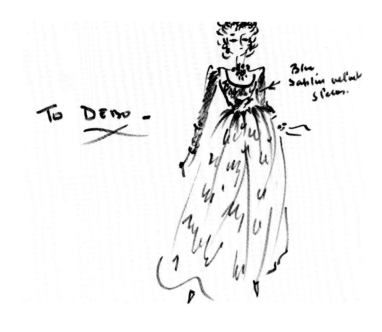

120 *(above)* Hubert de Givenchy's sketch of a circa 1960 evening dress given to Deborah Devonshire circa 2007. The sketch illustrates his suggestion of adding velvet sleeves, which was later implemented by Deborah Devonshire's seamstress, Christine Thompson.

121 *(opposite)* House sketch of 'Carmel' evening dress, Christian Dior Haute Couture, Spring/Summer 1953.

122 *(following pages)* Bruce Weber, Deborah Devonshire wearing a circa 1960 evening dress by Pierre Balmain, feeding her hens at Chatsworth, 1995.

carmel

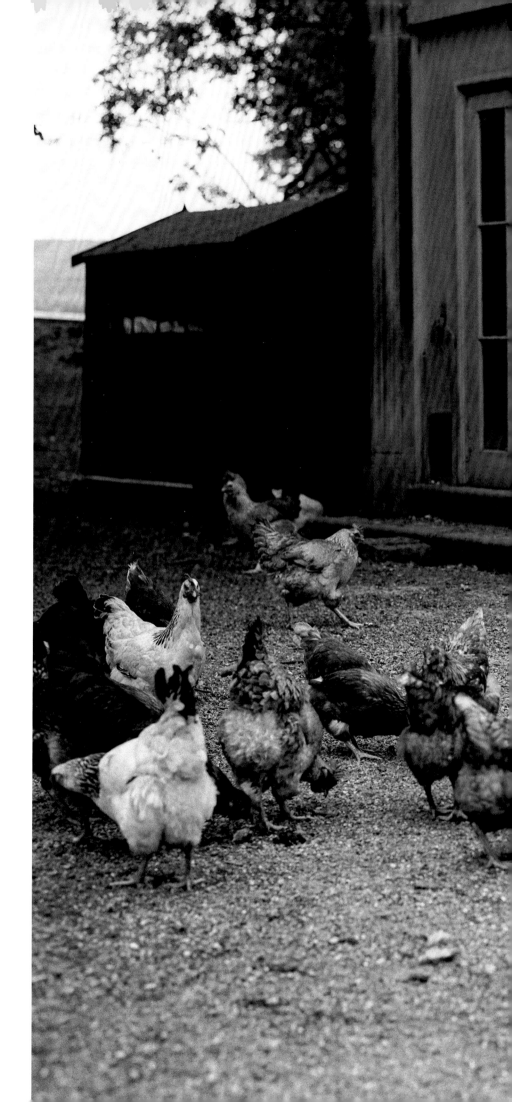

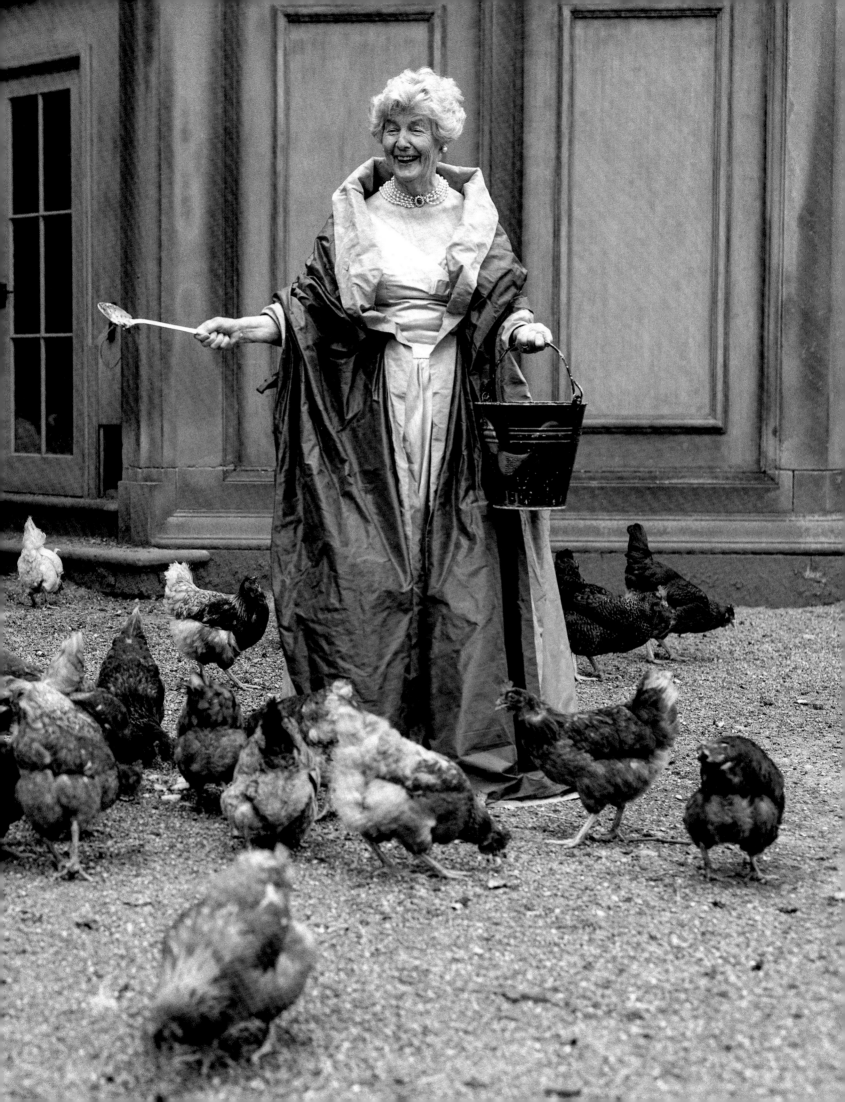

grumbled, 'was that it would join the permanent collection, so it was goodbye to my best dress, which is still there.'

Many of Deborah's favourite clothes came from Hubert de Givenchy (fig. 120) and Oscar de la Renta, who were both friends. She admired Givenchy's unerring eye and enjoyed visiting his boutique on the avenue George V, where 'Monsieur' wore a white coat, like a doctor, and would make tiny adjustments to a garment before allowing it to leave the premises. Oscar de la Renta's flowing silk evening gowns, often with a high ruff neck 'to hide the jowls', were an essential part of Deborah's wardrobe for the last 20 years of her life. She was photographed for *Vogue* with her granddaughter, the model Stella Tennant, in one of these dresses and described the results (fig. 119):

> They bound Stella's legs, up to where they join her body, in tartan. A Union Jack flag hung from her waist and her top was what my father would have called meaningless. Hair skewbald/piebald, all colours and stuck up in bits. Then they produced 'shoes' with 6-inch heels. More stilts – she could hardly put one foot in front of the other, wobbling and toppling, and being 6 feet tall she turned into 6'6". A prop was a big toy lamb, legs dangling as though dead. We looked just like that Grandville drawing of a giraffe dancing with a little monkey. I was the monkey.

Deborah admired and respected skilled workmanship in every field of enterprise, be it dressmaking or dry-stone walling, and appreciated the craft that went into making the clothes she wore. She was also a keen recycler and donated many of her clothes to charitable organisations. It was not unusual to see the three kings at the children's nativity play in her local church appear in gorgeous robes cut down from one of her dresses. The Mitford trait of making clothes last was as pronounced in Deborah as in her sisters, and the quality and timeless style of the great fashion houses meant that her clothes held their own for many years. She wore a pink satin Balmain ball gown that she bought in 1960 to her grandson William's coming-of-age party 30 years later (fig. 122). At her 80th birthday celebrations in 2000, she wore the costume designed by Worth for Louise, Duchess of Devonshire to wear as Queen Zenobia at the Devonshire House fancy dress ball in 1897 (fig. 94).

Deborah went on enjoying clothes and shopping well into old age. A photograph of her, aged 88, encapsulates the eclectic and dashing style she never lost: she wears a quilted cotton skirt, delicate white lace blouse, knee-high support socks (prescribed by her doctor after a mini stroke), grey velvet slippers emblazoned with Elvis Presley's portrait (fig. 81) and two strands of large pearls fastened by an aquamarine the size of a matchbox. 'Beautiful and always comfortable', which is what she said clothes ought to be.

123 *(opposite)* Deborah Devonshire's assorted Turnbull & Asser shirts in an armoire in a guest bedroom at Chatsworth.

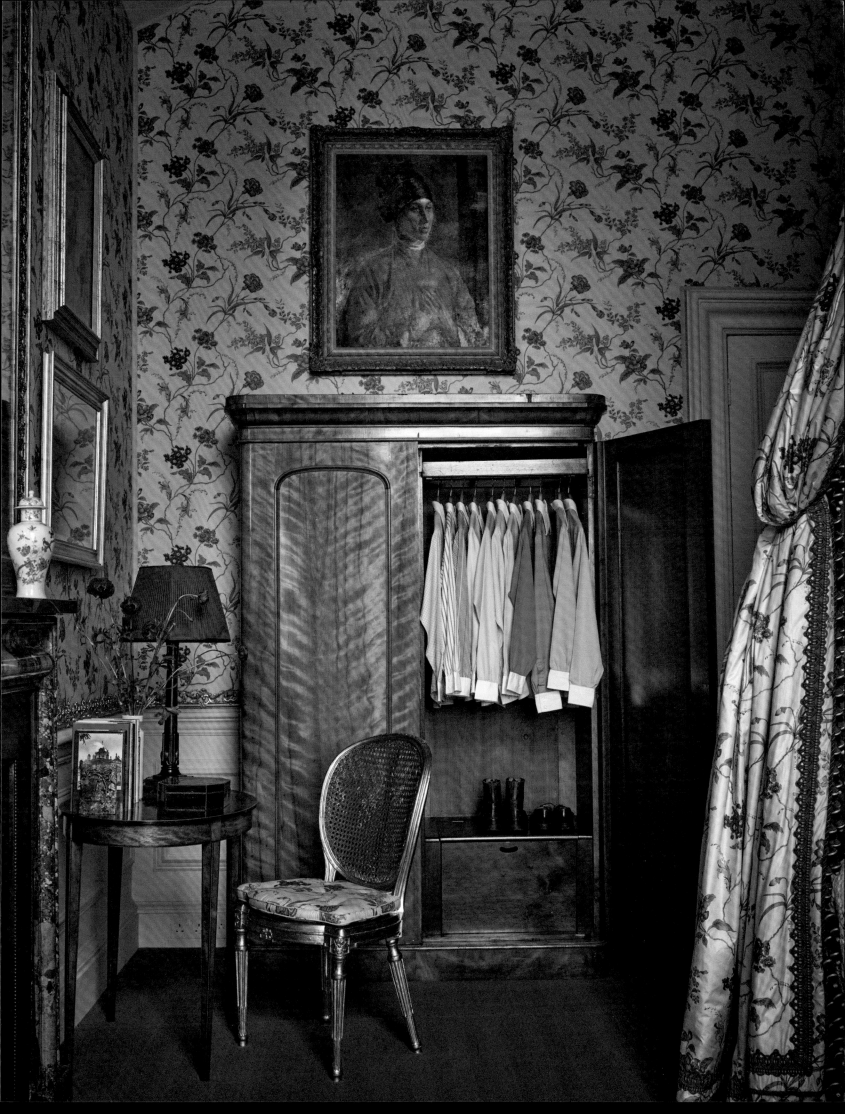

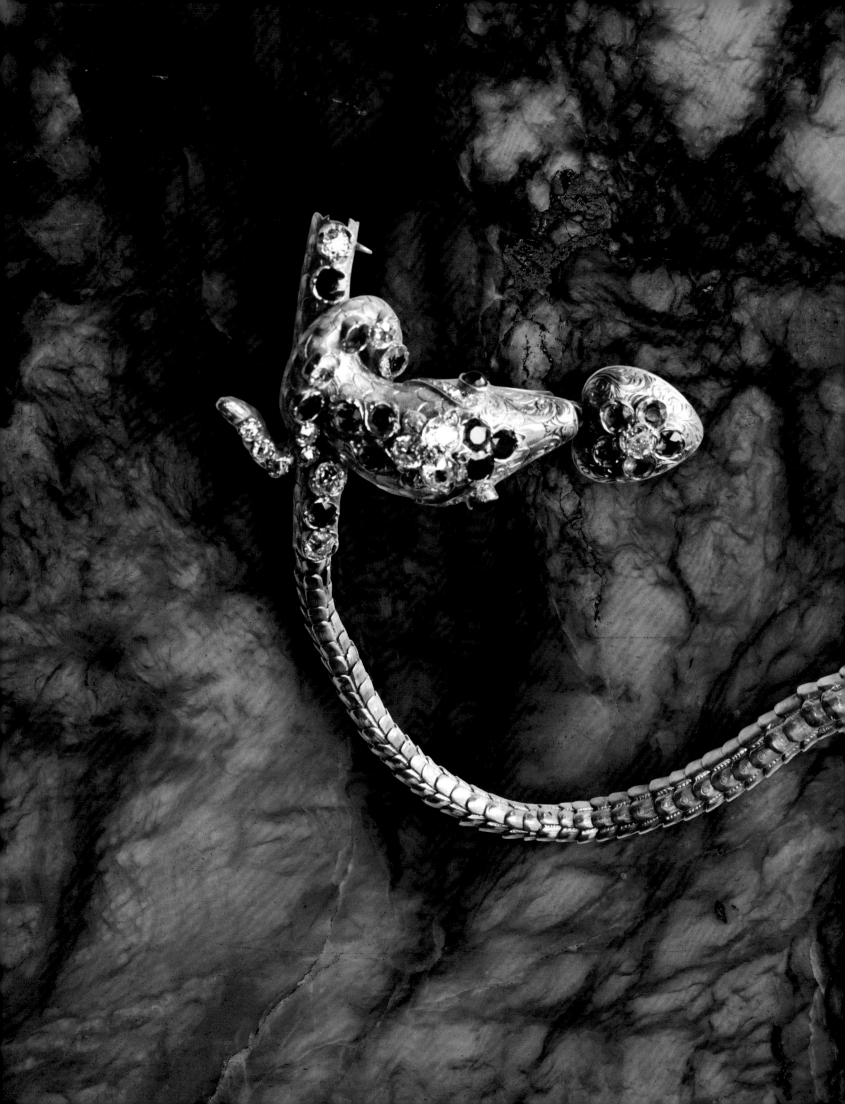

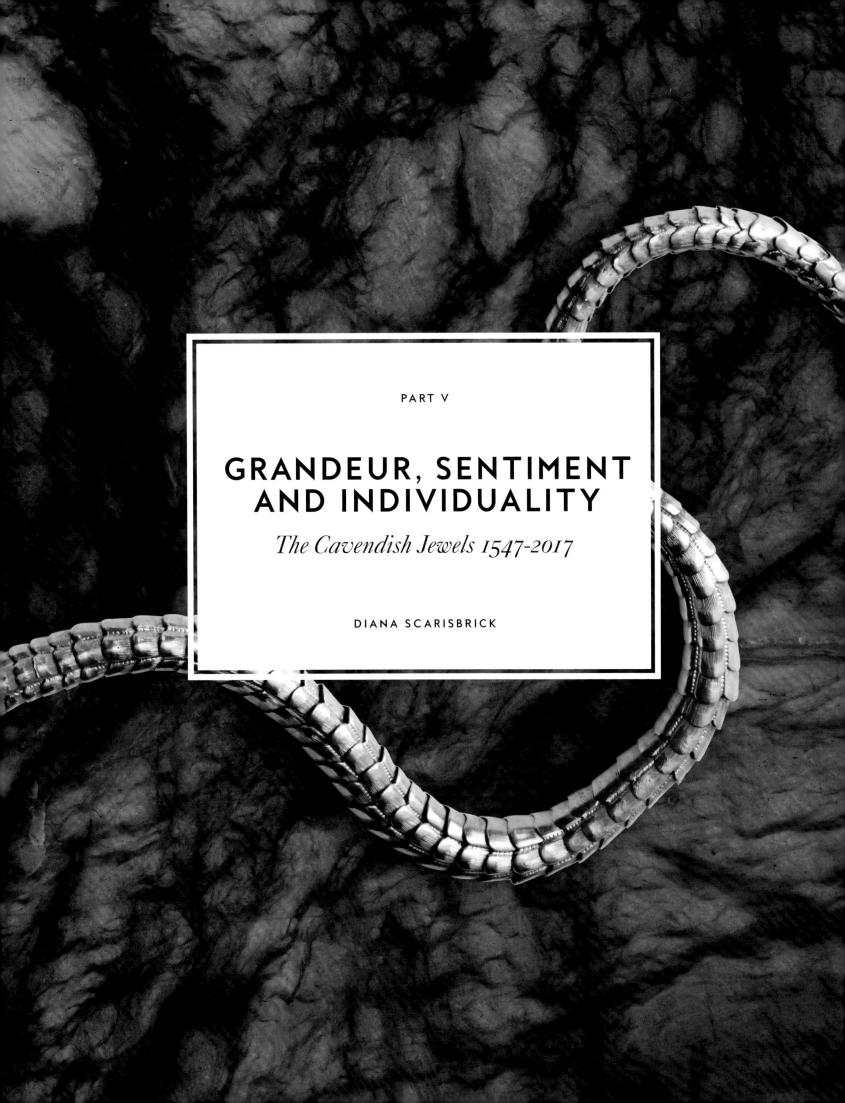

PART V

GRANDEUR, SENTIMENT AND INDIVIDUALITY

The Cavendish Jewels 1547-2017

DIANA SCARISBRICK

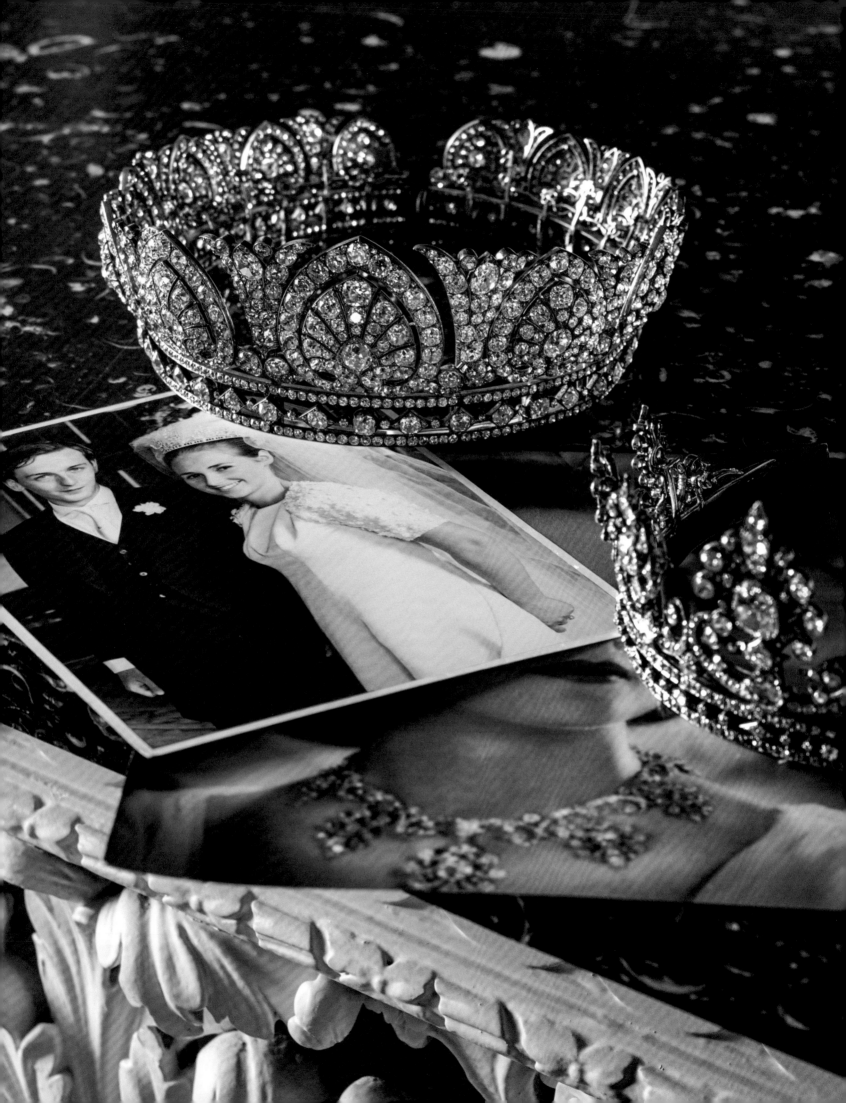

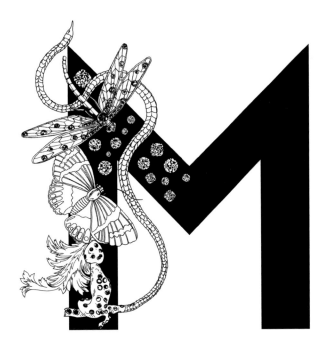

ore than any other works of art, it is the jewellery worn by successive generations of the Cavendish family which provides the key to their personal tastes, sentiments and friendships. This long story begins in 1547 with the wedding of Sir William Cavendish to the young Derbyshire widow, Elizabeth Barlow. After his death in 1557, she married again twice, and in her early 40s became Countess of Shrewsbury, proud and immensely rich, famous for her great houses at Chatsworth and Hardwick Hall. Appointed by Queen Elizabeth as custodian of Mary Queen of Scots, who had taken refuge in England, she received fine jewels – collars, bracelets, pomanders – as gifts from her grateful prisoner[1]. None of these mementos have survived, but portraits show her predilection for the ultimate Tudor status symbol: pearls, worn in long ropes set off by a black gown and white ruff (fig. 126). Ever since Bess of Hardwick's time the wives of her Cavendish descendants have demonstrated the same affinity for beautiful, milky white pearls.

She was followed by Countess Elizabeth, married to William, 1st Earl of Devonshire, who also displayed her rank and wealth resplendent in pearls – 'Persian, ragged and pear-shaped' – mounted in openwork coronets and a feather for the head, in necklaces, in ropes looped across the shoulders tied in a bowknot at the centre of the neckline, hanging from the ears, attached to diamond pendants and in dozens of diamond and pearl buttons highlighting the bodice and sleeves. Many more diamonds were set in a cross, a long chain and in a girdle, emphasising her high waist. Another girdle, threaded with barrel-shaped Virginia stones evoking the New World, was a gift from her husband, who was a great supporter of the colonies. As a loyal aristocrat, the Countess showed her support of Charles I by wearing his miniature enclosed in a diamond-studded case, and demonstrated family pride with a necklace of ruby and pearl clusters linked by 11 diamond-headed snakes, the Cavendish crest. Her attachment to her faith is reflected in bequests left to her beloved grandchildren. Each received a diamond ring inscribed with the admonition 'FEARE GOD' from the First Epistle of St Peter, in the hope that 'God would bless them all which shall follow the counsel contained in that posy to feare and truly to serve and value my love to them[2].'

In the next generation the diamond became the dominant factor in jewellery due to increased supplies of stones faceted in the rose ('fossett') and brilliant cuts, which released more light and fire than ever before. Recognising the power of diamonds to impress and sparkle, Christian (fig. 125), wife of the 2nd Earl of Devonshire, a good-looking redhead from Scotland, staunch royalist and patron of literature, dedicated her time and fortune to acquiring them. After the Civil War, during the Commonwealth (1649-1660), she felt free to buy Golconda diamonds and Persian Gulf pearls from the London dealers William Gumbleton and John Austin. Contrary to the popular image of that time, social life soon revived and women did not dress in drab Puritan grey, but instead, as she observed in 1653, were arrayed 'all in scarlet shining and glittering as

124 *(opposite)* (Left) Diamond tiara created for Duchess Louise, A E Skinner, 1893-1897. (Right) Diamond tiara created for Lady Louisa Egerton, daughter of the 7th Duke, 1870. Photographs of the Duke and Duchess of Devonshire on their wedding day, 1967, and Deborah Devonshire wearing the 1870 tiara as a necklace, 1951.

bright stars[3].' She had a penchant for earrings, both single and in pairs, of various designs combining diamonds of different cuts and coloured gems, such as her 'little pendant like a chaine for the ears' containing nine diamonds, two little fossett diamonds and at the end five pendant rubies and two table rubies, by two all-white pairs respectively set with 'six faire table diamonds, six large fossett' and 'one large middle stone and 35 small fosset (72) together with six paire of pendant pearls to hang in them.' Other rose- and table-cut diamonds radiating different accents of light were mounted into a great rosette for the breast, a stately chain, bracelets and a 'faire diamond locket the middle stone being a thick table cut stone weighing 7 carats, sett about with four faire table stones and four fossett diamonds of a bigger sort and 20 more of a lesser sort.' As this treasure epitomised family prestige, she therefore bequeathed 'for the use of the Heire Male of the Earls of Devonshire, the choyssest of my jewells and which I have collected, purchased and preserved with care and industrie[4].'

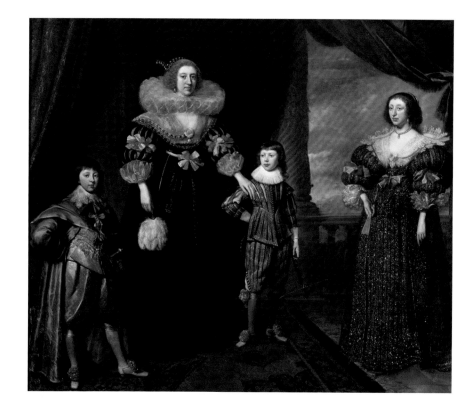

Amidst these heirlooms a new note was struck by the 2nd Duke, who assembled the famous collection of Roman and Renaissance cameos and intaglios, which still remains at Chatsworth. He took some of his favourites out of his cabinet to set in rings bearing his cipher and ducal coronet. Then, with the marriage of the future 4th Duke with Charlotte Boyle in 1748, another interesting ring came into the family, the signet of her ancestor, Richard Boyle, 1st Earl of Cork, who arrived in Dublin aged 22 in 1588 to make his fortune. With no other assets except his legal training, fine clothes, £27 in his pocket and this signet on his finger, he rose from the ranks of minor officialdom to Lord High Treasurer of Ireland. When Charlotte Boyle's wealth, estates and art collections passed into Cavendish hands, the family jewels assumed even greater importance.

Accordingly, after Georgiana Spencer married the 5th Duke, her first appearance at court in 1774 impressed Lady Mary Coke, who wrote that the 'drawing room was fuller than I ever saw it owing I suppose to curiosity to see the Duchess of Devonshire. She looked very pretty and happiness was never more properly marked in a countenance than hers. She was very properly fine for the time of year and her diamonds were magnificent. The girdle is a piece of finery so uncommon it made it all the more admired.' Georgiana became a national celebrity, and crowds gathered around her whenever she appeared in public, her head blazing with diamonds topped with the tallest ostrich feathers. Yet, although obliged to display her rank by wearing fine jewellery, she was happiest when wearing miniatures of her children and souvenirs enclosing locks of the hair of her friends. She also enjoyed showing off gifts from royalty,

125 (above) Daniel Mytens, *Christian Bruce, Countess of Devonshire and Her Children, William, 3rd Earl of Devonshire, Charles and Anne*, circa 1629.

126 (opposite) Probably Rowland Lockey, *Elizabeth Hardwick, Countess of Shrewsbury*, 1590.

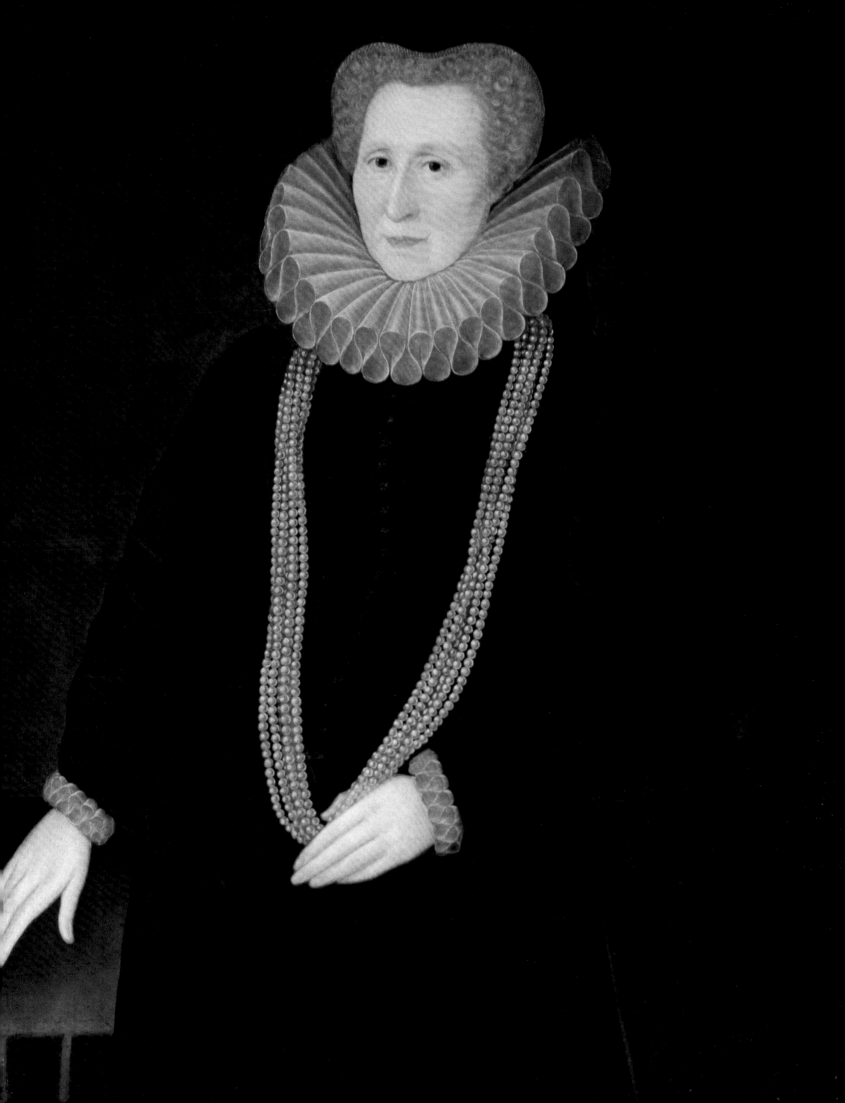

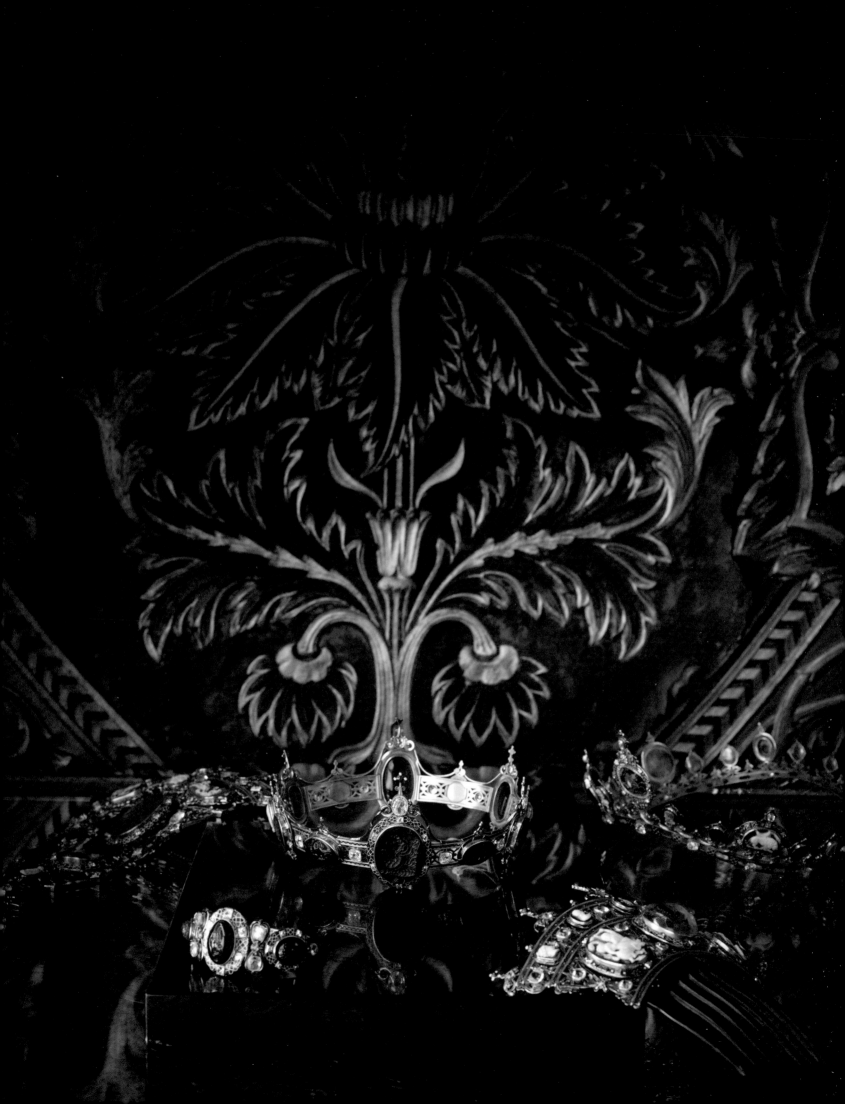

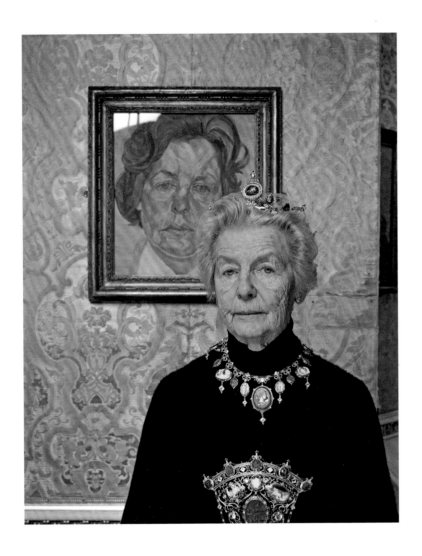

displaying a pearl buckle from Queen Marie Antoinette on the sash of a black-and-white dress at a French embassy ball and cherishing a diamond key brooch from 'her dearest, dearest brother', the future George IV in 1786[5]. Regarding it as a token of their friendship, she acknowledged 'with great pleasure the office you assign me and I shall wear the beautiful key with great pleasure and pride: it really is the prettiest ornament I ever saw.' She went on to promise that she would never, ever betray the secrets of his heart, assuring him that he was always in her thoughts, asking, 'Who can conquer hearts as well as you[6]?'

As a child, Georgiana's son, the 6th Duke, remembered playing with a large gold ring made in Alexandria, in the second century BC, embossed with heads of the great Egyptian divinities Jupiter, Serapis and Isis, which he believed to have belonged to the Emperor Nero and foreshadowed his future royal friendships. His prominent role at the coronations of George IV in 1821 and of Tsar Nicolas I in 1826 is recalled by gifts of rings from both monarchs, and his devotion to Princess Pauline Borghese by a bracelet she wore when mourning the death of her brother, Napoleon. Conscious of the rarity and artistry of the 2nd Duke's collection of engraved gems, he not only added to it and had four cameo theatrical masks reset into studs for his dress shirt, but also commissioned the famous parure (fig. 127) for Marie, the wife of his nephew the Earl Granville, representative of Queen Victoria at the coronation of Alexander II in 1856. Eighty-eight of the best cameos and intaglios were mounted by C F Hancock of Bruton Street into a coronet, comb, tiara and ferronière/bandeau for the head, and a necklace, stomacher and bracelet in Holbeinesque settings enamelled in sober red and black and encrusted with diamonds for sparkle[7]. The parure, one of the most celebrated creations of Victorian jewellery, was last worn by Deborah Devonshire who complained that it did not suit modern clothes and was prickly and uncomfortable (fig. 128).

The diamonds which lit up the above parure so effectively for the Countess Granville were removed for the high all-round crown (fig. 124) made by A E Skinner of Orchard Street for the German-born Dowager Duchess of Manchester, who married the 8th Duke in 1892. In addition, she dismantled all the other historic Devonshire jewels to obtain no less than 1,041 diamonds for this crown in which she held court, sparkling like a fairy tale queen. As London's leading political hostess, the tall and stately 'Double Duchess' was always perfectly dressed in white satin or black velvet, and, in the words of Benjamin Disraeli, 'always set everything on fire, including the neighbouring Thames[8].'

The next two Duchesses, Evelyn (fig. 41) and Mary (fig. 130), married respectively to the 9th and 10th Dukes, continued to represent the old order and appeared at national

127 *(opposite)* The Devonshire Parure, C F Hancock, circa 1852.

128 *(above)* François Halard, Deborah Devonshire wearing the Devonshire Parure, 2003.

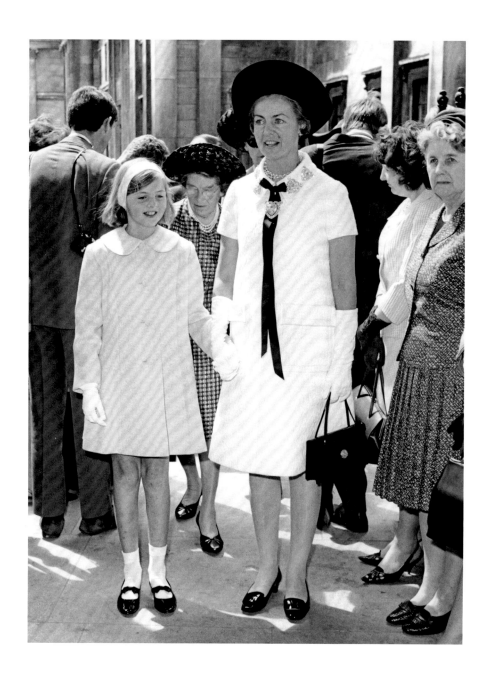

129 *(above)* Deborah Devonshire (wearing the A E Skinner tiara as brooches) and daughter Lady Sophia at the Duke of Devonshire's wedding, 1967.

130 *(opposite)* Cecil Beaton, Duchess Mary wearing the 1893-1897 diamond tiara by A E Skinner, 1953.

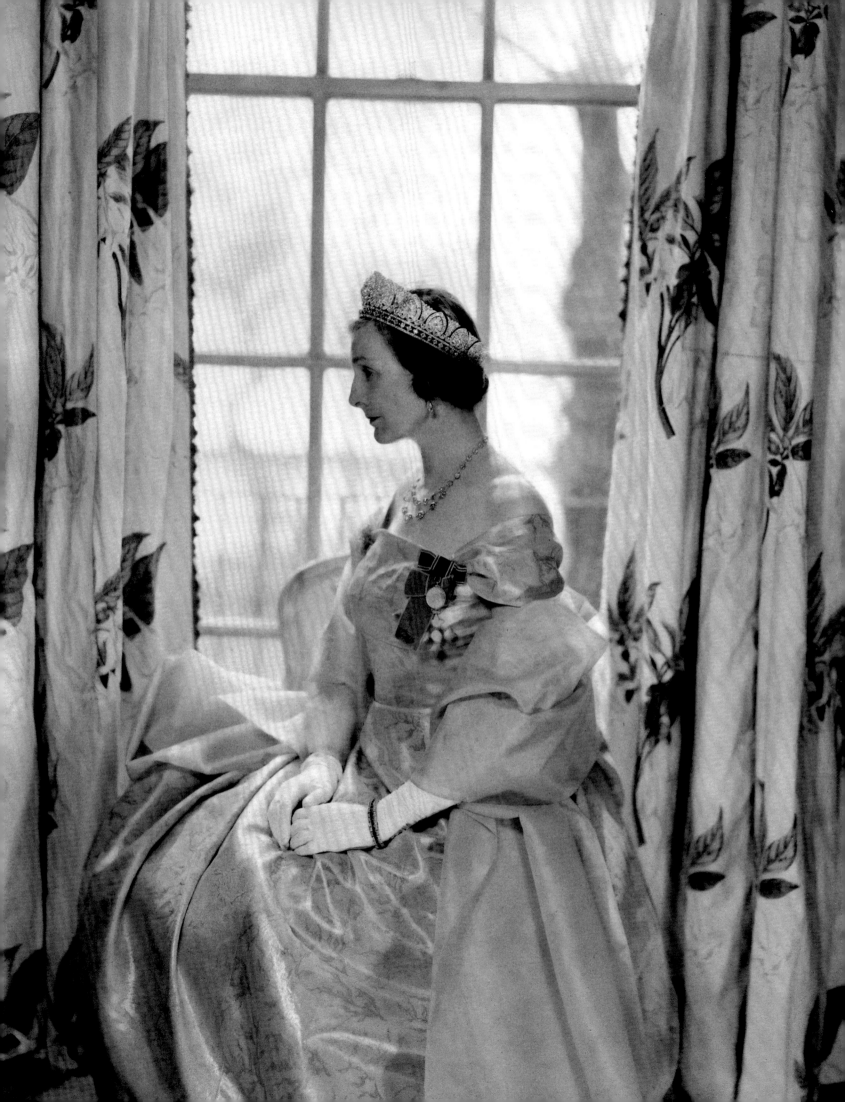

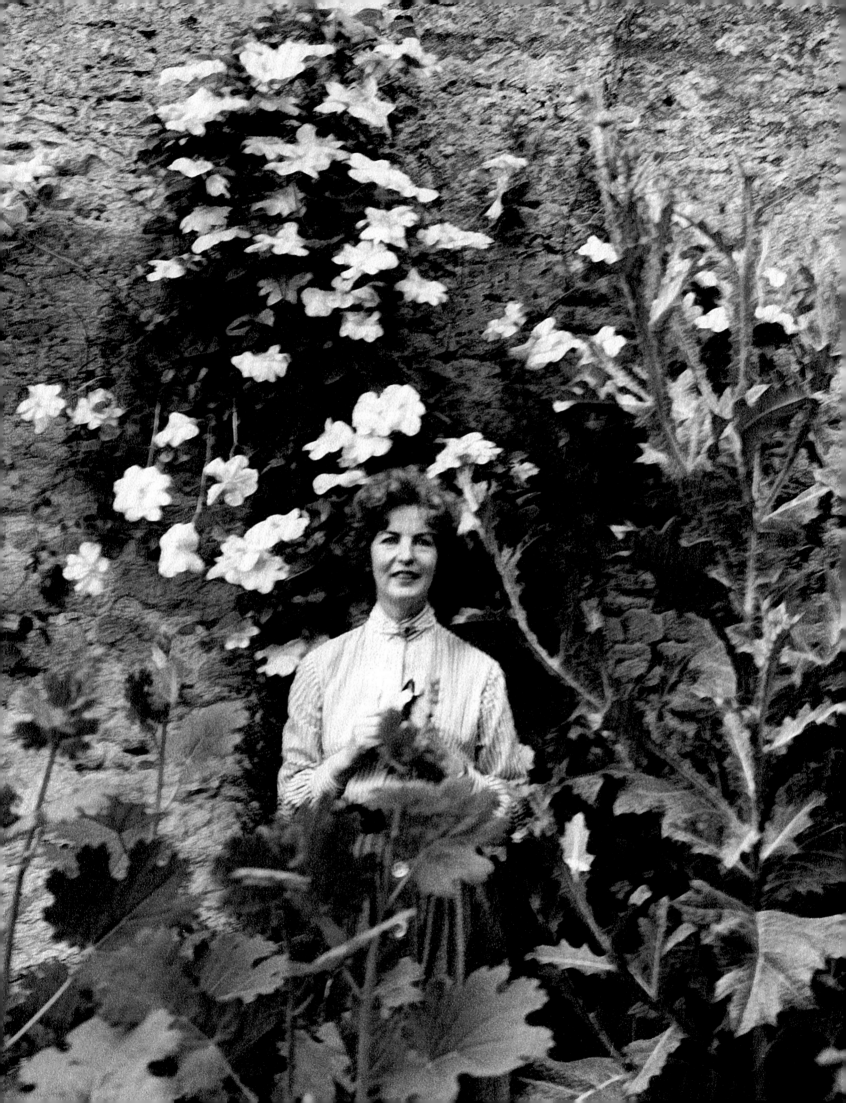

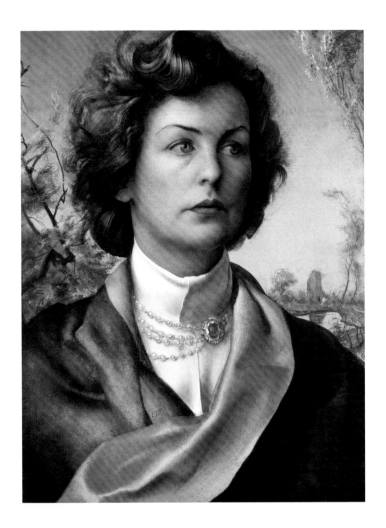

events resplendent in this magnificent crown, diamond necklace, earrings and ropes of pearls, their shimmering dresses weighed down with Orders and Badges. More personal is the serpent bracelet coiled around the wrist of Duchess Evelyn in her portrait by John Singer Sargent (fig. 34). Since the symbolism of the coiled snake holding a heart in its fangs signifies enduring love, it was the favourite Victorian jewel of sentiment, given to her as a bride by the future 9th Duke in 1892. A different, heraldic note is struck by the snake brooch which they gave their daughter, Dorothy, upon her marriage to the future Prime Minister, Harold MacMillan, in 1920. This rose- and brilliant-cut diamond snake, or 'serpent nowed', its coils twisted into a figure of eight, represents the Cavendish crest, and as the wife of a leading statesman Lady Dorothy wore it as a reminder of her own long family tradition of public service. In recognition of his achievement in continuing this tradition, as well as maintaining Chatsworth, she gave it to the 11th Duke, her nephew.

Because of her long reign as chatelaine of Chatsworth, we know more about Deborah Devonshire's collection than those of her predecessors. She seemed inseparable from her pearls with a Cavendish star ruby clasp (fig. 131), which she wore with a high white collar in her portrait by Pietro Annigoni (fig. 132), but during their long marriage the 11th Duke gave her many more jewels. They were almost all Victorian, beginning with a turquoise and diamond necklace and a sapphire and diamond twinned heart bracelet acquired at the auction sale of the American-born Countess Craven in 1961. Then followed a great collection of antique and modern jewelled insects – butterflies, dragonflies, moths, flies, bumble bees, hornets, wasps, spiders, beetles and grasshoppers – some all white, set with diamonds and pearls, others paved with coloured stones, including splendid rainbow-tinted opals (figs. 134, 136). These she wore in her own individual way (fig. 133). A fearsome spider might lurk on the shoulder of a jacket and varieties of insects swarmed on long narrow scarves reaching down to the hem of an evening dress, deliberately kept plain so as to show the jewels to best advantage. Always impressive, worn with taste and flair, they ensured that she would appear in public looking the model of a modern duchess. Important events in their life together were marked by further gifts of platinum and diamond bracelets, one inscribed with 'CHATSWORTH 7 JULY 1990' commemorating the coming of age of their grandson Lord Burlington, and another with the name of the 11th Duke's prize-winning race mare 'PARK TOP', both commissioned from London craftsmen. However, when shopping on her own, her greatest enthusiasm seems to have been for Joel Arthur Rosenthal, known as JAR. On the first visit to his Paris showroom she was quite overwhelmed by his genius: 'The more we saw the more we wanted to see – pieces so extraordinary, so beautiful and original that no words can describe their impact.' Further amazement followed when, by pinning a brooch onto her

131 *(opposite)* Cecil Beaton, Deborah
Devonshire, Haseley Manor, 1960.

132 *(above)* Pietro Annigoni, *Deborah
Devonshire*, 1954.

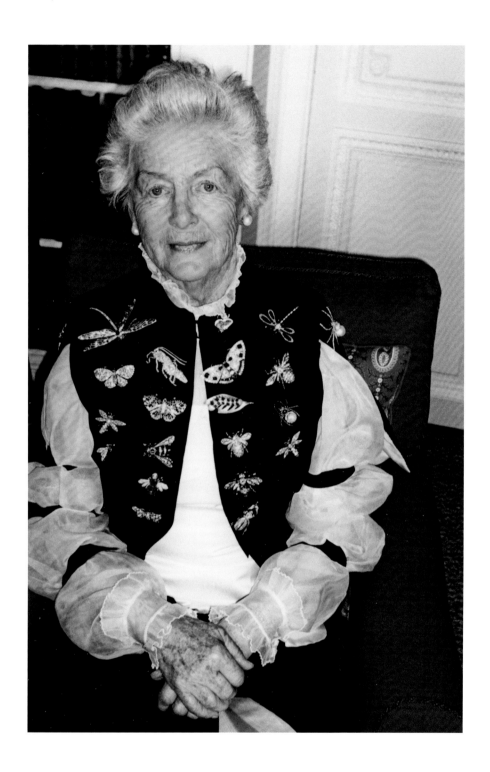

133 *(above)* Deborah Devonshire wearing her collection of insect jewellery, 1998.

134 *(opposite)* Deborah Devonshire's bug and insect jewellery atop *Metamorphosis Insectorum* by Maria Sibylla Merian, 1705.

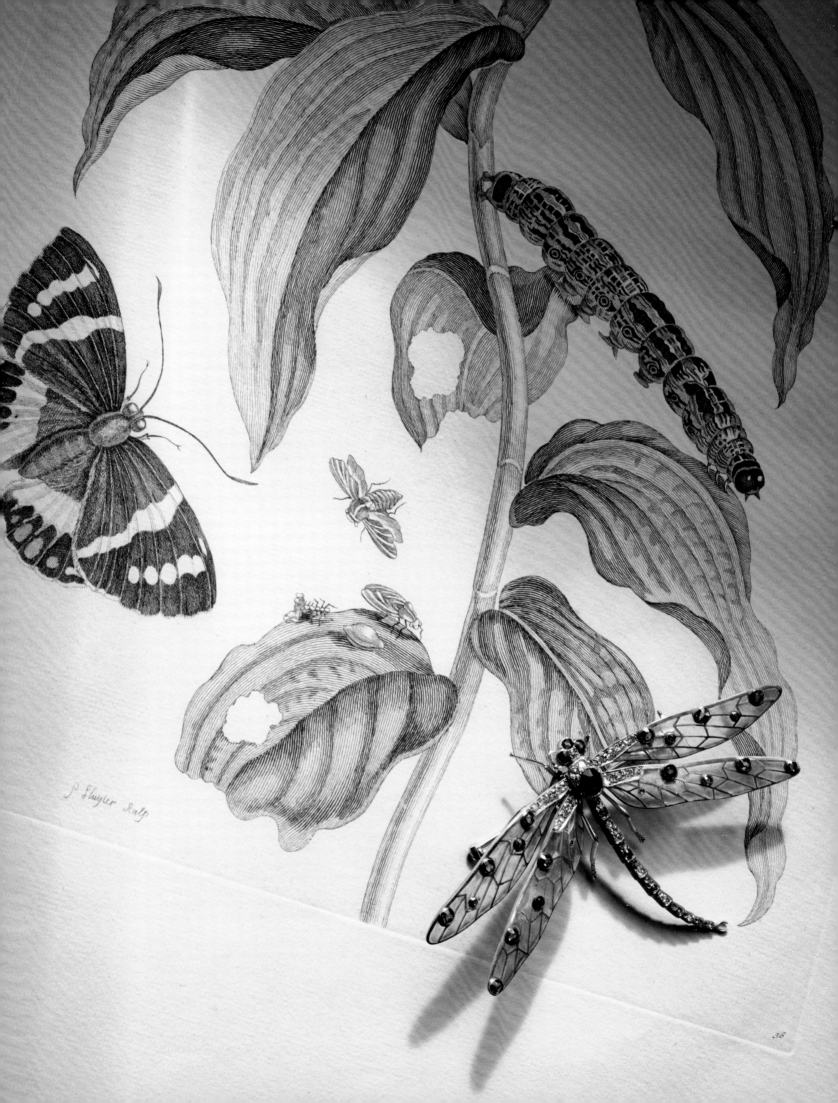

P. Sluyter Sculp

36

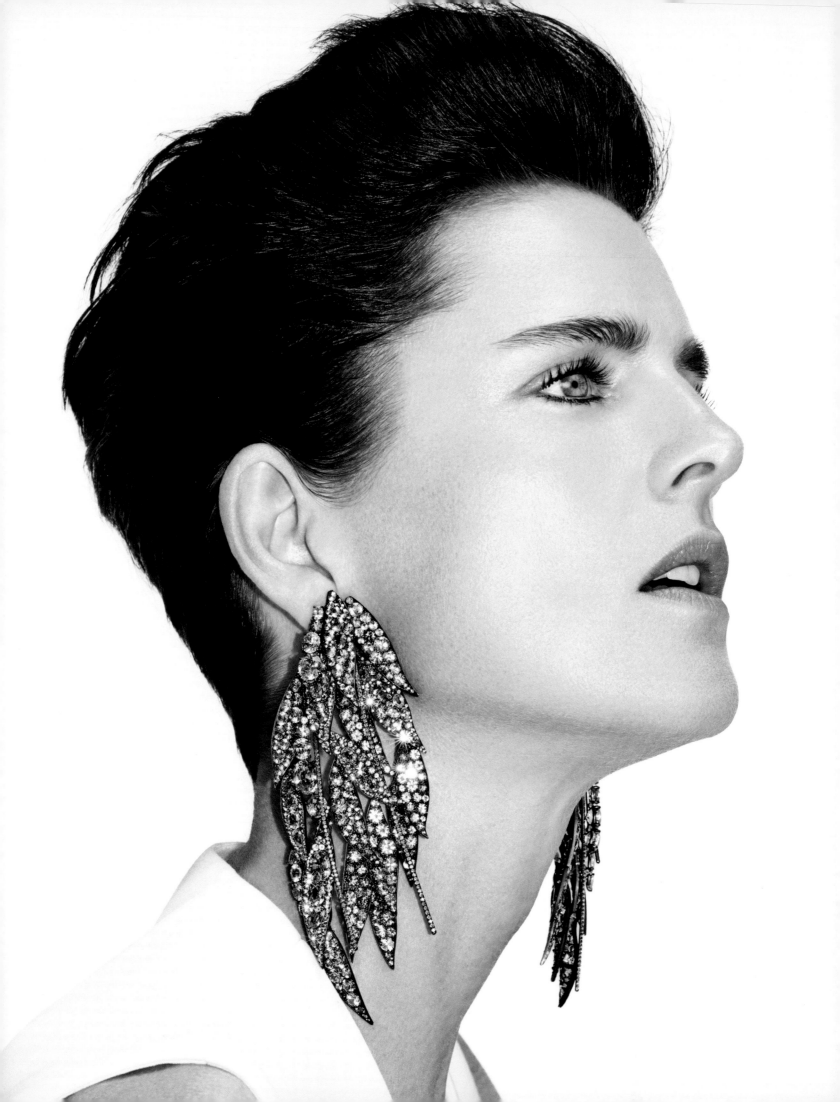

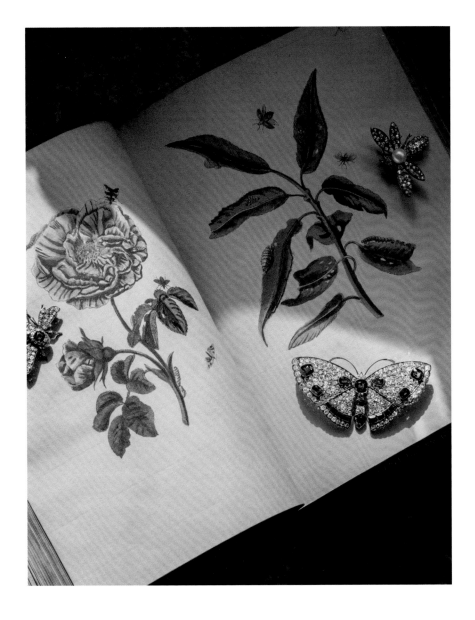

shoulder, he transformed an ordinary dress into something extraordinary; no other jewel had ever done that for her[9]. Another great JAR admirer is her granddaughter, the model Stella Tennant, who described a pair of his earrings for *Harper's Bazaar*: 'The ones I fell for hook, line and sinker were the willow leaved chrysoberyls and diamonds. I had never seen anything like them – the colours – subtle shades of blues and murky, watery greens, the sheer size and movement. Each leaf was articulated, allowing them to float in the breeze (fig. 135).'

The Duchess of Devonshire, the present custodian of the Cavendish hereditary jewels, is an accomplished horsewoman, who wears the PARK TOP bracelet and other trophies of family successes on the turf, an interest she shares with her husband, who was a leading figure in British racing. Echoing his contemporary art collection, she has also adopted a non-traditional style of her own. She wears designs by Andrew Grima (figs. 137-138), who won fame during the 1960s and 70s by following the new developments in sculpture pioneered by Elisabeth Frink. Grima began by rejecting conventional diamond and platinum jewels in favour of mere scatterings of diamonds and uncut semiprecious stones combined with yellow gold, roughly textured and reeded to a most attractive effect, and it was his choice of these less-expensive materials which allowed him the freedom to experiment with abstract forms, irregular outlines and meteoric shapes exploding dynamically into space, so as to create miniature works of art. Whereas the Devonshire pearls and diamonds represent the family history, these Grima jewels strike a thoroughly modern note, in keeping with the desire of the 12th Duke, like so many of his predecessors, to keep his ancient title abreast with the world of today.

135 *(opposite)* Kacper Kasprzyk, Stella Tennant wearing earrings by JAR. Originally published in *Harper's Bazaar*, September 2013.

136 *(above)* Deborah Devonshire's bug and insect jewellery atop *Metamorphosis Insectorum* by Maria Sibylla Merian, 1705.

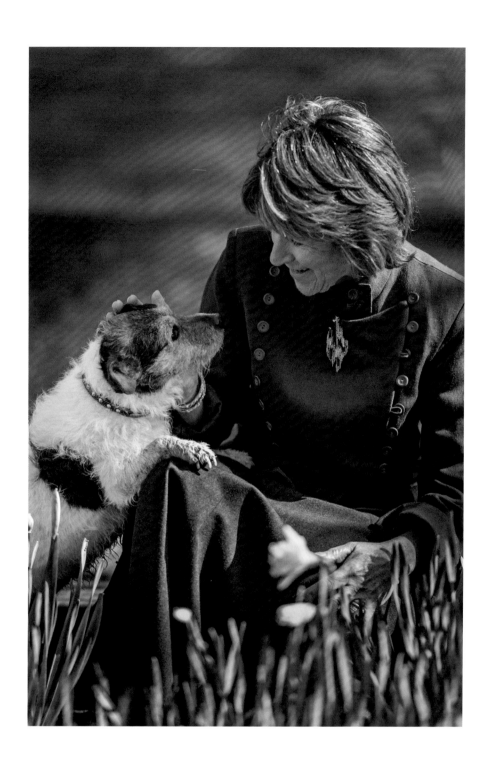

137 *(above)* The Duchess of Devonshire, wearing a brooch by Andrew Grima, with her dog Max, 2016.

138 *(opposite)* The Duchess of Devonshire's necklace by Grima, 2002.

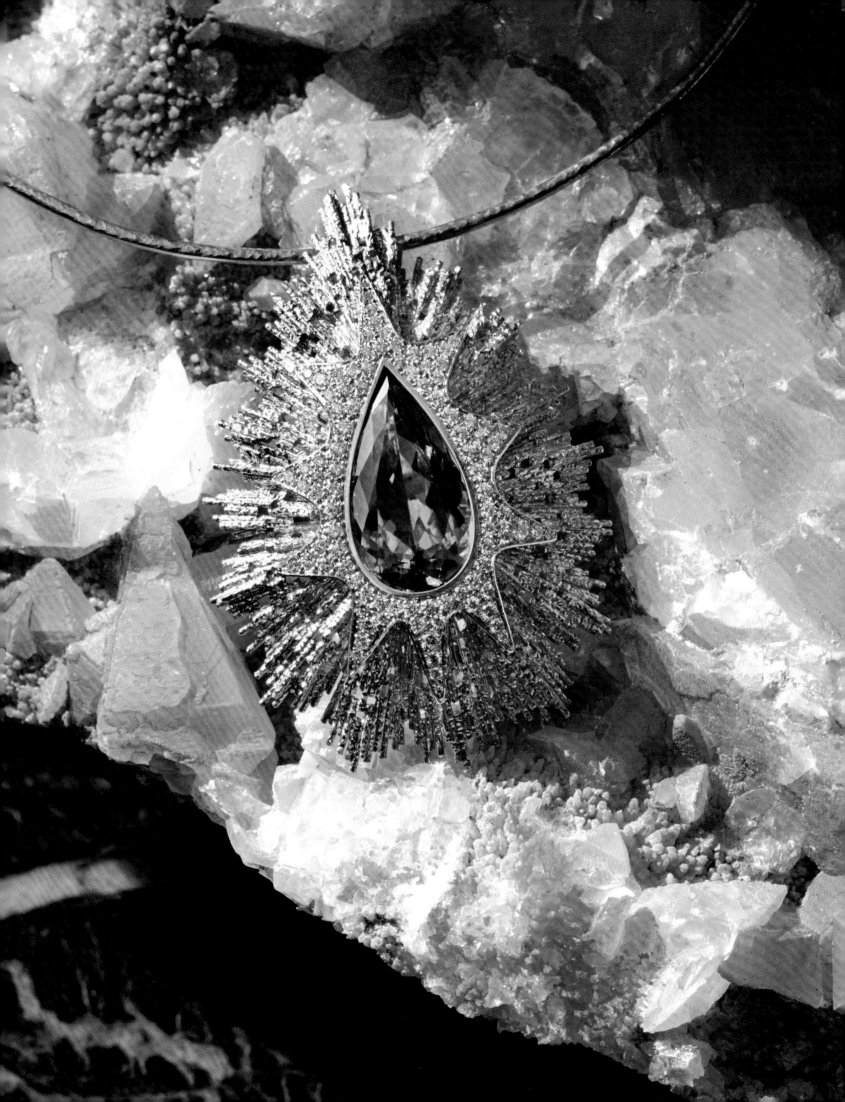

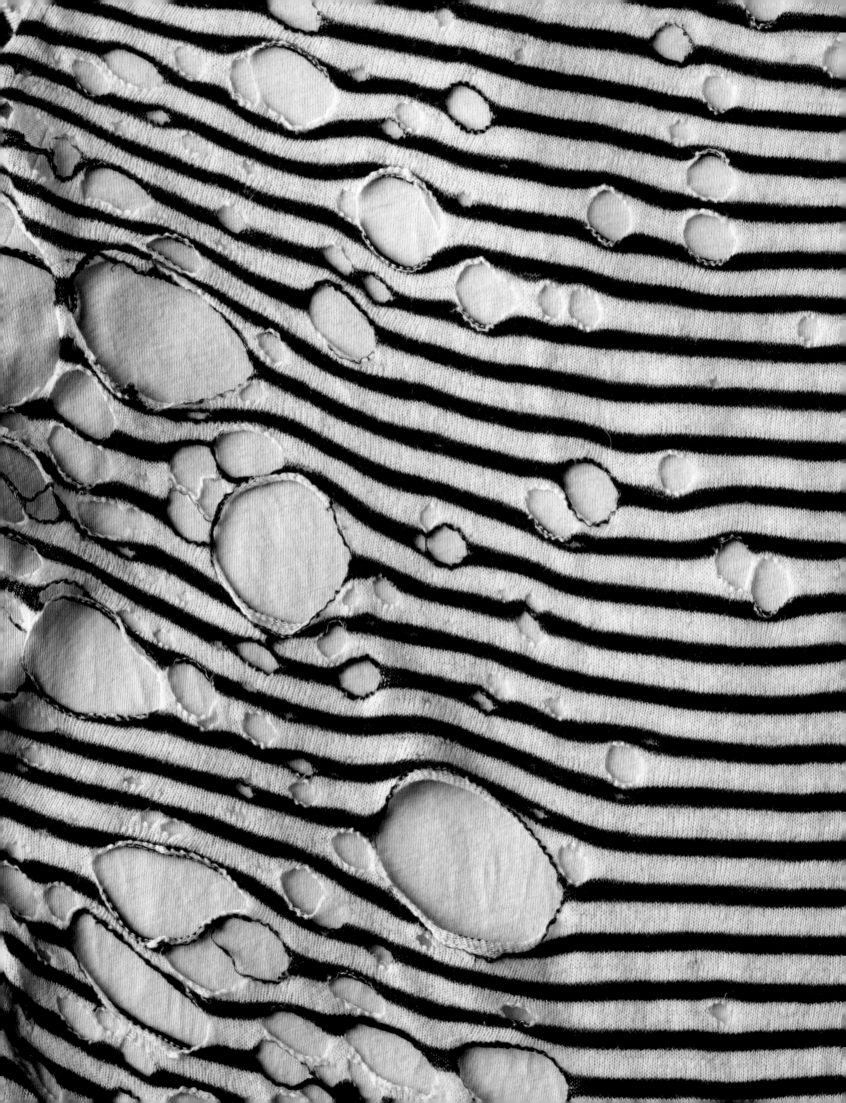

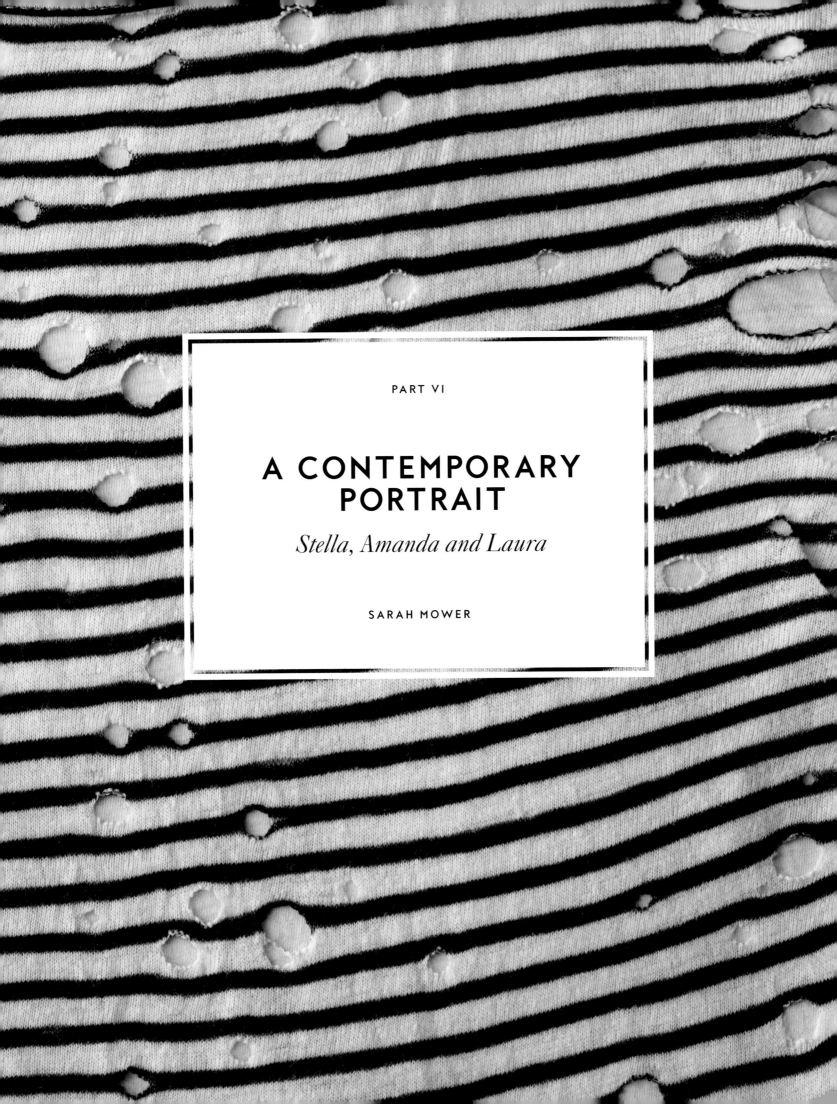

PART VI

A CONTEMPORARY PORTRAIT

Stella, Amanda and Laura

SARAH MOWER

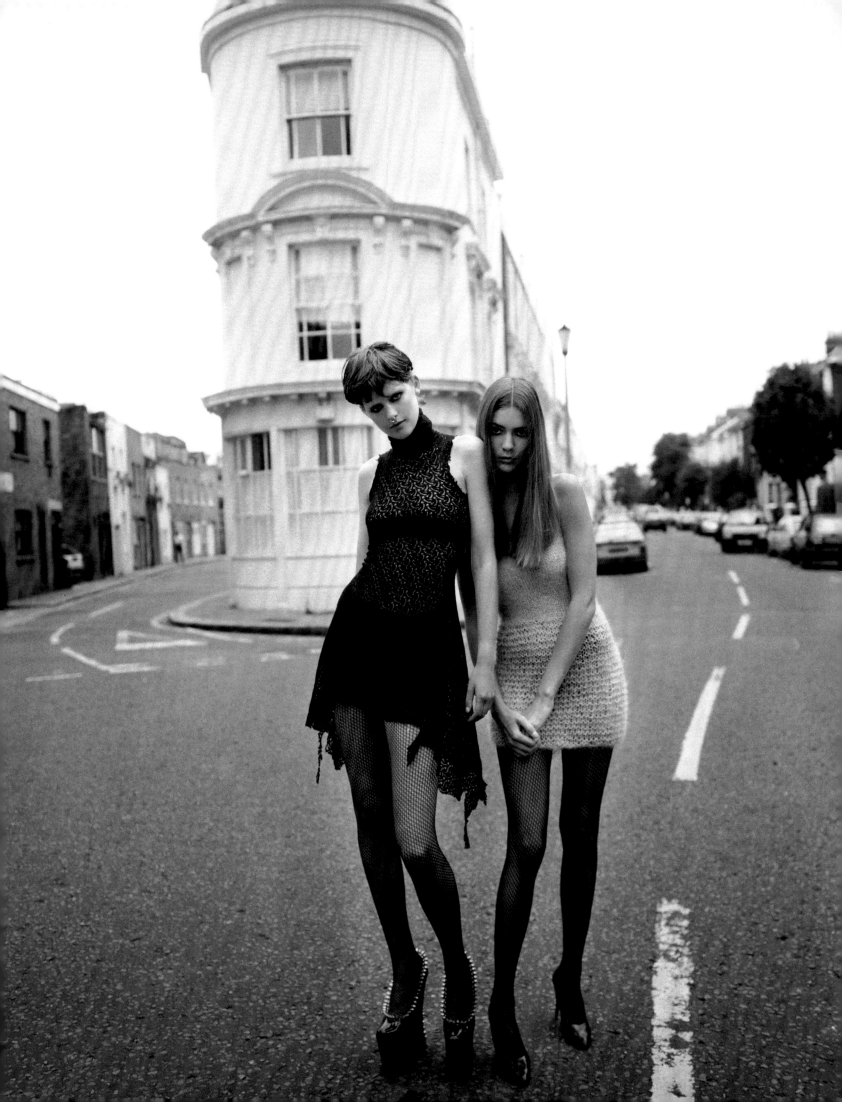

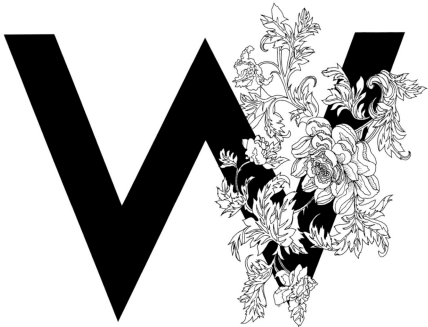

When it comes to the present day, Chatsworth's long history with fashion might have been a lot more evidently present if it weren't for a concerted attack of the carpet beetle. 'Oh', Stella Tennant is wracked by the memory, 'It was in my apartment, when I was living in New York. We had to have the fumigators in. All my clothes went into a pile on the floor, and they didn't warn me about what the chemicals would do', she groans. 'Everything with metal on it, zips and buttons, just melted.'

Perhaps it's best not to linger over exactly what might have been in the hoard which was annihilated that day, because it certainly contained quite a few gems whose loss would send collectors, archivists and costume historians into trauma at the mere thought. Like all models who were starting out in the 1990s, Stella Tennant was frequently paid in clothes by designers, and she began, as she has continued, with the very best. Chanel, Christian Dior (figs. 35, 85), Gianni Versace, Prada, Jil Sander, Helmut Lang, Martin Margiela, John Galliano, Dries Van Noten, Balenciaga, Giorgio Armani – there could scarcely be a list comprehensive enough to include all the designers who have asked Stella to channel their designs over a career which has spanned over twenty years.

Not that the garments that sadly met their end in her New York apartment would have matched up with many people's assumptions about the sort of clothes which are associated with Chatsworth. Some of them dated from the 'edgy' days of the 90s, when young, feistily challenging fashion was rising from London and Belgium. That was when Stella Tennant was singled out as an exceptional, angular girl who could look into a camera, walk the walk and elevate the underground attitude in a way which translated to the pages of *Vogue*.

Not all's lost, by any means, though. 'I'm a hoarder by nature', says Stella cheerfully. She has, for one thing, the very Alexander McQueen dress she wore in what she calls 'my first proper modelling job', the ground-breaking 'Anglo Saxon Attitude' shoot which was photographed by Steven Meisel on the streets around Portland Road, Notting Hill, for British *Vogue* 1993 (fig. 139). Captioned as, 'A black wool, bias cut, polo neck dress by Alexander McQueen', it was actually handmade by the designer himself. 'Wool lace', she remembers, 'with a bit of glue in it!'

In retrospect, that story was an historical turning point in the uprising of a generation of British fashion talent, including Stella's. McQueen, the ace-cutter and controversy-stirrer, had graduated from the Central Saint Martins MA Fashion degree just one year earlier. The reason Stella wore it that day was Isabella Blow, who had discovered and championed McQueen, and she was involved in realising the story for Meisel. It was Isabella who found Stella, too, through their mutual friend Plum Sykes, a young *Vogue* journalist. Sykes appeared in the story, too, as well as Bella Freud, Lady Louise Campbell and Stella's cousin Honor Fraser, who was also starting to model. 'Issy was collating people

139 *(opposite)* Steven Meisel, Plum Sykes and Stella Tennant in a dress by Alexander McQueen and shoes by Vivienne Westwood, originally published in British *Vogue*, December 1993.

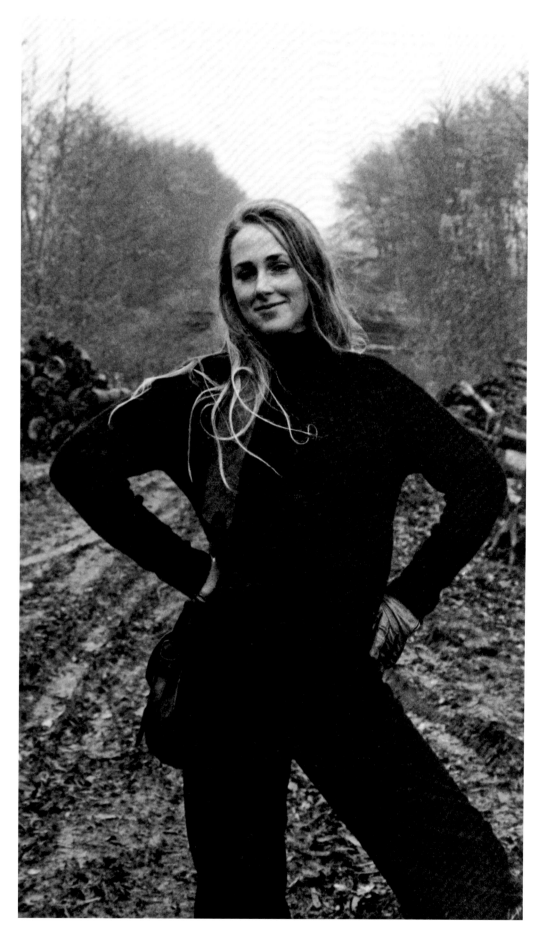

140 *(left)* The Duchess of Devonshire, 1968.

141 *(opposite)* Thomas Phillips, *Lady Caroline Lamb*, 1813.

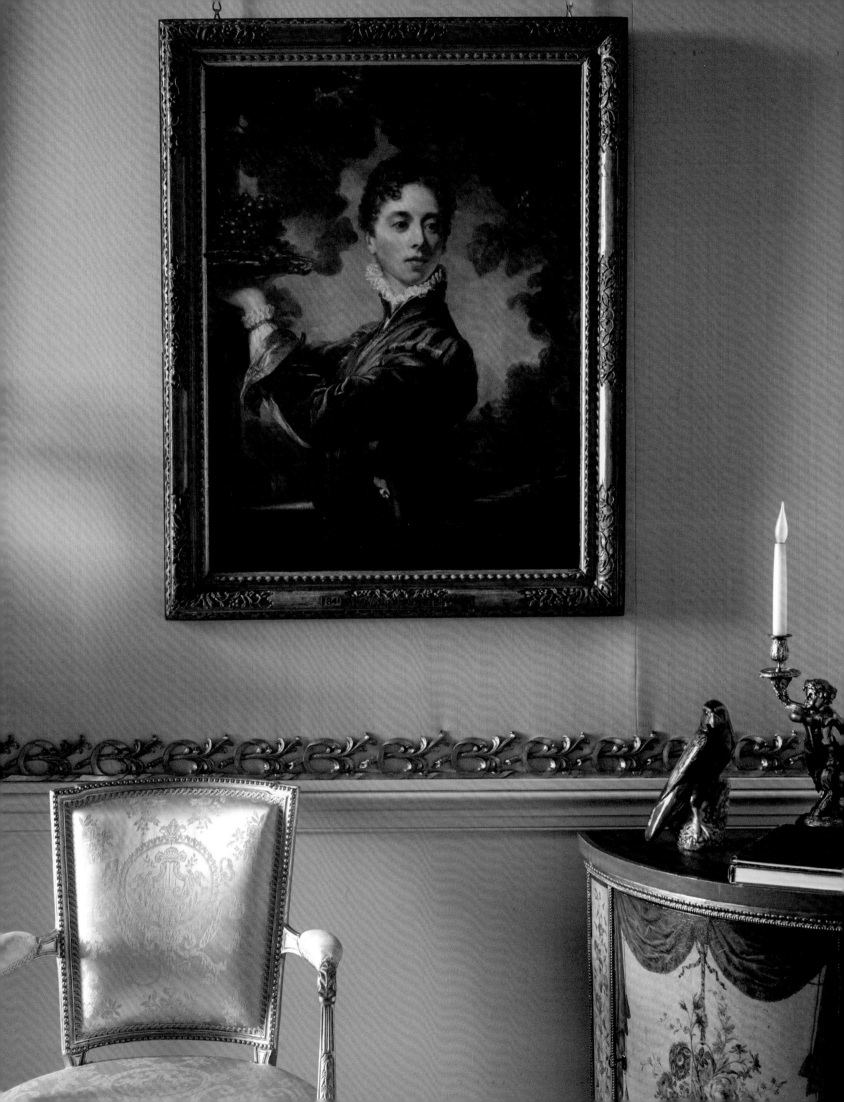

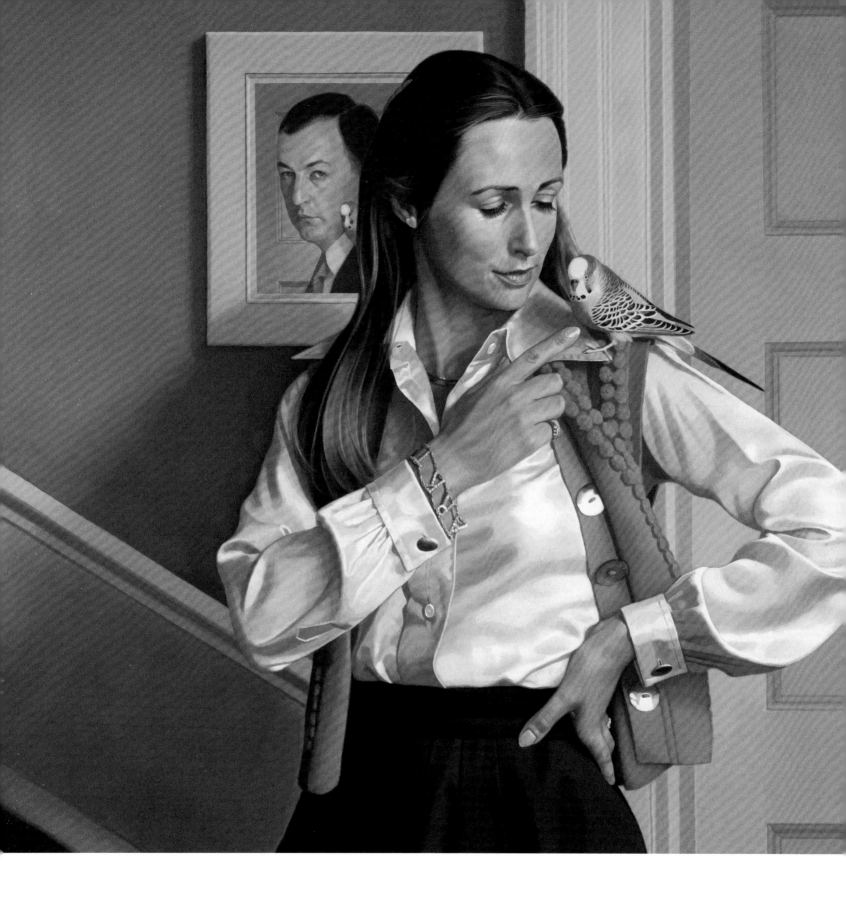

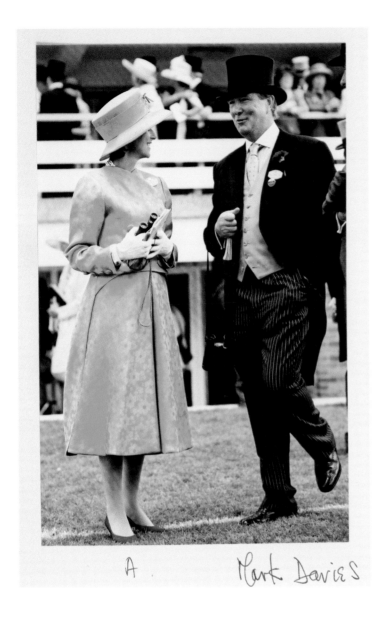

A.   Mark Davies

who weren't models for the shoot. I'd just finished art school, and I didn't know what I was walking into', Stella chuckles. 'I think my flatmate was more excited than I was.' One of the pictures has Stella wearing a pair of 'horse hoof' shoes by Fleur Oates, a jacket by Owen Gaster, hat by Philip Treacy and fishnets, looking straight into Meisel's lens. 'There is something very powerful about being photographed by Steven. I had never been observed before like that. It was very intense.'

In 1993, Stella was a recent Winchester School of Art sculpture graduate with a septum ring in her nose – an archetypical punk, by all appearances. The next thing she knew, Steven Meisel was booking her for a Versace advertising campaign which landed her plumb in the centre of high-flying supermodel-dom. 'My flatmate Jimmy Moffat negotiated it', she remembered. 'They were going to pay me £5,000. I turned up in Paris and they sent a stretch limo to collect me from the airport to take me to Le Meurice hotel, with a balcony overlooking the Tuileries and a marble bathroom. In the studio the next day, there was Garren the hairdresser, and Linda, Kristen and Shalom. I was totally freaked out', she laughs. 'There was *me* – and Linda Evangelista. We had to dance.'

Even when Stella began to appear in catwalk shows, it took time for the identity of the girl with the nose ring to dawn on fashion journalists – not perhaps, until the day they were astonished to turn around and notice that Debo, the then Duchess of Devonshire, was sitting next to them at an Ann Demeulemeester show. Stella's grandmother was looking in, on a trip to Paris. The two of them had lots of interests in common, from haute couture to chicken-keeping (fig. 122), plus a shared enthusiasm for collecting insect-shaped brooches, which Stella caught from her grandmother (fig. 133).

Stella is the daughter of artist Lady Emma Tennant and Toby Tennant. She was brought up with her brother Eddie and sister Isabel, with whom she now has an interior objets d'art company, Tennant & Tennant, on their father's sheep farm in Oxnam in the borders of Scotland. Stella and her husband, David Lasnet, were married there in June 1999. She was wearing a wedding dress Helmut Lang had made for her, incorporating an ivory skirt and vest top, loosely veiled in chiffon (fig. 60). It was the coolest possible fashion thing of the time, made at the height of Lang's fame, and his first wedding dress commission. She remembers her grandmother taking one look and greeting her with the words, 'Oh, darling – the bandaged bride!'

Shake the branches of the Cavendish family tree, and the various links between the fashion interests of the women relations start to fall out. Amanda Cavendish, Duchess of Devonshire, discovered her tastes through a British-based couturier, Franka

142 *(opposite)* Michael Leonard, *Lady With a Little Bird* (The Duchess of Devonshire), 1981.

143 *(above)* The Duchess of Devonshire wearing an ensemble by Franka with Mark Davies at Royal Ascot, circa 2003.

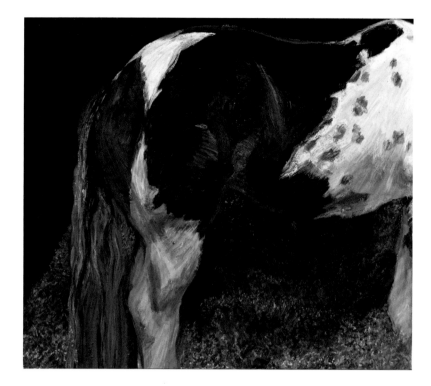

(fig. 143). Her daughter-in-law, Laura Burlington, who is married to her son William, trained with another British-based couturier, Inge Sprawson, worked with the French designer Roland Mouret (fig. 152) and also had a spell as a model (figs. 150, 153), like Stella, in the 90s. As individual as each one is, all three share a deep appreciation of craftsmanship, country clothing, tailoring, tweeds and textiles – an intrinsic part of the living culture of farming, fishing, shooting and hunting which goes deep into the history of British estates such as the Devonshires'.

Amanda Heywood-Lonsdale (fig. 142) had her first brush with the business of getting formal clothes made for her before she was married. Growing up in the 1960s, right in the middle of the free-thinking youthquake sweeping the world, she remembers not being all that enthusiastic when her mother, June Heywood-Lonsdale, took her off to a discreet address in Dover Street to see Madame Vernier (fig. 146), a milliner who had been placing her hats upon the lacquered hairdos of the British social world since the early 50s. 'I rather reluctantly had to find some clothes for Royal Ascot', she laughs. 'I'd just returned from Peru, and was rather grumpy.'

It was a fated appointment for the future Duchess, though. The advantage of Madame Vernier's business was that she cleverly offered a whole service, clothes as well as hats, so that clients needn't shop all over for things to match. If Amanda had any dread that she might be about to be manoeuvred towards dressing like her mother's generation, it lifted immediately, when 'the workroom door opened and a young person came out!' The designer behind the scenes was the Yugoslavian Baroness Franka Stael von Holstein, who had studied in Zagreb and come to London in 1961. She'd trained with the Queen's couturier Sir Norman Hartnell in his workrooms on Bruton Street, and understood all the nuances in the dress code book. 'Franka became a friend. She had a whole workshop, and made it so easy for me. She was very good at working out what shape flattered. When I married, she made most of my clothes. She designed and made me lovely things when I needed clothes for Ascot races (fig. 143), jackets for dinners and so on. I could say to her, "I like that, but can I have it in green?"'

In 1967, the year Amanda married Peregrine (Stoker) Cavendish, Madame Vernier recognised her protégé's contribution, and the company became Vernier/Franka. Later, Franka branched out on her own, becoming well known within British and European social circles. She conspired with Amanda to saturate her wardrobe with the colours she's always loved: chic clashes of pattern, cut into elegantly flowing shapes, indicative of the post-hippie mood of the 1970s.

When it came to choosing her wedding dress, the haute couture of Paris beckoned. 'I was 23 and my godmother Carmen Esnault-Pelterie, who worked with Givenchy, offered to give me my wedding dress as a present. I went to the Givenchy show – it was difficult,

144 *(above)* Lucian Freud, *Skewbald Mare*, 2004.

145 *(opposite)* The Duchess of Devonshire's riding boots and bridles in the tack room.

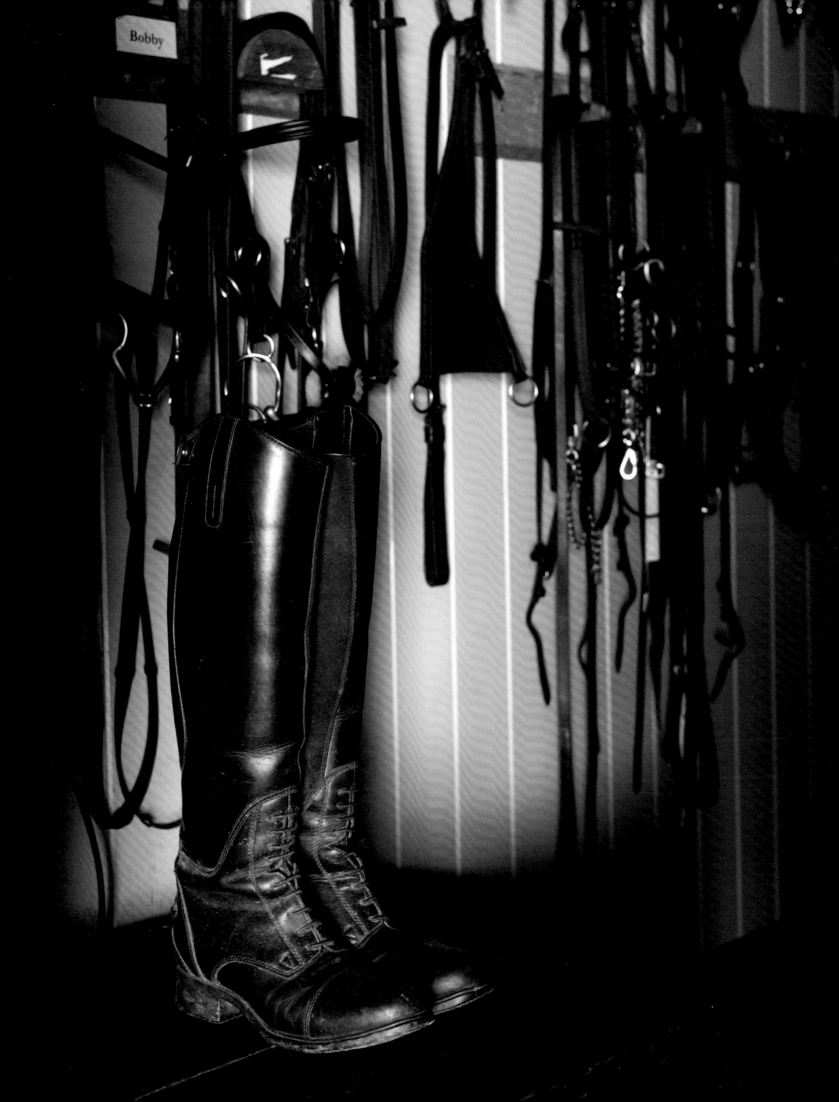

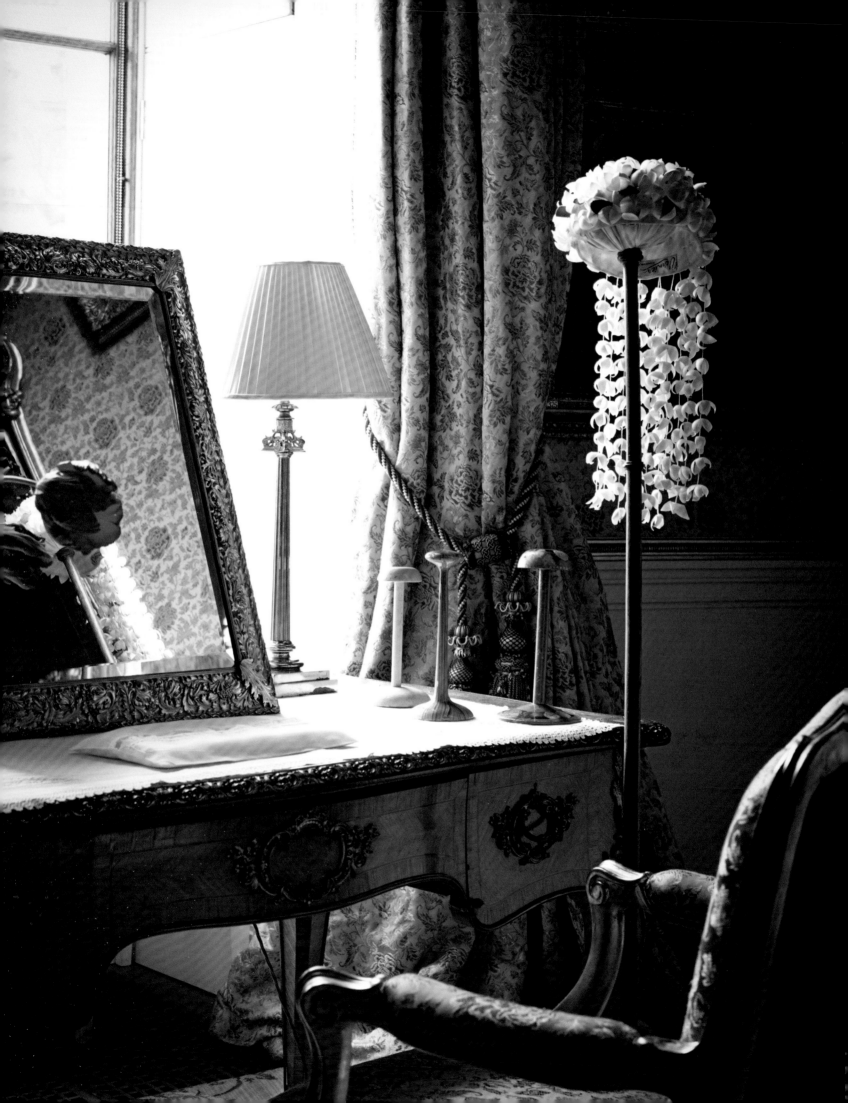

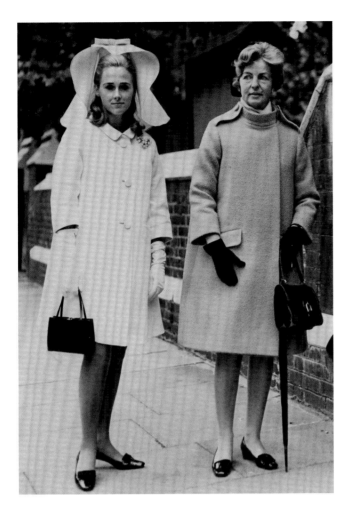

as long dresses had gone out of fashion. I waited and waited, and there at the end of the show was a beautiful dress.' On 28 June 1967, she walked down the aisle at St Martin-in-the-Fields wearing her Givenchy A-line dress in ziberline silk with a bolero picked out in 3-D organza flowers (figs. 57-58).

As a collector of the work of Andrew Grima (figs. 137-138), she also has an eye for the avant-garde in jewellery. She was introduced to the work of the man who radicalised postwar British goldsmithing with his uses of geological and natural forms almost by accident, after winning the prize of a Grima cyclamen-leaf brooch in a raffle at a charity ball at Blenheim Palace. Her fascination grew as she became able to purchase her own Grima, encouraged by her mother. 'Before my mother died, she said I should spend the money she left to buy nice jewellery, not day-to-day things', she remembers. 'Andrew Grima had a shop in Jermyn Street; it was like a cave, with dark grey slate on the outside. My collection started then.'

When Laura Cavendish, Countess of Burlington, married into the family in 2007, she came with a lifelong love of the skill of making clothes, learned at the knee of her grandmother Ann Roundell. 'She would have me to stay, and to occupy this child, she would set me up with her sewing machine, which I loved.' Young Laura became so engaged with making her own clothes at home in Cheshire that, on leaving school, she went to London as an apprentice to the exacting Austrian designer Inge Sprawson – herself taught at Chanel – who specialised in handmade couture for European royalty. There she learned to rehearse and perfect the correct techniques for constructing and finishing every detail of a garment; knowledge which she ended up bringing to Roland Mouret in the late 90s. 'I was introduced to Roland by the photographer Zanna, who had her studio in the Ragged School building in Bermondsey', she remembers. 'She said there was this Frenchman upstairs, who needed someone to sew.'

The reason Laura met Zanna in the first place was that she'd started modelling part-time, after being spotted whilst running an errand to buy thread from Peter Jones, Sloane Square, at the age of 16. She claims to have been a 'terrible, anxious' model and tells the story of once crashing to the ground in a faint while working for Hamish Bowles during a session for *Harper's Bazaar*. Laura's blonde, English-rose looks led to catwalk bookings for Helmut Lang, amongst others, in a phase just before Stella Tennant herself became a Lang favourite. Still, she jumped at Roland Mouret's offer to work behind the scenes rather than in front of the camera. 'I was fascinated by this man who was draping these incredibly modern dresses with no linings, and fixing them on the body with hat pins.'

Mouret, a butcher's son from Lourdes, was self-taught. His assistant brought him the insider arts of pin-hemming and French seams. 'At the beginning, it wasn't exactly mod-cons at the Ragged School', she hoots. 'Sometimes in winter, you'd have to choose between having the sewing machine on and the heater.' Three years later, Mouret's staff

146 *(opposite)* The Duchess of Devonshire's hat by Madame Vernier, 1965.

147 *(above)* Deborah Devonshire with the Duchess of Devonshire at the wedding of her brother David Heywood-Lonsdale and Victoria Wimbolt Lewis, 1967.

148 *(following pages)* Nick Knight, Stella Tennant in an evening ensemble by Christopher Kane, 2012. Originally published in British *Vogue*, September 2012.

149 *(page 194)* Military headgear, Chatsworth.

150 *(page 195)* Ellen von Unwerth, Countess of Burlington in an evening dress by Gianfranco Ferré, 1997. Originally published in Italian *Vogue*, March 1997.

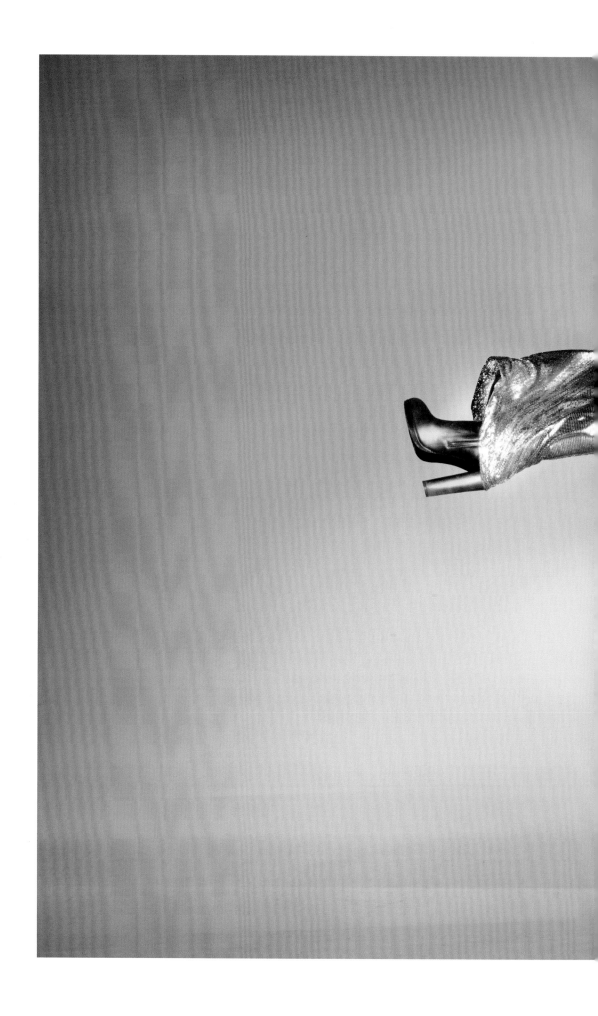

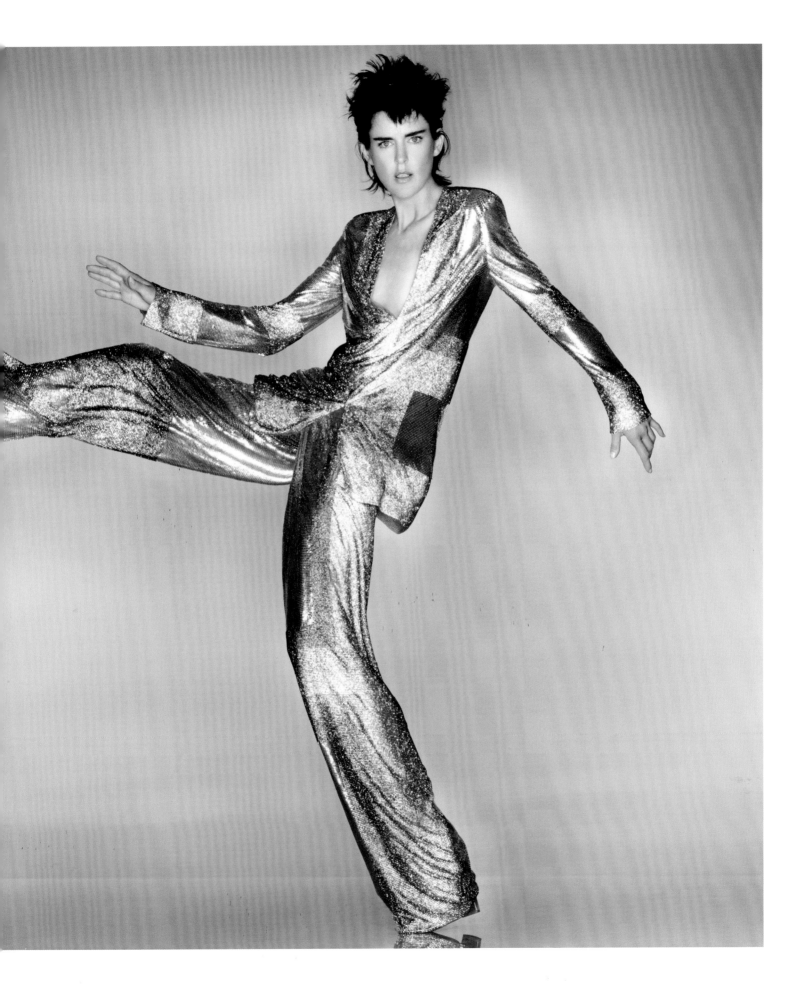

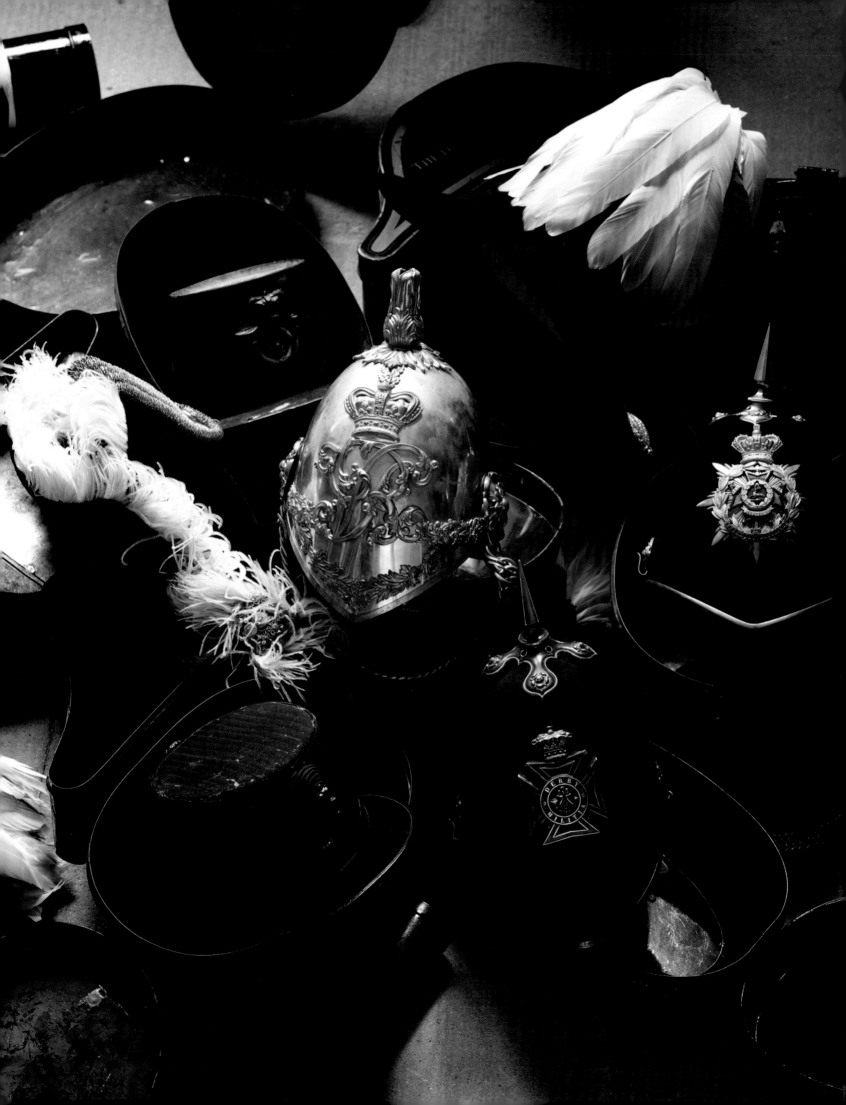

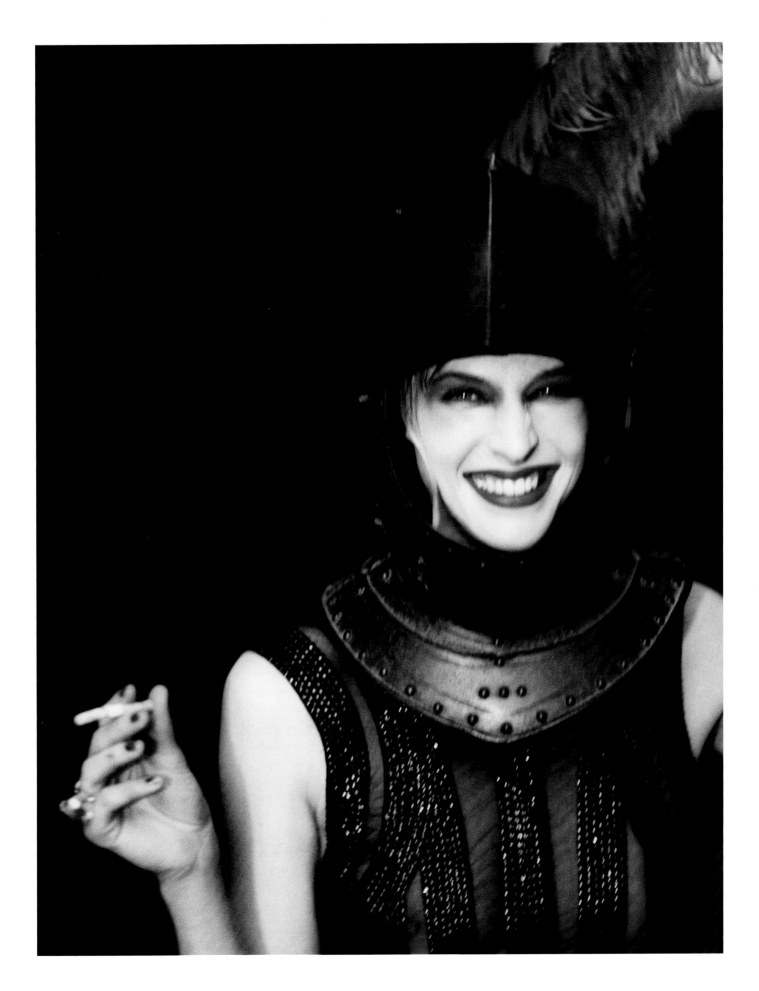

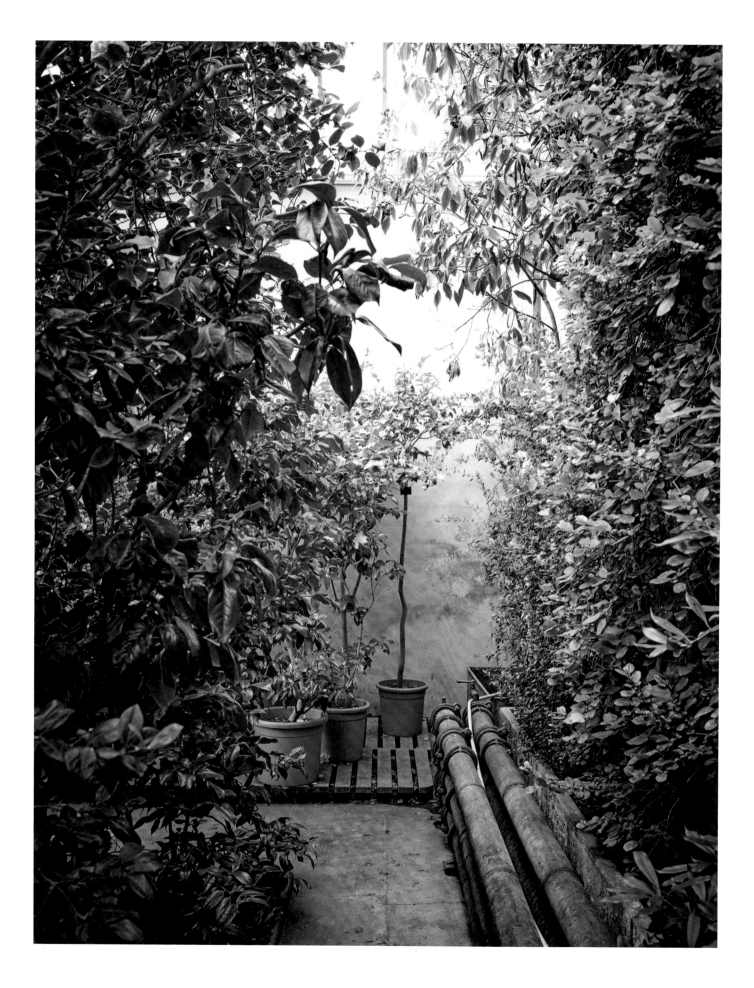

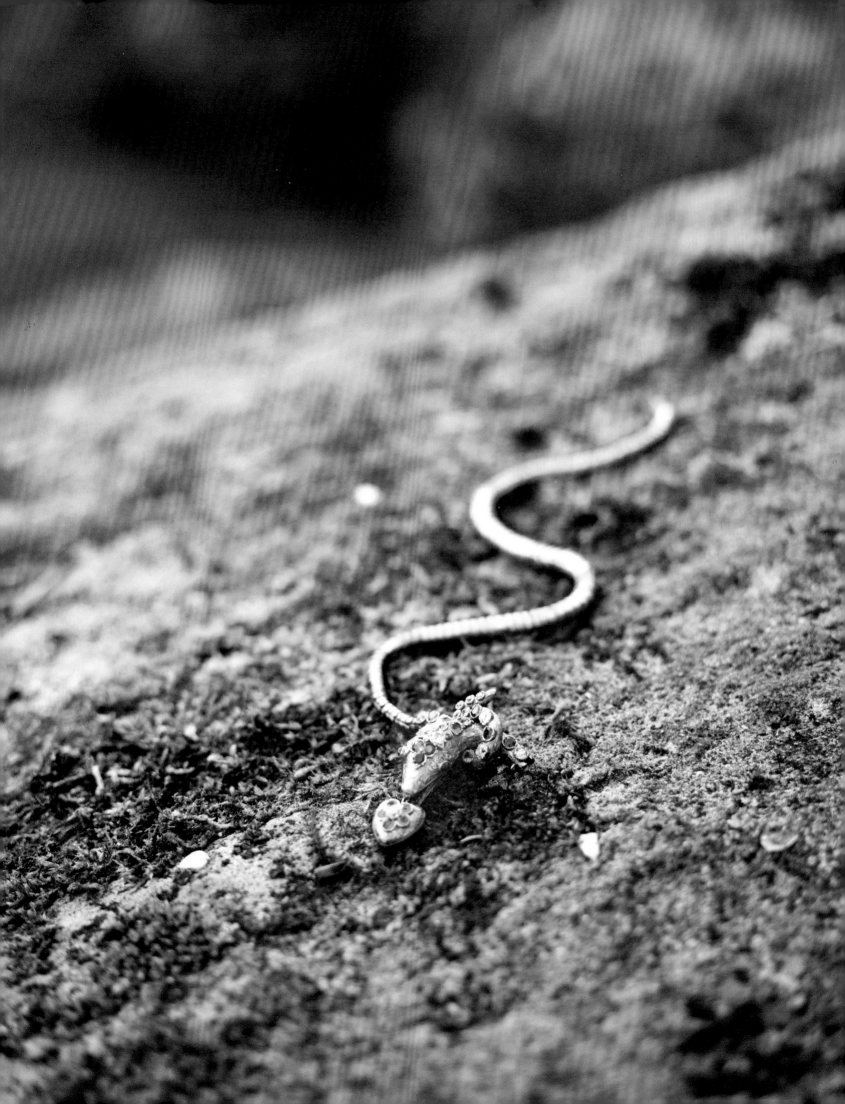

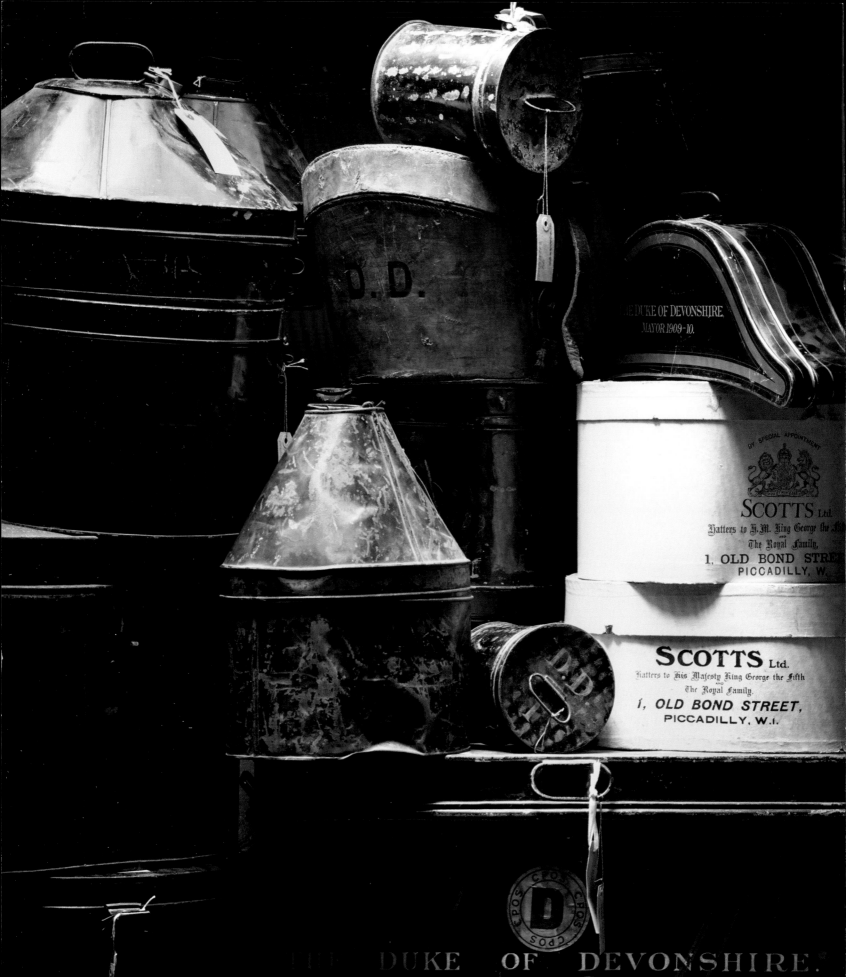

SCOTTS Ltd.
Hatters to H.M. King George the Fifth
The Royal Family,
1, OLD BOND STREET,
PICCADILLY, W.

SCOTTS Ltd.
Hatters to His Majesty King George the Fifth
The Royal Family,
1, OLD BOND STREET,
PICCADILLY, W.1.

THE DUKE OF DEVONSHIRE.
MAYOR 1909-10.

THE DUKE OF DEVONSHIRE.

THE EMPRESS OF FASHION: GEORGIANA, DUCHESS OF DEVONSHIRE, 1757-1806

1   J Friedrich Bielfeld, *Letters of Baron Bielfeld, Secretary of Legation to the King of Prussia*, trans. W Hooper, 4 vols., London, J Robson, 1768-70, 4.57.

2   H Walpole, *Letters of Horace Walpole, Earl of Orford, to Sir Horace Mann*, 2 vols., Philadelphia, Lea & Blanchard, 1844, 2.301.

3   See British Library Add [MSS 75754].

4   [D, 2.3769] British Museum.

5   See J Lister 'Twenty-Three Samples of Silk: Silks Worn by Queen Charlotte and the Princesses at Royal Birthday Balls, 1791-1794', *Costume* 37:1, 2003, pp. 51-65.

6   A Foreman, *Georgiana, Duchess of Devonshire*, London: Harper Collins, 1998, pp. 20-22, 22 n.1.

7   For a detailed discussion of Georgiana's role in popularising French fashions in England, and her personal influence on French style, see K Chrisman-Campbell, 'French Connections: Georgiana, Duchess of Devonshire, and the Anglo-French Fashion Exchange', *Dress* 31, 2004, pp. 3-14.

8   Lady Clermont to Georgiana, Duchess of Devonshire: Devonshire MSS, 27 November 1774. [CS5/52] Chatsworth.

9   M Granville Delany, *Autobiography and Correspondence of Mary Granville, Mrs Delany*, ed. Rt Hon Lady Llanover, 6 vols., London, 1861-62, 5.115.

10 J Harris, *A Series of Letters of the First Earl of Malmesbury, His Family and Friends from 1745 to 1820*, ed. Earl of Malmesbury, 2 vols., London, Richard Bentley, 1870, 1.296.

11 *Ibid*. 1.299.

12 W Whitten (ed.), *Nollekens and His Times*, 2 vols., London, John Lane, 1917, 1.55.

13 Lady L Stuart, *Lady Louisa Stuart: Selections from her Manuscripts*, ed. J A Home, Edinburgh, David Douglas, 1899, pp. 186-187.

14 *The Morning Post*, quoted in Foreman 38

15 *Galerie des Modes*, 27e Cahier de Costumes Français, 21e Suite d'Habillements à la mode en 1779.

16 It was probably on a 1775 visit to Paris that Georgiana first met Rose Bertin; she made her last purchase from Bertin in 1803, but the bill remained unpaid at the time of her death in 1806. See Rose Bertin, dossier VII, no. 716, fo. 7081. [MS 1] Fondation Jacques Doucet.

17 Rose Bertin, dossier I, no. 57, fo. 488. [MS 1] Fondation Jacques Doucet.

18 *Morning Herald and Daily Advertiser*, 21 October 1782, quoted in Foreman 97.

19 Foreman 121.

20 *Galerie des Modes*, 49e Cahier de Costumes Français, 43e d'Habillements à la mode en 1786.

21 Georgiana, Duchess of Devonshire, to Lady Elizabeth Foster: Devonshire MSS, 12 August 1783. [CS5/517] Chatsworth.

22 Lady L Stuart, *The Letters of Lady Louisa Stuart*, 29 November 1784, ed. R Brimley Johnson, London, John Lane, 1926, p. 71.

23 Georgiana, Duchess of Devonshire, to Lady Spencer: Devonshire MSS, 19 February 1785. [CS5/667] Chatsworth.

24 See K Chrisman-Campbell, *Fashion Victims: Dress at the Court of Louis XVI and Marie-Antoinette*, London, Yale University Press, 2015, pp. 172-99.

25 Georgiana, Duchess of Devonshire, to Lady Spencer: Chatsworth MSS, 5th Duke's Group, 14-18 August 1784. [no. 639] Chatsworth.

26 *Lady's Magazine*, 1787, 416, quoted in A Ribeiro, *Dress in Eighteenth-Century Europe, 1715-1789*, London, Yale University Press, 2002, p. 228.

27 J Gay, *The Guardian*, no. 149, 1 September 1713, p. 247.

28 S Richardson, Letter XC, 'Against a young Lady's affecting manly Airs; and also censuring the modern Riding-habits', in *One Hundred and Seventy-three Letters Written for Particular Friends, On the most Important Occasions*, London, C Hitch and L Hawes, 1764, p. 125.

29 Quoted in B Dolan, *Ladies of the Grand Tour*, London, Harper Collins, 2001, p. 179.

30 *Morning Post*, 18 July 1778.

31 *Morning Herald*, 1 May 1784.

32 Lady Spencer to Georgiana, Duchess of Devonshire: Devonshire MSS, 10 November 1790. [CS5/1074] Chatsworth.

33 C Chapman and J Dormer, *Elizabeth and Georgiana: The Two Loves of the Duke of Devonshire*, London, John Murray, 2003, p. 146; E Vigée-Lebrun, Souvenirs, ed. C Hermann, 2 vols., Paris, Les Femmes, 1986, 2.128.

34 *Morning Chronicle*, 31 March 1806, quoted in Foreman 391.

GRANDEUR, SENTIMENT AND INDIVIDUALITY: THE CAVENDISH JEWELS 1547-2017

1   Elizabeth Talbot, Countess of Shrewsbury, inventories and papers of Elizabeth Countess of Shrewsbury: List of jewels written out 'Geven by the Scotys queen to my lorde and me'. [NRA 23246] Sheffield City Archives.

2   Will of Elizabeth, Countess of Devonshire, Cavendish Wills and Inventories, 24 November 1642. [PRO Prob 10, Probate 7] Public Record Office, London.

3   Will of Christian, Countess of Devonshire, Cavendish Wills and Inventories, 10 June 1675. [PRO Prob 10] Probate Public Record Office, London.

4   Marquess of Ailesbury, Letter to Lord Bruce, 1898, p. 159. [HMC 43 18th Rept. Appendix VII] Historic Manuscripts Commission.

5   She placed the pearl buckle in the centre of the pearl necklace given to her daughter, Georgina, on her marriage to the Earl of Carlisle, who according to her will of 1848, returned the pearls to Chatsworth.

6   Letters of Georgiana Duchess of Devonshire to the Prince of Wales, December 1786. Chatsworth Archives.

7   D Scarisbrick, 'The Devonshire Parure', *Archaeologia*, vol. CVIII, 1986, p. 239-254.

8   B Disraeli, *Letters to Lady Bradford and to Lady Chesterfield*, 22 March 1877, vol. 2, 1929.

9   J A Rosenthal, *JAR Paris*, Suffolk, Antique Collectors Club, 2013, p. 2.

ACKNOWLEDGEMENTS

This book, and the exhibition that it celebrates, represent a great collective endeavour, and we are profoundly grateful to all those who have worked so enthusiastically with us to bring them to life.

House Style is published to celebrate an exhibition of five centuries of fashion at Chatsworth, and we would like to take this opportunity to thank those who have contributed to this show.

First and foremost, we would like to thank the exhibition's designers, Patrick Kinmonth and Antonio Monfreda, for their exceptional vision and dynamic creative direction. Working with their associates Mauricio Elorriaga and Annina Pfuel, with the assistance of Jack Henshall, Patrick and Antonio have conjured a thrilling exhibition quite unlike any other staged at Chatsworth. The exhibition has been realised in association with Factory Settings and lit with great imagination and artistry by Zerlina Hughes of Studio ZNA.

Our profound gratitude is due to the tireless Molly Sorkin and Jennifer Park, who have done a supreme job in realising our vision for both the book and exhibition, working with Chatsworth's similarly indefatigable duo of Denna Garrett and Hannah Obee, to bring the countless strands together. Janet Wood beautifully dressed many of the mannequins in the exhibition.

Our special thanks are due to those design houses who have lent significant examples of their work to the show, including Burberry, Chanel, Christian Dior, Erdem, Alessandro Michele for Gucci, Stella Tennant and Isabella Cawdor for Holland & Holland, Stephen Jones, Christopher Kane, Phillip Treacy, and Vivienne Westwood, as well as to Chris and Rebecca Sellors of C W Sellors, who painstakingly evoked the headdress worn by Duchess Louise to the Devonshire House Ball, and the two Devonshire diamond tiaras. Huntsman, meanwhile, recreated an ensemble originally made for Adele Astaire and detailed in their archives. T J Wilcox's film of Adele Astaire further enhances her story through the artist's eye.

Additional historic loans have greatly enhanced this exhibition and helped us to tell the story of fashion at Chatsworth. We would like to thank the following for lending their objects and expertise: Jenny Lister, Amy Higgitt, and Sara Mittica and all those at the Victoria and Albert Museum; Beatrice Behlen at the Museum of London; Rosemary Harden at the Fashion Museum, Bath; Fernanda Torrente at the National Trust; Diana Clements at United Grand Lodge; and Mona and Jenny Perlhagen of Chelsea Textiles for their donation of embroideries and their generous loan of an historic dress from the Chelsea Textiles Archive. We also thank Christian Lacroix; Olivier Saillard at the Palais Galliera, Musée de la Mode de la Ville de Paris and Robby Timmermans at ModaMuseum, Antwerp; Gainsbury and Whiting; and Nicholas Cullinan and the National Portrait Gallery; as well as all the individuals who have lent us their treasured belongings, among them the Duke and Duchess of Devonshire, William Burlington, Lady Celina Carter, Lady Jasmine Dunne, Lady Elizabeth Cavendish, Ava Astaire, Phyllis Posnick, Lady Emma Tennant, Isabel Tennant, and David Lasnet. We extend our deepest gratitude to Stella Tennant, who enthusiastically opened the treasury of her personal wardrobe to us, inestimably enhancing the breadth and style of our exhibition.

We applaud the gentle tenacity of Sarah Owen and the Development team in helping us all to realise our vision for the exhibition with their sponsorship outreach. We are very proud to have Gucci as our principal sponsor, and appreciate the support of their creative, publicity and marketing teams.

Our exhibition *House Style: Five Centuries of Fashion* was dependent on the generous support of Chatsworth House Trust and its Directors (John Booth, Cindy Chetwode, Mark Fane, Guy Monson, Edward Perks and Henry Wyndham) and highly valued partnerships with the following: Alessandro Michele, Robert Triefus, Alessio Vannetti and the wonderful team at Gucci; Chris and Rebecca Sellors, the father and daughter team at C W Sellors Fine Jewellery; Jonathan Wragg, Tom Street and Dawn Cowderoy of Investec Wealth & Investment; Jackie King from Sotheby's; and Ulrik Garde Due, Mariusz Skronski and Sally Warmington of Wedgwood. We would also like to thank Lucite International for their supply of Perspex® acrylic sheet for Patrick and Antonio's imaginative installation design.

Other supporters who have helped in many different and important ways include Jo Allison; Stefan Bartlett; Brooke Barzun; Fiona Browne; Alice Brudenell-Bruce; Ted Cadogan; Isabella Cawdor; Sarah Christie; Marianne Brown, Brett Croft, Gretchen Fenston, Cristina Palumbo, Paola Ranieri and Samantha Vuignier at Condé Nast Publications; Pauline Daley; Sydney Finch; Morgane Raterron and Jelka Music of Jean Paul Gaultier; Julian Hawkins; Anthony Kendal and Rossa Prendergast; Martina Mondadori; Justine Picardie, Lalitha Pillai; Kadee and Stefan Ratibor; Annette de la Renta; Richard Reynolds; the team at Scott and Co; Lisa Simpson; Phillip Varon; Jayne Wrightsman; and Lucy Yeomans. Lilah Ramzi was a vital link between Manhattan and Derbyshire. We are grateful to Anna Wintour at American *Vogue* for her interest in the project, and for her forbearance with Hamish's time.

For this tome itself, we are proud of the continuing support and enthusiasm of Charles Miers and his associate Gisela Aguilar and their colleagues at Rizzoli. The art director Jacob Wildschiødtz and his colleagues, Elina Asanti and Natalie Bergh, at NR2154 have given us a book beyond our imaginations, and we commend their inexhaustible creativity, and applaud the photographer Thomas Loof and art director Julie Lysbo who produced the contemporary images that provide such a dynamic counterpoint to the archival ones.

Other key members of the informed, enthusiastic and indefatigable team at Chatsworth were also essential in bringing this book to fruition. We applaud the photo librarian Diane Naylor, and archivists James Towe and Aidan Haley. Meanwhile, Susanna Stokoe and her textiles team, including the conservator Jo Banks, were vital to our understanding of the breadth of Chatsworth's textiles collection. Our deep thanks are also due to Charles Noble and Louise Clarke.

The reminiscences of Henry Coleman Sr, Helen Marchant and Christine Thompson, who worked with the late 11th Duke and his wife Deborah Devonshire, have proved invaluable to us all, as were the memories that their friend Hubert de Givenchy shared so generously.

The following distinguished writers and historians all provided insightful and fascinating essays for this book, and we are proud to include their contributions: Kimberly Chrisman-Campbell, Charlotte Mosley, Sarah Mower, Diana Scarisbrick and Sophia Topley. We would also like to thank Jonquil O'Reilly for her extensive research into the clothing of the Cavendish men.

The Devonshires have inspired artists and photographers across the centuries, and we had an embarrassment of splendid contemporary images to work with. We are indebted to the talent and generosity of: Julian Broad, Charlotte Bromley-Davenport, William Burlington, Walter Chin, Robert Fairer, François Halard, Rupert Hartley, Kacper Kasprzyk, Nick Knight, Thomas Loof, Glen Luchford, Steven Meisel, Diego Uchitel, Ellen von Unwerth, Tim Walker and Bruce Weber. We are delighted to have Mario Testino's stylish images in our book and gracing its cover. We would also like to thank the artists' studios, archives, museums and libraries who provided imagery, including Art and Commerce; Art Partner; The Cecil Beaton Studio Archive at Sotheby's; Christian Dior Couture; The Condé Nast Publications Ltd; The Elizabeth Day McCormick Collection at Museum of Fine Arts, Boston; Vanessa Fairer; Damien Hirst and Science Ltd, Huntington Art Collections, San Marino, California; Charlotte Knight; Lewis Walpole Library, Yale University; Museum of London; The Mitford Archive; Norman Parkinson Ltd / Courtesy of Norman Parkinson Archive; Trunk Archive; and the Victoria and Albert Museum, London.

Our greatest thanks must go to the Duke and Duchess of Devonshire for their unwavering faith in, support of and enthusiasm for this book and the exhibition that it celebrates.

—*Laura Burlington and Hamish Bowles*

PLATE 1 *(pages 10-11)* Chatsworth with the Emperor Fountain in the foreground.

PLATE 2 *(pages 12-13)* Great Dining Room, Chatsworth.

PLATE 3 *(pages 14-15)* Attributed to Bess of Hardwick, needlework of Elizabethan Chatsworth, 1590-1600.

PLATE 4 *(pages 16-17)* Detail of Cavendish family christening gown, late nineteenth century.

PLATE 5 *(pages 34-35)* William Hemsley's scenery on the stage of the theatre at Chatsworth, 1896.

PLATE 6 *(pages 106-107)* Lace panel including Duchess Georgiana's coat of arms, late eighteenth century.

PLATE 7 *(pages 122-123)* Detail of fancy dress costume by Jean-Philippe Worth for the House of Worth, after a design by Attilio Comelli, worn by Duchess Louise as Zenobia, Queen of Palmyra, 1897.

PLATE 8 *(pages 140-141)* Detail of dress worn by Deborah Devonshire, Oscar de la Renta, 2006.

PLATE 9 *(pages 162-163)* Gold- and gem-set necklace, 1840.

PLATE 10 *(pages 180-181)* Detail of shirt worn by Stella Tennant, Earnest Sewn.

PLATE 11 *(page 202)* Stack of hatboxes and metal trunks, Chatsworth.

Published on the occasion of the exhibition *House Style: Five Centuries of Fashion at Chatsworth*,
organised by and presented at Chatsworth, 25 March to 22 October 2017.

House Style: Five Centuries of Fashion at Chatsworth is made possible by the support of Chatsworth House Trust and Chatsworth Settlement Trustees.

SUPPORT FOR THIS EXHIBITION WAS PROVIDED BY

PRINCIPAL SPONSOR:

GUCCI

and

MAJOR SPONSORS:

  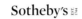

SUPPORTING SPONSOR:

LIBRARY OF CONGRESS CATALOG CONTROL NUMBER: 2016956367
ISBN: 978-0-8478-5896-5

FIRST PUBLISHED IN THE UNITED STATES OF AMERICA IN 2017 BY
Skira Rizzoli Publications, Inc.
300 Park Avenue South
New York, NY 10010
www.rizzoliusa.com

IN ASSOCIATION WITH
Chatsworth
Bakewell
Derbyshire
DE45 1PP
England
www.chatsworth.org

FOR SKIRA RIZZOLI PUBLICATIONS, INC.
Charles Miers, *Publisher*
Margaret Rennolds Chace, *Associate Publisher*
Gisela Aguilar, *Editor*
Victorine Lamothe, *Copy Editor*
Kaija Markoe, *Production Manager*
Kayleigh Jankowski, *Design Coordinator*

ART DIRECTION AND DESIGN BY NR2154
Jacob Wildschiødtz, Julie Lysbo, Elina Asanti, Natalie Bergh

JACKET
FRONT: Mario Testino, Stella Tennant in an evening dress by John Galliano for Christian Dior Haute Couture, Spring/Summer 1998,
set design by Patrick Kinmonth. Originally published in American *Vogue*, May 2006. © Mario Testino
BACK: Duchess Louise's silk and lace bag with gold work embroidery, 1890s, on a George III giltwood chair by François Hervé,
late eighteenth century. Photo by Thomas Loof © Chatsworth House Trust

CASE: William Hemsley's scenery on the stage of the theatre at Chatsworth, 1896. Photo by Thomas Loof © Chatsworth House Trust

ENDPAPERS: Venetian Point de Neige needlepoint lace, circa 1670. The Devonshire Collection © Chatsworth House Trust

2017 2018 2019 2020 / 10 9 8 7 6 5 4 3 2 1
Printed in Italy

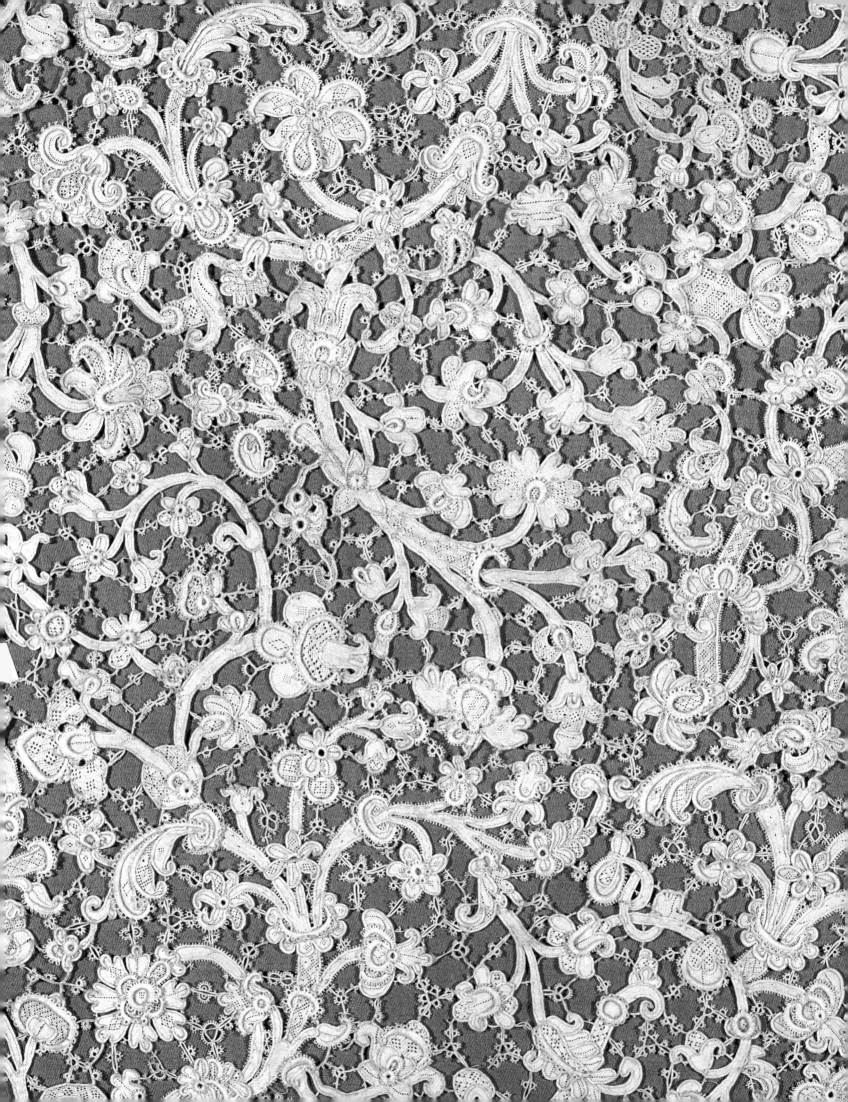